PRAISE FOR
Recipes for Change

"High-quality, delicious food is one of the best medicines
available to us—not only for treating health problems but for
preventing them in the first place. Bon appetit!"
—Christiane Northrup, M.D.,
author of *Women's Bodies, Women's Wisdom*

"*Recipes for Change* addresses the nutritional needs of menopausal
women in a helpful and comprehensive way—with inspiring
recipes to boot. Bravo!"
—Dolores Riccio, author of *Superfoods for Women*

"Much more than a cookbook, *Recipes for Change* offers unique
and effective advice for treating menopause holistically."
—Dana Jacobi, contributing editor, *Natural Health*

LISSA DEANGELIS was the Associate Director of the Natural Gourmet Cookery
School in New York City for seven years. She holds a master's degree in Human
Nutrition, has a private nutrition consulting practice, leads corporate seminars,
and teaches cooking at the professional level and in workshops. She lives in
North Edison, New Jersey.

MOLLY SIPLE is a registered dietician with a master's degree in nutrition, a former
caterer, and now a consultant on women's health and nutrition to Los Angeles
hospitals. A former editor at *House Beautiful*, she is a staff writer on female health
for the Holistic Book Project in Los Angeles, where she lives.

RECIPES
for
CHANGE

Gourmet Wholefood Cooking for
Health and Vitality at Menopause

Lissa DeAngelis
and Molly Siple

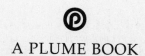

A PLUME BOOK

A NOTE TO THE READER: The ideas, procedures, and suggestions contained in this book are not intended as a substitute for consulting with your physician. All matters regarding your health require medical supervision.

PLUME
Published by the Penguin Group
Penguin Putnam Inc., 375 Hudson Street, New York, New York 10014, U.S.A.
Penguin Books Ltd, 27 Wrights Lane, London W8 5TZ, England
Penguin Books Australia Ltd, Ringwood, Victoria, Australia
Penguin Books Canada Ltd, 10 Alcorn Avenue, Toronto, Ontario, Canada M4V 3B2
Penguin Books (N.Z.) Ltd, 182–190 Wairau Road, Auckland 10, New Zealand

Penguin Books Ltd, Registered Offices: Harmondsworth, Middlesex, England

First published by Plume, an imprint of Dutton Signet, a member of
Penguin Putnam Inc. Previously published in a Dutton edition.

First Plume Printing, May, 1998
10 9 8 7 6 5 4 3 2 1

 REGISTERED TRADEMARK—MARCA REGISTRADA

The Library of Congress has catalogued the Dutton edition as follows:

DeAngelis, Lissa.
Recipes for change : gourmet wholefood cooking for health and vitality
at menopause / Lissa DeAngelis and Molly Siple.
p.   cm.
Includes index.
ISBN 0-525-94102-9 (hc.)
ISBN 0-452-27293-9 (pbk.)
1. Menopause—Nutritional aspects.   2. Menopause—Complications—
Diet therapy—Recipes.   3. Middle aged women—Nutrition.
I. Siple, Molly.   II. Title.
RG186.D43   1996
618.1'750654—dc20   95-25810
                                                         CIP

Printed in the United States of America
Set in Palatino and Bauer Bodoni
Designed by Eve L. Kirch

This book is dedicated, with love, to our parents.

ACKNOWLEDGMENTS

We'd like to thank the many professionals who gave us the benefit of their knowledge by granting interviews and answering questions: Nicholas Gonzalez, M.D.; Serafina Corsello, M.D.; Hugh Riordan, M.D.; Christiane Northrup, M.D.; Alan Gaby, M.D.; Nan Kathryn Fuchs, Ph.D.; Nancy Appleton, Ph.D.; Susan M. Lark, M.D.; Katherine A. O'Hanlan, M.D.; Udo Erasmus, Ph.D.; Russell Jaffe, M.D.; Forrest H. Nielsen, Ph.D.; Claude L. Hughes, Jr., M.D.; James Jackson, Ph.D.; Yewoubdar Beyenne, Ph.D.; Bruce McLucas, M.D.; Harriet Beinfield, L. Ac.; Laurie M. Aesoph, N.D.; Vasanto Melina, R.D.; W. B. Milliman, N.D.; Betty Ballantine; Noela Evans; Joanna Poppink, M.F.C.C.; Angeline Vogl; Beverley Russell, Ph.D.; Lois Brown; and Carol Mann, who brought our work to Dutton. Special thanks to Annemarie Colbin for introducing Molly to Lissa.

Thanks to our editorial team, for their commitment to the book and their wise guidance: Carole DeSanti, Julia Moskin, and Amy Mintzer.

Our many thanks to our family members: Esma Shaw for all her help; Adolph and Dorothy DeAngelis for lifelong encouragement and support; and Cosmo Guarriello for his undaunting support and guidance in making this book possible. And a big thank you to Robert, Helene, Joshua, and Kimberly Nahm, and Victor, Al, Betty, and Jean Guarriello; and to Jack, Dianna, Sharayah, Victor, Joshua, Theresa, Dawn, Lisa, and Jennifer.

Thank you to all our friends who rallied around us while we worked, keeping us company and cheering us on: Joan and Bob Axelrod, Sally Beaudette, Andy and Michelle Blum, Vincent Carreri, Felix and Yelena Chalyavsky, Richard Coons, Linda and Bruce Seiden, Bea and Jim Fitzpatrick, Bruce Gamradt, Alex and Inna Gorelik,

Elsa Hart, Henry Hilton, Chris Hardy, Garry Isenstadt, Debra Italiano, Paula Jackson, Richard Jeffery, Lex Lalli, Rich Lieberman, Lynn Matherson, Ed Michalove, Alain Montour, Dion Neutra, Ann Marie Nolan, Ugo Polla, Sonny Rivera, Cori Santiago, Chris and Mark Seasly, Mark and Tatyana Shvartsapel, Savva and Mila Spektor, Bruce Seiden, Jim Tribe, Ann Videriksen, Toni Wechsler, M.P.H., and Dee Yalowitz.

And for our photos we thank photographer Tom Doran of Westbury, New York, and Fresh Fields Market. Finally, special thanks to remembered family and friends Janet Wilhelmson, Frank Accuri, and Andrew Lederman.

CONTENTS

Recipes for a Healthy Menopause

PREFACE

This book was born when Molly Siple had her first hot flash. It came during a big, traditional Thanksgiving dinner; the kind with plenty of sweet, rich side dishes and desserts and lots of wine and coffee alongside. The flashes continued for weeks afterward, accompanied by fatigue, fits of rage, and a fuzzy-headed feeling she couldn't shake off. Molly was already doing an internship in clinical dietetics as part of her training to become a registered dietician, but she didn't know what to make of these changes. Her own body felt strangely unfamiliar.

When these feelings were identified as signs of menopause, Molly first went the usual route: hormone replacement therapy. But the fuzzy-headedness continued, and she could tell that the hormones were masking, rather than curing, her symptoms. She decided to put her training in nutrition to work. In addition to a program of exercise, meditation, and alternative therapies like acupuncture and Chinese herbalism, she changed her way of eating to reflect what she knew about the healing potential of food.

Molly's life and health were transformed by this decision. She called her longtime friend Lissa DeAngelis, and with their shared commitment to women's health, as well as a fascination with food and its healing properties, they planned this book. Lissa's education in food, cooking, and nutrition had begun in childhood. She grew up in a house filled with Mediterranean tastes and smells: the lasagna, roasted peppers, and stuffed artichokes her Italian grandmother made; her Greek grandmother's spinach pie, egg-lemon soup, roast leg of lamb, and sweet walnut baklava. At nineteen she owned her own whole grain bakery; she went on to become a restaurant chef and, ultimately, associate director of the Natural Gourmet Cookery School in New York City.

As we worked on this book, sampling and perfecting exciting new dishes and munching on the healthy snacks you'll find in the recipe pages, Molly's menopausal symptoms abated dramatically. And years earlier, Lissa had changed her way of eating to these natural foods, and put an end to her premenstrual problems. We know that eating health-supportive foods can make an enormous difference for any woman, at any stage of life. You'll learn exactly how the food you eat affects your body, your health, your mood, your mind—everything that makes you what you are! The recipes give you the tools you need to put that knowledge to work. We are thrilled that *Recipes for Change* is in your hands at last.

—Lissa DeAngelis
Molly Siple

INTRODUCTION

This is a book for women. Written by women, it is about the bodily processes and changes all women experience as they mature.

We are here to add a powerful tool to your store of knowledge—a greater understanding of the relationship between what you eat and how you feel, which will enable you to make more educated food choices. The recipes that follow give you delicious ways to put these foods on your table. Why do food choices matter? Because what you eat actually *becomes* your body, profoundly affecting your health. As mother, wife, or life-partner, you probably also feed those close to you, and what you place on the table makes a difference in their health as well.

You may have picked up this book because of a general interest in nutrition, cooking, or health, but chances are you picked it up because you're experiencing hot flashes, fatigue, or mood swings. If you have several more years before menopause, so much the better. The way in which food is used in this book and our recommendations for what to eat also alleviate menstrual problems. You don't need to wait until menopause to incorporate these eating changes into your diet and to benefit from the powerful results they can bring. But if your menopause is in full swing, you'll find not only a new approach to eating, but specific recommendations for the symptoms that are bothering you: what's in your diet that may be exacerbating or even causing that symptom and what you should add to your diet to alleviate the symptom. Eating the unprocessed, nutritious whole foods described here and eliminating certain foods that can unbalance your blood sugar, hormones, and emotions can curtail the miseries of menstruation and menopause. When you remove foods from your diet that rob nutrients from your body and replace them with foods that contain the vital nutrients your body requires, day by day your body will feel and look better. This way of eating transforms people's lives, as it has ours, and is a wonderful and powerful way to achieve health and vitality throughout your life as your body goes through its many changes.

All women experience the monthly cycle of menstruation. The average age at the onset of menstruation varies widely from culture to culture: Menstruation continues until it stops naturally, usually between the ages of forty-seven and fifty-five. (Menses can also stop due to excess weight loss from radical dieting, or strenuous athletic training, or because of medical interventions such as chemotherapy or a hysterectomy in which the uterus is removed.) The transition phase between having regular periods and no periods at all is called perimenopause. In most women, perimenopause begins around age forty-seven and lasts anywhere from a few months to several years. The first symptoms of what we call menopause—which may include heavy bleeding, exaggerated PMS (premenstrual syndrome), and hot flashes—can appear during perimenopause. Technically, menopause is the actual cessation of menstrual periods. A woman is not menopausal in scientific terms until she has gone twelve months without a menstrual period. This book and the recipes in it are designed to get you eating great food for maximum health and well-being all along the road from regular menstruation, through perimenopause, into menopause and beyond.

Besides addressing the special nutritional needs of our bodies as they acclimate to the hormonal changes of menopause, taking care of ourselves nutritionally can also reduce the likelihood of various diseases—some fatal—that women can be prone to over the age of fifty; you'll find detailed discussions here of nutritional tools for preventing and combating hypothyroidism, heart disease, osteoporosis, and breast cancer. Other lifestyle changes can also make a difference. Exercise, various methods of detoxifying the body, stress control, meditation, unloading personal stories that keep anguish within, and working on self-esteem are all ways we can take care of ourselves. Aging consciously can be a wonderful process, especially when it comes with good health.

In the following pages, we will introduce you to the nutrients you need to move through this change with maximum vitality. Then we will look at the symptoms that are a part of many, but not all, women's experience of menopause. Within each topic we will present foods to avoid and foods to choose for nutritional support in averting, minimizing, and combating that particular symptom. You will find a wide range of food sources for each essential nutrient and delicious recipes to nourish you. Each recipe includes an introductory note focusing on a particular nutrient or special benefit of each dish.

Once you have established a pattern of eating well, you'll find it's something that cannot be put aside. It happened this way for both of us and we know it will happen for you. One way to insure that you continue your good habits is to gather the support of others who have already made a change in their way of eating. You can meet these new allies in local natural food stores and cooperatives, organizations promoting healthy eating, and natural food restaurants. There are already millions of people who eat this way. Look around a little and ask—they are usually pleased to share their knowledge.

Making Changes . . . It's Not All or Nothing

For some of you, the foods and ideas about cooking and nutrition we promote are going to be brand new; others of you who already eat a more natural, whole foods–based diet will find some fresh tips. Our grand purpose is to educate you about the healing properties of whole, unprocessed food and the importance of eating these. If you eat a typical American diet, we realize that our recommendations may be a complete turnaround from how you've eaten so far in life. Given this, we suggest you make one change at a time. Replace your converted white rice with brown rice. Try a slice of whole wheat toast with almond butter and a piece of fruit in place of just black coffee and a bagel for breakfast. Get comfortable with this change and then make another. It may take longer for you to see all the results when you make changes incrementally, yet slow change is often an easier way of incorporating new habits into a busy life, and this approach may make it more likely that you'll keep these new ways forever. However, if you're enthusiastically ready for a total overhaul of your eating habits (or if you're suffering from intolerable hot flashes, mood swings, and sleepless nights), then don't hesitate to make radical changes right away.

There's no question that quitting smoking, cutting down on or eliminating coffee and alcohol, and exercising will give your health a boost. But whether you're ready to make those changes or not, eating foods that are health-supportive is still a good place to start. Taking better care of yourself is a lifelong process that you can begin today.

Here's how to proceed: Read a little of the book, cook a couple of the recipes, and eat. Order out and eat. Take a nutritionally focused cooking class for fun and eat. Just keep eating! Note how foods affect you each day. What did you eat? Do you have more energy and a longer attention span? Or do you feel more tired than usual and especially cranky? Feel warmer or cooler? Think back to what you ate. It can take anywhere from as little as several minutes to as much as two or three days for food to affect the way you feel. Monitoring your eating this way will allow you to start sorting out the foods that don't work in your body from those that do. Discovering what foods make you feel bad is as important as learning what foods will make you feel good. We know food can cause a shift in your vitality, and we know that feeling well matters. So, if living a life of health and vitality is what you want . . . read on!

The Sooner the Better

When you make changes in your eating habits, you set yourself up for a healthy future, and the earlier you start, the sooner you will benefit. Women who are still menstruating can prepare themselves for the future and clear up their PMS symptoms at the same time. Your experience of your monthly menstrual cycle is dramatically affected by what you eat and your resulting state of health. In our work as nutritional counselors, we've seen many women with premenstrual difficulties (cramping, bloating, breast tenderness, and general malaise) who changed their food choices and immediately noticed a lessening in their monthly symptoms and eventually stopped having difficulties altogether. With a change in diet, other women became fertile after years of attempting unsuccessfully to become pregnant. And after improving their diets, most clients report a higher level of energy and general good health, with fewer colds, allergies, skin problems, and unwanted weight gain.

Women who have had severe menstrual difficulties throughout their lives tend to have a worse menopause. A change in diet in the perimenopause years can minimize the unwanted symptoms of menstruation and the discomforts of menopause, too.

❧ 1 ❧

Food First:
The Basics for Menopause

How does food relate to menopause? Menstruation and menopause are initiated and accompanied by changes in hormone levels. These changing hormone patterns affect all of your body systems, including your heart, nerves, skin, and bones. The discomforts of menopause are caused by the body's attempts to adjust to fluctuating hormone levels and are greatly exacerbated by what we do and don't eat.

Eating delicious foods that are also nutritious is one of the most effective ways of supporting yourself through all of your body's transitions. There are vitamins, minerals, and other important nutrients essential to good health during menopause that are largely missing from the standard American diet, which relies on foods that are overly processed and nutritionally deficient. Happily, nature offers all the necessary nutrients in the form of glorious foods for you to benefit from and enjoy.

Our approach is based on the research of many investigators—from doctors to anthropologists—who have studied the eating habits of women around the world and their experience of menopause. The foods we use contain vitamins and minerals that alleviate PMS, reduce fatigue, and lessen hot flashes. They are known for their long-term benefits in increasing bone mass, lowering cholesterol, and preventing cancer. Some nutrients maintain skin suppleness and sexual vitality, while others keep your mind alert. While enjoying tasty and healthful meals, you'll be providing yourself with the protection offered by the natural pharmacy of nutrient-rich foods.

What's Good for the Goose . . . Men and Menopause

The foods we recommend for a woman's menopause are good for everyone else, too. Men can benefit from the nutrients these foods contain, nutrients which their aging bodies need as well.

Men do experience hormonal changes as they age, but there is no true male equivalent of menopause. Under normal conditions, men do not undergo a precipitous change in the concentration of the male hormone testosterone, but a number of recent studies have shown that testosterone levels do drop off gradually with age, perhaps as much as 30 to 40 percent between the ages of forty-eight and seventy. And there is fallout from this change, symptoms that may be attributed to lowered testosterone as well as to the general aging of the body and to the psychocultural experience we call midlife angst. These symptoms include a decline in muscle mass and strength, a buildup of body fat, flagging energy, lowered fertility, decreased libido, balding, and a slowing of the body's ability to heal after injury. Some men may also experience sexual dysfunction.

Men are also threatened by the same degenerative diseases as women—heart disease, cancer, and even osteoporosis. Men lose bone mass later in life than women, but the damage can be more severe. The nourishing foods used in these recipes can revitalize a man's aging body. For both sexes, eating well contributes to the possibility of having a long and healthy old age.

We've Cooked a Feast and You're Invited

The foods of nature—whole grains and beans, fresh vegetables and fruits, nuts and seeds—are seductive by themselves with their sweet juices, rainbow of colors, and mouth-watering tastes. They need no massive advertising campaigns to captivate and encourage you to eat them. Some foods that we cook with may have been on your "not to be eaten" list (especially eggs and nuts), yet looking closely at their nutritional makeup, we strongly believe that they have a place in your diet, and we'll explain why. We've created menus that are completely vegetarian and ones that include animal foods. We have found that not everyone can or necessarily should sustain a vegetarian way of life, so whatever your persuasion, we've made sure there will be plenty of appetizing and scrumptious foods to eat when you cook from this book.

As in the diets of traditional cultures worldwide, we rely on a predominance of plant foods, and all our ingredients are from fresh, unprocessed, and unrefined foods. Persian-Style Peppers Stuffed with Lentils and Bulgur, accented with cinnamon and mint, or Moroccan Chicken with Cashews and Chick-peas Served with Couscous, are a sampling of what you will find. The dishes are delicious, simple to make, easy to like, and are built from the foods that offer a strong foundation for your good health to rest upon.

Why do we steer you away from processed foods? Processed and refined foods no longer have many important nutrients that you need to stay well and often include ingredients that may be making you feel worse. Processed foods are prevalent in the supermarkets, yet the processing of food only began about 100 years ago. Up to then, the preserving and transporting of food had remained the same since ancient times and the ingredients came straight from the fields, pastures, and streams.

Why do we recommend whole foods? Whole foods have all of their nutritious parts with nothing edible removed. An apple is a whole food; apple juice has had all of its fiber removed and, calorie for calorie, has fewer nutrients. Brown rice is a nutrition-packed whole food; white rice is missing its bran and germ and is nutritionally deficient even when enriched. Whole foods have rich and full flavors, often requiring only a few condiments to fully bring out their sumptuous tastes. The whole foods used in our recipes can easily be found in supermarkets and natural food stores.

Medical Science Meets Traditional Wisdom: Good Nutrition Is Becoming an Alternative Therapy

The current medical wisdom says that since the problems of menopause are caused by a loss of production of estrogen and other hormones, the only solution for the alleviation of perimenopausal and menopausal symptoms is hormone-replacement therapy such as estrogen (ERT) or a combination of estrogen and progesterone (HRT). If this is all that's been offered to you, you haven't been given the full spectrum of choices available. Without rejecting what western medical science has to offer, we want to educate you more fully about the role of nutrition in aggravating and alleviating the symptoms of menopause. For years, researchers have noted that women in many parts of the world describe fewer menstrual, premenopausal, and menopausal complaints in comparison to what is currently experienced by American women. There are studies and reports of women in Japan, India, Africa, the Mediterranean, Indonesia, and other cultures documenting menopause to be a relatively untroubled transition. Numerous conclusions have been drawn from women's globally varied experience. One theory is that negative attitudes toward our bodies explain our menstrual and menopausal miseries. Some hypothesize that in cultures where a woman's status increases as she ages, women have a less troubled experience of menopause. Another theory is that menopausal symptoms depend upon how many children a woman has and at what age she had them. But in recent years, as doctors and health researchers have looked more closely at what different cultures eat and the role food choices might play in the rates of various diseases, this is what has emerged: Though standard of living, the status of women, parity, and diet vary widely from Japan to India to Africa to the Mediterranean, a common characteristic is that women in all these cultures eat a predominantly traditional diet comprised of nutrient-rich foods, the bulk of their calories come from plant foods, and they don't eat large quantities of processed foods, loaded with sugar, preservatives, and many other additives.

Our experience as nutritional counselors supports these observations: In general, women who over their lifetime have eaten a diet that has included grains, beans, fresh vegetables, and fruits have not had a difficult menopause. Women who have relied on processed and refined foods depleted of nutrients have had a fair amount of trouble. Essentially, the intensity of menopausal difficulties may be linked to nutritional deficiencies and not necessarily to hormonal changes and aging.

Active Ingredients

Science is finally beginning to understand why certain foods are good for your health during menopause. First, food can directly affect your hormone levels. Doctors now know that high-fiber, low-fat diets can reduce circulating estrogens, and some compounds such as bioflavonoids, which are plentiful in citrus, can help regulate this hormone. Soybeans and soy products, which have been touted for their possible cancer-fighting properties, are rich in phytohormones—plant hormones that mimic and modulate the action of your own hormones. Phytohormones, sometimes called phytoestrogens, are also found in oatmeal, cherries, and many other foods. Second, certain vitamins and minerals widely available from food sources but which most of us don't get enough of have a role to play, too. It's the B vitamins in whole grains such as whole wheat, brown rice, and millet that assist in reducing fatigue. The magnesium in molasses can prevent unexpected heart palpitations. Sexual vitality and skin suppleness depends on the presence of niacin, zinc, and essential oils, which are present in fish and shellfish.

Later, we'll provide detailed discussions of how these nutrients work, and we'll look at each of the celebrated symptoms of menopause and tell you how you can use food to counteract each one. But the general principle is this: There are foods present in excess in our diet that at best are nutritionally deficient and at worst actively undermine health. These foods are "Off the Menu." There are other foods—fresh, nutritious, and delicious—that support women's health and minimize the discomforts of menopause. These foods are "On the Menu." Eliminate as many of the off-the-menu items from your diet as possible, and incorporate as many of the on-the-menu foods as you can. Once you've turned on to the glorious whole foods "on the menu," you won't want to turn away.

Off the Menu

- Refined sugars
- Caffeine and coffee
- Processed oils
- Refined white flour and refined grains

Why sugar is off the menu: Refined sugars are completely devoid of vitamins, minerals, and fiber, and have no nutritive value. They stress your body and deplete it of vitamins and minerals. Refined sugar consumption can lead to calcium loss and increased overeating, and contributes to weight gain, diabetes, tooth and gum disorders, nervous disorders, low blood sugar, and fatigue. Refined sugars include cane and beet sugar, brown sugar, corn syrup, dextrose, glucose, maltose, and fructose. But cutting out sugar doesn't mean that you have to give up sweetness. Maple and grain syrups like barley and rice malt, date sugar, and fruit juices provide sweetness and contain all the vitamins and minerals needed for body functions—but of course use these with moderation. Fruits are a natural source of sugar, and whole fruit provides fiber. Honey is a concentrated sugar, but is acceptable for occasional use when maple and grain syrups are unavailable. Artificial sweeteners, including aspartame, sorbitol and saccharine, can produce many undesirable side effects and are to be avoided completely.

Why caffeine is off the menu: Caffeine quickens respiration, increases blood pressure, stimulates the kidneys, excites the brain's functions, and temporarily alleviates fatigue and depression. It can also create vitamin and mineral deficiencies, prevent iron absorption, irritate the stomach lining, aggravate the heart and arteries, and increase nervous symptoms. The most well-known caffeine-containing beverage is coffee. What many people don't realize is that coffee is also a diuretic. It has few nutrients but stimulates the excess excretion of urine along with the vitamins and minerals this urine contains. This is just as true of decaffeinated coffee, including the water-processed kind.

Caffeine is also found in teas that are not marked "caffeine-free," in chocolate, and in many sodas and soft drinks.

Why processed oils are off the menu: Liquid fats that come from seeds, beans, or nuts are known as oils. After oils are removed from plants they are treated with chemicals and heat to refine and deodorize them. All refined oils have had the flavorful elements and natural color of the original food they were pressed from removed, to make them tasteless and keep them from smoking at high temperatures, and deodorized oils have had their smell eliminated. Most oils that you probably cook with (including corn oil, canola oil, safflower oil) are refined. Refined oils contain toxic substances and should be avoided. Hydrogenated fats, such as shortening and margarine, are made from liquid oils that have been combined with hydrogen to make them solid at room temperature. Consumption of hydrogenated fats, which raise triglycerides and cholesterol, is strongly linked to heart disease. When you eat these types of fats and oils, you take in unnecessary toxins and miss out on the beneficial elements that are in unrefined fats and oils.

Why white flour and grains are off the menu: Just like white rice, wheat that has been processed to make white flour has had its bran and germ removed. Most commercial baked goods and pastas are made with only white flour, and when the bran and germ are missing, so are B vitamins, fiber, essential oils, and the other vitamins and minerals that these parts contain. In fact, when grains are processed, over twenty vitamins and minerals are removed and only four or five are returned. You can significantly improve the nutrition power of your diet just by replacing processed grains with whole, unrefined ones.

All whole grains are correctly called complex carbohydrates consisting of the bran, germ, and starchy endosperm. (Refined grains, which consist of just the endosperm, are simply called carbohydrates.) Throughout the recipes, we cook with only whole grains and whole grain pastas. If you are new to whole grains, you're about to be introduced to a world of culinary delights.

On the Menu

There are certain foods that are particularly full of the nutrients women especially need. These are your staples and the ingredients that are featured in the recipes.

MASTER LIST OF FOODS FOR CHANGE

Grains:
whole wheat, brown rice, buckwheat, millet, cornmeal, oatmeal, whole grain pastas

Beans:
navy, black, adzuki, chick-peas, lentils, pinto, kidney, soy

Vegetables:
dark leafy greens, asparagus, potatoes, yams, mushrooms, napa cabbage,
bok choy, cabbage, broccoli, carrots, beets, garlic, butternut squash,
artichokes, seaweed

Fruits:
berries, citrus, figs, black currants, avocados, apples, plantains, apricots

Nuts and Seeds:
almonds, walnuts, chestnuts, hazelnuts, cashews; sunflower, sesame,
and pumpkin seeds

Fish:
salmon, mackerel, herring, tuna, trout, oysters, shrimp, clams

Meats:
chicken, beef, lamb, game, plus organic liver

Fats and Oils:
extra-virgin olive oil, flax seed oil, unrefined sesame oil, unsalted butter

---

Whole grains top the list because they are full of fiber, vitamins, minerals, and other nutrients. As you can see, there are many to choose from, offering a variety of taste and texture. All of them can be prepared as a simple side dish in place of white rice, but we'll give you lots of recipes for using these great foods in more interesting ways. Since we eat a lot of grain in the form of flour (in bread and pasta), it's important to choose products made with whole grain flours. Most commercial pasta is made from a refined durum wheat, or semolina flour. This type of flour has had the bran and germ removed and is missing important fiber and nutrients. There are many packaged dry pastas (including brands imported from Italy and Japan) made with whole wheat, brown rice, and buckwheat. (A list of our favorite brands is in the Appendix.)

Beans, next on the list, are recommended especially for their fiber—the soluble variety, which is soft and less woody than vegetable and grain fiber. Beans contain a wide range of vitamins and minerals and, especially when coupled with whole grains, are a healthy source of protein. Beans come in all sorts of colors and shapes and can be made into many delicious foods or eaten by themselves. Beans are an essential food—and we will tell you how to eat them and be gas-free!

Topping the **vegetable** list are the dark leafy greens—collards, kale, turnip greens, dandelions, mustard greens, chicory, escarole, and broccoli rabe. They are high in minerals, including calcium and magnesium, both of which are good for the bones and heart. There are also equally important root and vine vegetables.

The **fruits** on the "Master List" have been chosen because they are rich in many nutrients. Their juiciness restores fluids that can be lost with hot flashes and resupply the body with vitamins and minerals lost in perspiration.

Nuts and seeds contain essential oils and protein and are a good food source. Many women have stopped eating these great and universal foods because of a fear of fat and its attendant calories, but poor information has generated an irrational anxiety. The kinds of fats in nuts and seeds are healthy, needed fats. Walnuts contain the same kind of oil as fish. Almonds contain the same oil as olives. Nuts and seeds also contain an abundance of necessary minerals. We encourage you to integrate them into dishes and main meals, rather than just eating them as occasional snacks. Nuts and seeds should be everyday foods.

If you are a vegetarian, you may be surprised to see meat and fish on the "Master List." If you're not a vegetarian, you may be surprised at how far down the list meat appears. Our own philosophy is that eating moderate amounts of animal foods is acceptable, but vegetarians and meat-eaters each have special nutritional challenges. Meat-eaters need to make sure that fatty animal foods are not crowding lean, fiber- and nutrient-rich plant foods like whole grains, beans, and vegetables off their plates. Vegetarians need to make sure that they are not subsisting solely on carrots and carbohydrates (even high-quality, complex ones!) and missing out on protein. It's quite possible to eat a vegetarian diet and still get the protein you need, but getting adequate amounts of protein is absolutely essential.

Fish is ranked above meat as a source of protein due to the special oils it contains and for its light and easy-to-digest protein. We recommend certain fish and shellfish for the oils they contain and their high mineral content.

Meats, which encompass poultry, beef, lamb, and pork, are included because they are a good source of iron and vitamin B_{12} and also because some people do feel better when eating animal foods. We recommend organic meats, those that have been raised without antibiotics or added hormones.

Fats and oils: There is much confusion about the use of fats in our daily diet, and what kinds and how much are healthy to eat. The American diet is high in saturated fat and most people need to cut back on this. Refined and hydrogenated fats are poor quality and can lead to heart disease and impair liver function; however, everyone needs some fat in their diet because fats play a role in the health of tissues, organs, and cells throughout the body. It's time we stop being "fat phobic" and learn which fats are the important ones to include.

It is of utmost importance to use cooking oils that are fresh, unrefined, free from heat processing, and not hydrogenated. Any oils of lesser quality can be toxic when eaten in even normal quantities over time and can help initiate degenerative diseases. Quality oils contain oil-soluble vitamins, lecithin, essential fatty acids, phytohormones, some minerals, and their own preservatives, anti-oxidants such as vitamin E, that keep oil from going rancid. Fresh, unrefined fats and oils, as they've been used for centuries, are the healthiest and much research supports this. Extra-virgin olive oil, unrefined sesame oil, flax seed oil, and unsalted butter all belong in your kitchen.

Extra-virgin olive oil is the only unrefined oil sold on the mass market. It contains phytohormones, chlorophyll, magnesium, vitamin E, and carotene. It's an excellent source of mono-unsaturated fat, which has been linked to low rates of heart disease. For daily use keep some extra-virgin olive oil in a small container that is completely lightproof, and keep the rest in the refrigerator. (When cold, it will solidify, but will quickly become liquid at room temperature.)

Unrefined sesame oil is a polyunsaturated oil that is available in the natural-food store and is not to be confused with dark sesame oil, which is made from sesame seeds that are roasted before pressing the oils from them. Unrefined sesame oil can be used in cooking, whereas the dark sesame oil with its robust taste is most healthfully added to a dish after cooking and used as a condiment for flavor.

Fresh flax seed oil was used widely in Europe until the turn of the century and is being revived as a super-nutritious food, especially for female health. It is high in omega-3 fatty acids, which are especially abundant in the brain cells, nerve relay stations, visual receptors, adrenal glands, and sex glands—the most biochemically active tissues in our body. Omega-3's have been found to lower triglycerides, expand arteries, decrease clotting, and prevent the growth of new cancer cells. (Canola has been promoted for its high omega-3 content, but it has far less than flax seed oil.) The American diet is low in these omega-3's and using flax seed oil is a good way to boost your supply.

Flax seed oil goes rancid very quickly and must be stored in the refrigerator. Here it will keep for at least four weeks, and in the freezer it will stay fresh for several months. Use it in a salad dressing and as a flavor accent drizzled over cooked vegetables. Some people are put off by the smell of flax seed oil in the bottle, but we urge you to try it on food, where most people find it delicious. Fresh flax seed oil has a buttery taste.

Unsalted butter, which is made from cream, is a fat that remains a solid at room temperature. (Because of the strong salt flavor of salted butter, it's hard to tell when the butter has gone rancid, so we only recommend using unsalted butter.) Unsalted butter can be stored refrigerated for up to two or three weeks and frozen for several months.

When butter is heated to high temperatures, it does not readily break down into dangerous transfatty acids, making butter an excellent choice for sautéing and baking, superior to any other fat. It is minimally processed and contains a natural antioxidant, vitamin E. We use butter when we bake cakes and cookies. It has a wonderful smell and taste, adds richness, and lightens the texture of a baked product. We all need some saturated fat and unsalted butter is a good source.

High-quality fats and oils are important to women throughout their entire lives. When extreme low-fat diets are adhered to for long periods of time there can be many subtle signs that show up as we mature. Some of the more obvious ones are dry skin, brittle hair, and peeling nails. These symptoms can easily be reversed with the addition of fresh, high-quality fats. More information on fats and oils appears in the Appendix.

Variety: More Foods, More Nutrients

Eating a wide range of fresh foods will provide you with a broad range of nutrients, the full spectrum that you need as a woman, monthly and over the years. There may be no single wonder food that can quench a hot flash or revive a fading memory, yet eating a range of nutrient-rich foods can.

A simple way to assure yourself that you are getting that broad range of nutrients is to shop for foods of different colors—red, orange, yellow, green, dark brown, deep purple, black, and white. Eat a range of colors and you get a range of nutrients. It's true!

	Off the Menu	On the Menu
Grains	White rice and refined flour (found in white bread, bagels, crackers, cookies)	Whole grains, including brown rice, buckwheat (kasha), millet, cornmeal, oatmeal, whole wheat
Fats and Oils	Refined and processed oils, margarine, hydrogenated oils	Healthy oils, such as extra-virgin olive oil, flax seed oil, unsalted butter, unrefined sesame oil
Vegetables	Frozen and canned vegetables	Fresh vegetables, especially yams, winter squash, sweet potatoes, carrots, bok choy, asparagus, Chinese napa cabbage, mushrooms, and dark leafy greens (i.e., kale, collards, and turnip greens)
Nuts and Seeds	Commercially roasted nuts and seeds	Raw nuts and seeds, especially walnuts, almonds, hazelnuts, sesame and pumpkin seeds, and chestnuts
Beans	Canned baked beans	Dried beans, including black beans, adzuki beans, chick-peas, pinto beans, navy beans, and lentils
Fish and Shellfish	Deep-fried fish and shellfish	Baked, broiled, and poached fish and shellfish, including salmon, sardines, mackerel, herring, roe, tuna, trout, and oysters, shrimp, and clams
Poultry and Meats	Fried chicken, luncheon meats, non-organic liver	Baked, broiled, or roasted chicken, duck, beef, lamb, game, and organic liver
Fruit	Canned fruit, sugar-coated fruit	Fresh and dried fruits (preferably unsulphured), especially avocados, berries, citrus, currants, figs, apples, cherries, plantains, and apricots
Sweeteners	Refined and processed sugars (white sugar, dextrose, fructose, table sugar)	Natural sweeteners, such as maple syrup, molasses, rice syrup, barley malt, fruit juice
Beverages	Coffee (with and without caffeine), caffeinated teas, alcohol, sodas with phosphates (sugared and diet), sugared drinks	Filtered water, fresh juice, grain coffee substitute, herbal tea

Why Organic?

Organic foods are the best choice for your health and well-being and for the planet as a whole. These include all plant foods grown without chemical fertilizers, pesticides, and herbicides, and animals raised on organic feed and not given antibiotics and hormones. When farmers have been certified by at least one third-party organization to verify that these standards are maintained, their produce can be labeled "certified organic." Organic practices maintain the purity of the earth's water supply. When buying organic, you also support American farmers working on small, family-owned farms.

As often as possible, buy foods that have been produced free of chemicals. It is easy to begin by purchasing organically grown whole grains and beans available in most natural food stores. Organically grown onions and carrots are commonly found in many grocery stores as well.

The label "natural" tells you nothing about whether the food was produced with or without the use of chemicals, antibiotics or hormones. If a farm is producing food without chemicals but has done so for less than three years (the minimum required for certification in most states), its produce may be labeled "natural," but usually when a farm is going for organic certification, the produce label will state this. On animal foods, "natural" means only that the animals have been taken off all antibiotics and hormones fifteen days before slaughter.

"Naturally" raised animals are better than commercially raised animal foods, but when there is a choice, choose organic.

❧

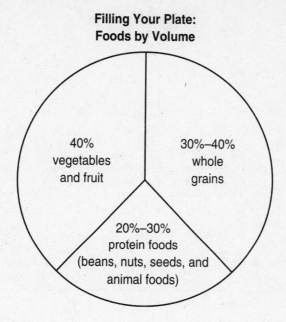

**Filling Your Plate:
Foods by Volume**

40%
vegetables
and fruit

30%–40%
whole
grains

20%–30%
protein foods
(beans, nuts, seeds, and
animal foods)

Filling Your Plate

For maximum health and vitality, you should be eating: 30 to 40 percent whole grains, 20 to 30 percent protein foods (beans, nuts, seeds, and animal foods), and 40 percent vegetables and fruit.

This is an overall guideline that doesn't have to be met at every meal or even on a daily basis. The volumes can change from day to day, allowing you to choose more or less of something as you feel the desire for a certain food. One day you may eat more protein, the next day more vegetables, and another more whole grains or fruit.

If you translate this into actual foods, here's what you'd see on your dinner plate: a cup of cooked grain and a cup of vegetables, with a 4-ounce portion of meat (the size of the palm of your hand) or half a cup of beans, plus a salad with dressing and a healthful dessert topped with some nuts.

With this kind of eating you can be assured that you will have enough protein, which is in whole grains, beans, nuts, seeds, and vegetables, as well as animal foods. And you'll be getting a lot of vitamins, minerals, and fiber in all the plant foods.

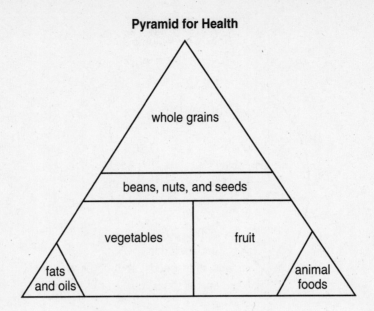

Pyramid for Health

Here is a pyramid showing the relative importance of each food group. We place plant foods high and central and animal foods and fats to the side. The smaller "fat and oils" and "animal foods" sections contribute more calories than appears, because fats are more calorie dense than fruits and vegetables. This food group pyramid gives you a quick overview of our "recipes for change."

❧ 2 ❧

Special Nutrients for Women

As scientists begin to discover what foods are good for women, new nutritional stars are making their debut. Bioflavonoids, boron, phytohormones, and essential fatty acids (as well as special fats and oils) are coming to the forefront. These nutrients, which are found in countless foods, play numerous roles in supporting your body during the many changes of menses. Because some of these nutrients might be less familiar and all are important to your health as a woman, we have provided an overview of what they are and how they work in your interest. Charts containing comprehensive lists of foods rich in each of these nutrients, as well as foods high in all the specific vitamins and minerals, appear in the back of the book.

Bioflavonoids: This group of compounds (which includes citrin, hesperidin, rutin, and flavones) has a structure and chemical activity similar to estrogen. By mimicking estrogen and modulating estrogen fluctuations, the presence of bioflavonoids in the body has been shown to control hot flashes and the psychological symptoms of menopause, including anxiety, irritability, and mood swings. They lessen heavy menstrual bleeding in premenopause, strengthen capillary walls, and help to keep the skin healthy and supple. Some of the foods that contain bioflavonoids include **green peppers, cherries, buckwheat (kasha), rose hips,** and especially **citrus,** which contains the complete bioflavonoid complex. The central white core of a citrus fruit has the most, but there are also bioflavonoids in the pith and membranes. (See Appendix, page 376, for a complete list of foods containing bioflavonoids.)

Bioflavonoids are better absorbed when consumed along with vitamin C. Fortunately, these two nutrients often come naturally paired, as in oranges. When cooked, bioflavonoids are stable and not destroyed.

Boron: Throughout your life, sufficient boron is needed for metabolizing calcium as well as for maintaining motor skills and mental alertness. Two large **apples,** a cup of **broccoli** florets, or a handful of **nuts** supplies about 1 mg of boron, a start for the 1 to 3 mgs of boron per day required for good health. Interestingly, a recent study of women on estrogen replacement therapy seems to indicate that boron can mimic and enhance the action of supplemental estrogen. (See Appendix, page 379, for a complete list of foods containing boron.)

Phytohormones: Sometimes called phytoestrogens, phytohormones are substances found in plant foods that affect your hormone status. They are present in dozens of foods that we commonly eat, and these foods have been shown to have an effect on hormonal balances in the body. Phytohormone potencies are considerably weaker than the estrogen that is produced in your ovaries, called estradiol, but although these plant hormones are 1/400th to 1/100,000th the potency of estradiol, they can mimic and modulate estrogens and can help stabilize hormone fluctuations, thus reducing the symptoms of menopause. Some of the foods that contain phytohormones are **brown rice, beans, flax seeds, radishes, tofu,** and **pomegranates.** They are also found in **rhubarb, potatoes, fennel,** and **green tea.** (See Appendix, page 386, for a complete list of foods containing phytohormones.) Vegetarian women can have phytohormone levels one hundred times greater than women eating the typical American diet.

Consuming foods rich in phytohormones may also lower your risk of heart disease and breast cancer. Japanese women eating a traditional diet have fewer incidences of hot flashes and lower rates of breast cancer. Scientists have suggested that the consumption of soybeans and soy products like tofu which are high in phytohormones is part of the reason. However, the traditional Japanese diet is also low in processed and refined foods and high in mineral-rich seaweed and fresh fish oils—all of which may be important factors. When Japanese women change their eating habits to the standard American diet, their incidence of heart disease and cancer parallels the current American levels.

Herbalists have successfully used plant hormones for thousands of years. The herbs dong quai and black cohosh—frequent ingredients in the herbal medicines used to treat the symptoms of menopause—contain these plant hormones.

Essential fatty acids: Also known as EFAs, the essential fatty acids are indeed essential to a woman's health since they make up the components of many organs and tissues. They bring oxygen to our tissues, help prevent premenstrual symptoms, improve the condition of hair, nails, and skin, and help prevent all major degenerative diseases, including heart disease and cancer. They are vital to your health throughout your entire life.

There are two families of EFAs, called omega-6 and omega-3. We need about twice as much omega-6 as omega-3. However, most of us are already getting so much omega-6 that we need to seriously boost our consumption of omega-3 fatty acids (in which the standard American diet is very low) to get that 2:1 ratio. Toward this goal, we've included many recipes that feature **walnuts**, **flax seed oil**, **dark leafy greens**, and **fish**, all of which are high in this essential nutrient. The average healthy adult requires 4 teaspoons of essential oils per day, but a woman in menopause, especially with dry skin, hair, and vaginal tissue, may need up to 2 to 3 tablespoons per day before her symptoms will improve.

Why Not Get What You Need from Vitamin Supplements?

It is generally agreed that if we consumed the recommended minimum five servings a day of fruits and vegetables and if we varied those vegetables, we might indeed have good levels of vitamins and minerals in our bodies. It is currently estimated that less than 9 percent of the population eats this many servings of fruits and vegetables, and thus many women throughout their entire lives are missing adequate vitamins and minerals. Many women enter menopause depleted and missing important nutrients.

You can ask your doctor or nutritionist to test your vitamin and mineral levels, and if you then decide to take supplements, these need to be taken in conjunction with nutrient-rich foods. Vitamin and mineral supplements are only useful if taken with carbohydrates, proteins, and quality fats. Together with these foods, they build and fuel a depleted body. Taking supplements without accompanying food is like giving water to a flowerpot that has no plant.

⚜

3

The Signs of Menopause:
Typical Problems and the
Foods That Fix Them

The signs of menopause usually occur for several months or years before you actually cease menstruation. They can include hot flashes, fatigue, weight gain, heart palpitations or flutters, mood swings, and forgetfulness. Changes in your glandular and hormonal systems can affect everything from your thyroid and the quality of your skin to your sexuality. In the perimenopausal phase, before menstruation has fully ended, some women experience premenstrual difficulties with exaggerated symptoms.

While the symptoms of menopause are not universal, about 85 percent of American women report experiencing some symptoms ranging from mild discomfort to very bothersome problems. Only 5 percent of menopausal women have symptoms more severe than this. Although the general dietary recommendations for combating all these symptoms are similar, there are specific foods that can lessen and prevent individual symptoms.

You can feel better just by eating better. Whether you're among the 5 percent who are seriously suffering or you have a symptom or two, in this section you'll find bottom-line advice—what to eat and what not to eat in order to feel better and to avoid producing additional symptoms. In fact, if you are relying on a lot of nutritionally depleted foods, it may be these foods that are causing the problems. Eliminate them from your meals and see what symptoms clear up that you blamed on menopause or menstruation. And then whatever other discomforts remain, handle these by consistently eating meals made with foods high in nutrients.

You'll see that we've highlighted certain vitamins and minerals that treat each condition. (In the Appendix you'll find comprehensive lists of foods rich in each nutrient.) At the end of each segment there are carefully selected lists of the foods that benefit and relieve specific symptoms. Pay special attention to the "Foods to Avoid," which can make your symptoms worse. Each symptom section also contains two days' worth of menus for three meals plus snacks. You can begin rejuvenating yourself with your very next bite.

The Estrogen You Make: It's Not Over Yet

Menopause is the conclusion of menstruation but not the end of all estrogen production. Even after menopause, the body still makes several kinds of estrogen. Before menopause your ovaries make estradiol, and even after menopause your ovaries continue to make some. But after menopause your adrenal glands become the major site for hormone production and they produce a hormone that converts to estrone, a weaker form of estrogen. This conversion occurs in fat tissue, muscle, and bone marrow. Some estrogen is also produced in your intestines when bacteria act on fatty acids. A third type of estrogen, called estriol, arises mainly from estrone that is converted in the liver. In other words, you're not totally out of estrogen with menopause.

Premenstrual Syndrome

The bad news is that some women experience worse PMS during perimenopause than they ever did earlier in life. The good news is that the symptoms of premenstrual syndrome whenever they occur can be reduced or eradicated by feeding the body the foods it needs. PMS, which can affect menstruating women one or two weeks before their menstrual cycle begins, can include cramping, water retention, skin eruptions, headaches, breast swelling and tenderness, joint pain, nervousness, and emotional ups and downs.

PMS symptoms are often traced to hormonal imbalances—excessive levels of estrogen and inadequate levels of progesterone, a situation that is typical of the irregular cycles of perimenopause. Because of this, women in perimenopause may experience PMS even if they've never had symptoms before. Abnormal hormone levels can also produce low blood sugar (hypoglycemia) and hypothyroidism with resulting PMS-like symptoms.

If a change in your diet does not correct your PMS, check with a health practitioner. Allergies, candidiasis, and malabsorption difficulties can also produce PMS-like problems.

What to Avoid to Beat PMS

Dairy: Dairy products are best avoided completely. Women who eat high amounts of animal fat and dairy products are known to become more affected by the symptoms of PMS. Consumption of dairy products such as ice cream, cottage cheese and other hard and soft cheeses, and processed cheese foods can cause swelling, cramping, and breast tenderness in many women. After several months to several years of avoiding dairy products, many women have reported shrinking or disappearance of fibroids, less menstrual bleeding and for fewer days, and reduction or absence of all other PMS symptoms. Butter is the only dairy product that is still recommended since it is primarily fat and contains very little milk solids or protein.

Salt and sugar: High salt intake can cause fluid retention. If fluid retention is a problem, reduce your salt intake. (Actually, if you start consuming fewer processed foods, you'll dramatically reduce your sodium intake without even trying. It's virtually impossible to add as much salt to home-cooked foods as is present in processed foods.) Refined sugar intake can destabilize blood sugar, causing irritability, depression, and a general feeling of malaise, often connected to PMS. You may think that a chocolate bar will make you feel better, but it will probably make you feel worse.

In our work as nutritional counselors, we sometimes find a case in which what not to eat is as important as what to eat. Amanda had experienced cramping, swelling, and breast tenderness throughout her life. Even in high school her PMS would bother her to the extent that she would miss at least one day of school per menstrual period. We suggested that she stop all dairy products. Each month she noticed a significant reduction of stressful PMS symptoms. Within six months of eliminating all dairy foods, she no longer had PMS complaints.

What You Need to Beat PMS

High fiber, low fat: The basic PMS dietary guidelines are to eat a diet that is high in fiber and low in fat. This means plenty of fresh **vegetables** and **fruits**, **beans** and **whole grains**, including whole grain cereals and breads. The fats from **nuts** and **seeds** are preferred, and also those from **fish** and **poultry**. Eating a high-fiber and lower-fat menu can decrease estrogen levels, which, when high, may lead to cramping, excess bleeding, and fibroids. With a lower animal-fat intake, less estrogen is consumed and produced.

Bioflavonoids and vitamin C: These are successful in reducing heavy menstrual bleeding. Bioflavonoids, especially when used with vitamin C, decrease capillary fragility and consequently decrease menstrual flow. Bioflavonoids also steady your own estrogen levels, tempering the symptoms of PMS caused by hormonal ups and downs. In Asian cultures, women eat a lot of bioflavonoid foods such as soba (buckwheat) noodles and papaya, and they don't tend to have premenopausal PMS problems. Coupling bioflavonoids with a vegetarian diet is really optimal.

Phytohormones: The plant foods that contain phytohormones, such as **brown rice**, **soybeans**, **oatmeal**, **green beans**, **cucumbers**, **cherries**, and **citrus**, can help reduce the swings in estrogen levels that cause many of the PMS symptoms.

Magnesium and other minerals: A wide spectrum of minerals are needed to keep PMS at bay. Whole grains, such as **buckwheat**, **whole wheat**, and **cornmeal**, with their fibrous bran offer both magnesium and the kind of fiber that helps to sweep the unused estrogen out of your body. **Beans**—especially soy, adzuki, and all white beans—are high in this important mineral as well as other needed minerals.

Essential fatty acids: These components of dietary oils help regulate the menstrual cycle, reducing PMS cramps, tender breasts, water retention, and mood swings. The omega-6 fatty acids found in most **nuts, soybeans, brown rice,** and **sesame seeds** are especially helpful.

Foods to avoid: fatty red meats; dairy products; refined grains; commercial salted foods; refined sugar; caffeine; alcohol; processed foods; also avoid cigarette smoking.

Cigarettes and Menopause

Smoking has a toxic effect on the ovaries. In premenopausal women, smoking is antiestrogenic, causing egg production to stop prematurely: Women who smoke reach menopause about one and a half years earlier than nonsmokers. Smoking and the byproducts of nicotinic acid can exacerbate symptoms and problems that may accompany menopause. Smoking can cause irregular and heavy bleeding and has been linked to hot flashes. Smoking ages the skin, depriving it of oxygen. It is also associated with higher risks of cardiovascular disease and osteoporosis. As the scientific papers point out, the mechanisms of these actions are not clear. The dangers, however, are perfectly clear.

FOODS FOR HEALING PMS

- Whole wheat, bulgur, whole wheat couscous, brown rice, wild rice, whole rye, buckwheat (kasha), millet, oatmeal, cornmeal, whole grain pasta, soba noodles (buckwheat)
- Pinto beans, black beans, white beans (Great Northern, navy, lima, cannellini), chick-peas, adzuki beans, soybeans
- Seaweed, mushrooms, Jerusalem artichokes, spinach, broccoli, potatoes, dark leafy greens, sweet potatoes, beets and beet greens
- Avocados, peaches, watermelon, all berries, all citrus, mangoes, dried currants, plantains
- Almonds, chestnuts, pine nuts, Brazil nuts, walnuts, pistachios, sunflower seeds, flax seeds, pumpkin seeds, sesame seeds
- Tuna, mackerel, trout, salmon, clams, oysters, roe, shrimp, halibut, chicken, chicken livers, quail, eggs, beef liver, venison, game, pork, lamb, organ meats
- Miso, yogurt, rose hips, blackstrap molasses

Menu Suggestions for Combating PMS

Here are two days of menus—one vegetarian, one non-vegetarian—designed to reduce the symptoms of PMS. Each "day" starts with dinner and proceeds through the next day's breakfast, lunch, and snacks. The menus include "do ahead" tips (like soaking beans at dinner for the next day's lunch) and use leftovers to build new meals.

Vegetarian	*Non-vegetarian*
Dinner: Black Bean Soup with Orange and Cinnamon; Millet-Rice with Peas and Tomato; Turnips with Tops in Creamy Sauce; Your Basic Green Salad	**Dinner:** Hearty Rigatoni with Sausages, Garlic, and Broccoli; Your Basic Green Salad with escarole *(soak chick-peas)*
Dessert: Light Lemon Pudding Parfait with Kiwi Slices	**Dessert:** Peach Crumble
Breakfast: Black Bean Soup with Orange and Cinnamon; whole-grain bread	**Breakfast:** Old-Fashioned Oatmeal with black currants, blackstrap molasses, and sunflower seeds *(cook chick-peas)*
Snack: almonds and berries	**Snack:** watermelon chunks and mango
Lunch: Millet-Rice with Peas and Tomato; Turnips with Tops in Creamy Sauce; Grated Beet and Hiziki Slaw on salad greens *(make Peach Crumble)*	**Lunch:** rigatoni, garlic, and broccoli with chick-peas; Fast Salad
Snack: pear and orange	**Snack:** baked sweet potato or Peach Crumble

Hot Flashes

A surge of heat that moves through your torso and expands to your arms and face is called a hot flash. Your first one may be a surprise, and you might think it's the room that's overheated or that you're wearing too many clothes. Hot flashes can begin during perimenopause or menopause, and may occur for several years.

Although the series of physiological events that produce a hot flash are not completely understood, it is known that estrogen plays a role. Flashes can be triggered by stress or emotional situations, hot weather, a confining space, and they can be caused by eating certain foods.

What to Avoid to Beat Hot Flashes

Common triggers: The most common hot-flash food triggers are **spicy foods, caffeine, chocolate**, and **alcohol**. Even a warm drink or a hot meal can activate a hot flash. If you have a hot flash, think back to what you've had to eat or drink in the last few minutes or hours, and often by avoiding these stimulating foods you can avoid triggering another. If you're not sure which foods will have this effect on you, eliminate the suggested trigger foods for a week and then add them back to your meals one at a time to see which produce effects. Experiment with this several times until you are sure which foods, and in what quantity, are causing the hot flashes.

Over Marla's lifetime she had never developed the habit of drinking coffee or alcohol and wasn't a big chocolate eater. She changed jobs at around forty-nine and started having hot flashes soon after. When we looked at her eating patterns, we saw that with the stress and responsibility of her new job she had begun to drink small amounts of coffee each day, thinking she would get more energy, and she would have an occasional glass of wine or other alcoholic beverage with clients. On top of this, she was eating chocolate at night. We asked her to experiment and on the days she had no coffee, alcohol, or chocolate, all of her hot flashes disappeared. She tested this several times and finally decided that ridding herself of symptoms was more important than her reasons for eating this way and now she is hot flash free.

Irregular eating: Irregular eating can cause hot flashes by destabilizing your blood sugar. If you see a pattern between dips in your energy, food intake, and hot flashes, then make sure to eat at regular intervals. (For a more complete discussion of blood sugar, see page 30.)

What You Need to Beat Hot Flashes

Vitamin E: Extensive research has proven that vitamin E—contained in **whole grains, nuts**, and **seeds**—can reduce hot flashes. Refined grains, such as white flour and white rice, and refined cooking oils are low in vitamin E. Heating, frying, and storing foods also destroys this vitamin. To maximize the effectiveness of vitamin E, you need to combine it with selenium. These two nutrients work together and both are found in **lamb, cabbage, molasses**, and **eggs**.

Bioflavonoids: These are in **green peppers, buckwheat**, and especially **citrus** fruit. When you eat an orange, include some of the pith, the membranes, and the soft white core—all the places where the bioflavonoids are stored.

Magnesium: Magnesium helps quench the heat of hot flashes, assisting the body in maintaining a level temperature. This mineral is found in **beans**, **spinach**, and **sunflower** and **sesame seeds**.

Phytohormones: These plant hormones are needed to balance your estrogen supply, preventing extreme highs and lows that may initiate flashes. **Soybeans** and the tofu and tempeh made from them have exceptionally high amounts. There are also many foods common to American cooking that have some estrogenic activity—**oats**, **potatoes**, and **apples** to name a few.

Water: With hot flashes, you can lose significant amounts of body fluids, even if you're not aware that you are perspiring. We suggest that you keep a glass of water nearby and drink six to eight glasses a day. Other beverages such as fruit juices, herbal tea, and bouillon should not be included in your count.

Minerals: When you perspire, you can also lose minerals—especially sodium, potassium, chloride, and magnesium. The loss of these minerals along with the accompanying water adds to the feeling of exhaustion that hot flashes can cause. To replace minerals, munch on **fruits**, **nuts**, and **seeds**, and drink **bottled waters** that contain minerals. After a night of hot flashes, in the morning you can replenish your mineral supply with a breakfast of creamy **brown rice cereal** made in salted water (see Brown Rice Congee), topped with a **banana** and a drizzle of **blackstrap molasses**.

We counseled Anne, who was in perimenopause and having rampant hot flashes. She usually quenched her thirst with colas and coffee and rarely drank water. We encouraged her to keep a pitcher of water on her desk and a water bottle in the car to remind herself to drink water throughout the day, and to eat watery foods such as **melon**, **cucumbers**, and **mushrooms**. She was amazed to find that she could keep her stamina and energy even while her temperature rose and fell, and she also noticed that she now has less frequent episodes of flashing.

Exercise: Physical activity can sometimes be beneficial in reducing hot flashes. Exercise is also a great way of reducing stress, which often can act as a powerful hot-flash trigger.

Foods to avoid: warming and overly stimulating foods; caffeine drinks including coffee; black tea; all alcoholic beverages, including beer and wine; desserts made with white sugar; spicy chili and curry; chocolate; black and white pepper.

FOODS FOR REDUCING HOT FLASHES

- Whole wheat, bulgur, whole wheat couscous, brown rice, whole oats, kasha, whole rye, cornmeal, quinoa, whole grain pasta
- White beans (Great Northern, navy, lima, cannellini), soybeans, chick-peas, split peas, adzuki beans
- Green peppers, broccoli, kale, seaweed, tomatoes, cucumbers, potatoes, green and snow peas, garlic
- Mangoes, all citrus, dried currants, cantaloupe, figs, papayas, cherries, blackberries
- Brazil nuts, almonds, hazelnuts, sunflower seeds, sesame seeds, flax seeds
- Shrimp, oysters, mackerel, perch, haddock, flounder, chicken, eggs, beef liver, pork
- Rose hips, fennel seed, blackstrap molasses, sauerkraut, water

MENU SUGGESTIONS FOR FIGHTING HOT FLASHES

Here are two days of menus—one vegetarian, one non-vegetarian—designed to quench hot flashes. Each "day" starts with dinner and proceeds through the next day's breakfast, lunch, and snacks. The menus include "do ahead" tips (like soaking beans at dinner for the next day's lunch) and use leftovers to build new meals.

Vegetarian	*Non-vegetarian*
Dinner: bowl of Antipasto; Whole-Grain Pasta with Tofu Alfredo Sauce (*soak chick-peas; make Sunflower-Nori Snack*)	**Dinner:** Flounder Rolls Stuffed with Salmon and Lemon; Puréed Cabbage and Potatoes; Steamed broccoli and snow peas; cucumber slices (*make Chick-pea Hummus, pot of brown rice*)
Dessert: tangerines and Hearty Oatmeal-Apple Muffins with apple butter	**Dessert:** Zen Punch and California Waldorf Salad made with fresh figs
Breakfast: Brown Rice Congee with banana, blackstrap molasses, and almonds (*cook chick-peas*)	**Breakfast:** fresh orange sections; Salmon and Rice Patties; tomato slices
Snack: Sunflower-Nori Snack with black currants; Rose Hip Cooler	**Snack:** Hearty Oatmeal-Apple Muffins; cup of herbal tea
Lunch: cooked and raw vegetables with dressing; Tofu Alfredo Sauce on whole grain bread or crackers	**Lunch:** Chick-pea Hummus sandwich with whole wheat pita; Fast Salad made with steamed broccoli and snow peas, with raw green pepper and cucumber
Snack: cantaloupe slices	**Snack:** California Waldorf Salad with figs

Fatigue

Feeling very tired, if not exhausted, is one of the most common and annoying discomforts of menopause. There are numerous causes of menopause fatigue, but they can all be addressed by eating better. First, make sure you are eating. It sounds silly, but you may be depleted simply because you're running on empty and all you need to do is make sure you're not skipping meals. Start the day with a hearty breakfast and keep a healthy snack in your purse or car. Fatigue can also be a symptom of hypothyroidism (see page 45).

What to Avoid to Beat Fatigue

Refined sugar: Found in many prepared foods and snacks besides candy, refined sugar causes your blood sugar to rise and then, after a short period, quickly fall, which you may experience as fatigue. Refined sugar can also deplete your system of vitamins and minerals and in this way, too, leave you feeling exhausted. Stabilize your blood sugar by eating three meals a day, plus a healthy snack between each meal. For best results, make sure each meal contains some complex carbohydrates, protein, and fat. Add **yams**, **winter squash**, and **fruit** to your meals to satisfy your craving for sweets and you'll be steadying your blood sugar as well.

When you have a craving for sweets, you may just be craving calories. Give yourself some protein and fat, and then see if you still want a sugar snack.

Monique was accustomed to skipping breakfast and lunch. She'd have a cookie or a piece of fruit while running from one place to another, although she always had dinner with her husband. After she turned fifty, she started complaining of extreme exhaustion. We had her eat small, regular meals and snacks throughout the day and her fatigue went away, except on the days that she forgot to eat! And, even though she ate more food, she didn't gain any weight.

Substances that deplete your adrenal glands: Fatigue can be caused by adrenal gland exhaustion. Caffeine causes the adrenals to trigger the release of glucose, which is then converted into energy, giving you a momentary lift. In this way, the caffeine in coffee, tea, and chocolate can make you feel energized, at least briefly, but the process is very wearing on these important glands. Nourish your adrenals with foods that contain riboflavin, vitamin B_5, vitamin B_6, and vitamin C, all present in familiar foods such as **potatoes**, **broccoli**, **whole grains**, and **beans**.

Allergens: Fatigue can be caused by allergies, especially allergies to molds. Other common allergens are corn, wheat, rice, milk, chocolate, and food additives. A medical professional specializing in the treatment of allergies can test your sensitivities to certain substances.

What You Need to Beat Fatigue

B vitamins: This large vitamin group is necessary for the conversion of food into energy. A range of B vitamins can be found in **whole grains**, **beans**, **vegetables**, **fruits**, **nuts**, **seeds**, **fish**, **poultry**, and **meat**. Your body's supply of B vitamins needs to be replenished on a daily basis.

Iron: Heavy menstrual bleeding can result in iron deficiency anemia, which causes fatigue as the iron-poor blood is unable to deliver oxygen to the cells. Iron is found in **blackstrap molasses**, **seaweed**, **liver**, **beans**, and **raisins**.

Sleep and rest: Yes, to beat fatigue, you must get enough sleep. Unfortunately, several other symptoms—especially PMS and hot flashes—can make it difficult to get a good night's sleep. If you are experiencing any of the symptoms that result in sleep deprivation, use the foods that counteract them to help reduce fatigue. Periodic moments of just sitting back in a chair and taking a few deep breaths or a midafternoon nap can also be revitalizing, especially in a room with fresh air.

Sue-Anne was feeling tired and looking depressed. Everyone in her office started questioning her about what was wrong. When she told us of her hot flashes and sleepless nights we knew immediately what could be causing the problems. Close evaluation of her diet showed that she drank decaffeinated coffee (which still has some caffeine) with several cookies in the evening before bedtime. We suggested that she eliminate these two items and instead eat a bowl of oatmeal at bedtime to help her sleep. (Carbohydrates cause the body to produce its own tranquilizer, a great sleep aid. Enjoy some whole grain bread or cereal and snooze.) She soon called to report sleep-filled nights and no hot flashes. Within a week she looked and felt like herself again.

Exercise: Even brief and easy activity will bring fresh oxygen into the system and having this is as important as ample rest. Of course, exercise can lead to reducing to a normal weight and this, too, can lessen fatigue.

Foods to avoid: all refined sugars and concentrated sugars; refined flour products; fast foods; black tea; coffee and decaffeinated coffee; also avoid cigarette smoking.

Blood Sugar

Many symptoms in menopause—hot flashes, mood swings, and fatigue—can be worsened by blood sugar that swings between highs and lows. To stabilize your blood sugar, eat three meals a day plus snacks in between, or have frequent mini-meals throughout the day. As much as possible each meal should contain some complex carbohydrate, some protein, and some fat because each provides energy within a different time span. The complex carbohydrates give you energy for the first hour and a half after eating, then the protein begins to be used, and after three hours the fat has been broken down and becomes the final source of fuel. Eating all three at the same meal gives you a supply of energy that lasts three to four hours.

Avoid white sugar and concentrated sweets which give you a boost of energy followed by a drop. Our dessert recipes use small amounts of sweeteners such as maple syrup that don't affect blood sugar as dramatically, especially when used with whole grain flours and some fat. Instead of fruit juice, which assimilates into the blood quickly, choose a piece of fruit, which takes longer to digest.

Chromium, magnesium, and niacin are also necessary to keep blood sugar steady; you'll find all three in brown rice and broccoli.

FOODS THAT FIGHT FATIGUE

- Whole wheat, bulgur, whole wheat couscous, brown rice, millet, cornmeal, wild rice, kasha, whole grain pasta
- Navy beans, chick-peas, pinto beans, black beans, lima beans, soybeans
- Seaweed, asparagus, mushrooms, potatoes, dark leafy greens, beets and beet greens, green peas, broccoli, kuzu, spinach, yams
- Mangoes, avocados, watermelon, prunes, plantains, peaches, grapes, figs
- Almonds, Brazil nuts, cashews, chestnuts, hazelnuts, sunflower seeds, flax seeds, pumpkin seeds
- Tuna, salmon, oysters, trout, clams, shrimp, caviar, haddock, quail, chicken, eggs, turkey, beef liver, venison, game, pork
- Yogurt, miso, tahini, blackstrap molasses

Menu Suggestions for Combating Fatigue

Here are two days of menus—one vegetarian, one non-vegetarian—designed to fight fatigue. Each "day" starts with dinner and proceeds through the next day's breakfast, lunch, and snacks. The menus include "do ahead" tips (like soaking beans at dinner for the next day's lunch) and use leftovers to build new meals.

Vegetarian	*Non-vegetarian*
Dinner: Black Bean Loaf; Greens Four Calcium; Wild Mushroom Sauce; Composed Salad of Oranges, Avocado, and Endive	**Dinner:** Braised Chicken with Kale; Asparagus Mimosa with Lemon and Flax Seed Oil; Wild-Rice Ring with Almond Romesco Sauce; Your Basic Green Salad
Dessert: Peach Cobbler with herbal tea *(make Almond and Apple Butter Spread)*	**Dessert:** mixed fruit compote with yogurt
Breakfast: whole grain toast with Almond and Apple Butter Spread; soft-boiled egg	**Breakfast:** Homemade Granola with Tahini Milk
Snack: hazelnuts and cashews	**Snack:** Baked yam
Lunch: Black Bean Loaf sandwich on whole grain bread; avocado slices and endive	**Lunch:** chicken and kale sandwich on whole grain roll
Snack: watermelon chunks *(make compote with dried prunes, peaches, figs, raisins, and almonds)*	**Snack:** slice of Wild-Rice Ring with mustard; Peach Cobbler

Heart Palpitations

In menopause some women experience heart palpitations, an unexpected quickening of the heartbeat. Eating nutritious foods helps prevent these from occurring. *If you do experience anything more dramatic, see a physician immediately, as heart palpitations could be a sign of something more serious.*

Our friend Rose Mary was quite unsettled by the little flutterings of her heart she experienced as she began menopause. She would suddenly be aware that her heart skipped a beat or momentarily speeded up. Our advice was to eat foods especially high in minerals, and avoid those that deplete them, such as foods with refined sugar and coffee, and the heart palpitations stopped recurring.

What to Avoid to Calm Heart Palpitations

Caffeine and sugar: Caffeine can cause fluttering and heart palpitations even in young people, but if you thought you were never sensitive to caffeine before, you may not recognize what it's doing to you now. Cut out the caffeine and you'll save yourself not only the discomfort from the palpitations but the strain on your heart as well. Refined sugar makes trouble on several fronts: the "rush" immediately after eating it can cause palpitations, and swings in blood-sugar levels that result from eating refined sugar can do this too. Keep your blood-sugar levels as stable as possible to avoid this unpleasant sensation. (For more information on the role of blood sugar in many of the symptoms of menopause, see page 30.)

What You Need to Avoid Heart Palpitations

Minerals: Magnesium and calcium are needed to maintain a regular heartbeat, and sodium, potassium, and phosphorus are also necessary for heart health. **Dark leafy greens**, **beans**, and **fruits** are good sources of all of these minerals.

Liquids: Fluid imbalances can trigger palpitations. It's important to keep yourself well-hydrated, drinking six to eight glasses of **water** throughout the day, especially if you are having hot flashes, which can cause sweating.

> ***Foods to avoid:*** coffee (including decaf) and all caffeinated drinks; refined and processed foods; refined grains; refined sugars.

FOODS THAT WILL ASSIST WITH HEART PALPITATIONS

- Kasha, whole wheat, bulgur, whole wheat couscous, brown rice, millet, quinoa, whole grain pasta
- Soybeans, white beans (Great Northern, navy, lima, cannellini), chick-peas, adzuki beans, lentils
- Spinach, seaweed, dark leafy greens, beets and beet greens, potatoes, carrots, artichokes, bok choy
- Figs, plantains, avocados, papaya, all berries, pears
- Almonds, Brazil nuts, hazelnuts, pistachios, sesame seeds, sunflower seeds, flax seeds
- Mackerel, sardines (with bone), clams, pompano, shrimp, lamb
- Blackstrap molasses, tofu, tempeh, sauerkraut, pickles, goat cheese, water

MENU SUGGESTIONS FOR AVOIDING HEART PALPITATIONS

Here are two days of menus—one vegetarian, one non-vegetarian—designed to reduce heart palpitations. Each "day" starts with dinner and proceeds through the next day's breakfast, lunch, and snacks. The menus include "do ahead" tips (like soaking beans at dinner for the next day's lunch) and use leftovers to build new meals.

Vegetarian	*Non-vegetarian*
Dinner: Kasha Loaf with Yam; Marinated Arame Salad with Horseradish; Tempeh, Green Beans, and Carrots with Mustard Sauce	**Dinner:** Broiled Mackerel in Lime Juice; Quinoa Risotto; Collard Greens with White Onions; Carrot and Cabbage Slaw
Dessert: Strawberry Tart with Walnut Crust	**Dessert:** Beverly's Cantaloupe with Freshly Grated Ginger *(make Sunflower-Nori Snack)*
Breakfast: Strawberry Tart with Walnut Crust; grain coffee substitute	**Breakfast:** Quinoa Risotto with almonds
Snack: slice of Kasha Loaf with Yam	**Snack:** goat cheese with whole-grain crackers
Lunch: tempeh sandwich on whole grain bread with lettuce, tomato, sprouts, and pickle	**Lunch:** mackerel sandwich with mustard and sauerkraut on whole grain bread; Carrot and Cabbage Slaw
Snack: fresh pear	**Snack:** Sunflower-Nori Snack

Memory

There is a possible biochemical link between memory and estrogen, which appears to have a highly selective effect on memory functions. Estrogen improves verbal but not visual recall. It can revive short-term memory, and the ability to acquire or retain new associations. Though the research is inconclusive, scientists hypothesize that estrogen may affect an enzyme in the brain that's needed for memory function, and the adrenal glands may also be involved. Most significantly, though, much perceived "memory loss" at menopause is actually due to fatigue and low blood sugar. You'll find that these spells of forgetfulness lessen as the body is fed nutritious foods and learns how to manage its hormonal changes.

What You Need to Maintain Memory

Steady blood sugar: The brain depends upon a steady supply of blood sugar to function clearly, and when blood sugar drops, remembering things may become more difficult.

Virginia came to us complaining primarily of a poor memory. She had developed a system to remember things by posting notes all over her apartment, desk, and refrigerator, but sometimes she would even forget to look at these. When she came in for her appointment, we asked her what she ate for breakfast. She reported having had coffee and a piece of toast, same as every other day. She also mentioned that by 11 A.M. she was especially light-headed and unable to think straight or remember details. To us, the solution seemed simple. We suggested she spread a little almond butter on her toast and eventually eliminate the coffee. We also suggested that she add an egg or some oatmeal with sunflower seeds for protein to get her through the morning. As soon as the next day, and in the weeks to come, on the days Virginia ate a hearty breakfast she found herself remembering more and writing fewer notes.

Quality fats and essential fatty acids: Fat is a major component of cell walls and is necessary for the transmission of impulses that carry thought. The brain cells are composed of 60 percent fat. The majority of these fats are built from essential fatty acids—omega-3 and omega-6—that are not manufactured in the body and must be supplied on a daily basis. In a healthy brain, the omega-3 fatty acids predominate; these are plentiful in **oily fish**, **walnuts**, and **flax seed oil**. Omega-6 fatty acids are in **vegetables**, **wild game**, and **seeds**. Organic, free-range, or fertilized **eggs** are also a good source of these quality fats. (This is one instance where it's really worthwhile to find a source for noncommercial eggs, as supermarket eggs may not actually contain the fats you need because of how the chickens are raised.)

Anti-oxidants: Much has been made in recent years of the possible role of anti-oxidants in fighting cancer. What anti-oxidants do is to protect the fragile structures of essential fatty acids, keeping them from breaking down into toxic substances. As you increase your consumption of EFAs, you also need to increase your consumption of the anti-oxidants and the vitamins and minerals that play a role in their function—beta-carotene, vitamin C, vitamin E, selenium, the bioflavonoids, vitamins B_5 and B_6, thiamin, copper, manganese, and zinc. Anti-oxidants also help in cell-to-cell communication. To include anti-oxidants in your meal, serve yourself **winter squash**, **oranges**, **grapefruit**, **whole grains**, and **shrimp**.

Lecithin: The brain needs lecithin—contained in **egg yolks, beans,** and **cabbage**—to produce chemicals that act as messengers for thoughts and memories. This biochemical process also requires vitamin B_5 and the hormone DMAE, found in **sardines** and **anchovies**.

Vitamins: The B vitamins fuel brain chemistry; a deficiency manifests itself as memory loss and mental confusion. **Whole grains** and **breads, cereals,** and **pasta** made with them contain a wide variety of these vitamins. (Eating whole grains, which are complex carbohydrates, is also a good way to maintain blood-sugar levels.) Folic acid, an important B vitamin, in particular is necessary for proper brain function.

Minerals: Sufficient magnesium, potassium, phosphorus, and boron are important to mental alertness. **Millet, dark leafy greens,** and **figs** are full of minerals.

Exercise: The brain needs oxygen. Daily exercise is a good way of increasing your supply.

Foods to avoid: refined oils; a predominance of saturated fats rather than polyunsaturates; refined sugars; processed and fast foods.

❧

A build-up of heavy metals can cause memory loss. Mercury, cadmium, and lead are the most common of the heavy metals that don't belong in our bodies and that can enter from a variety of sources, including gasoline combustion fumes, industrial pollution, and possibly dental fillings. The most common source of these metals in the food supply is fish. These materials can build up in your body, which has difficulty filtering or excreting them, and they can displace other minerals. If your memory loss has persisted for a long time, have a hair analysis to rule out heavy metal toxicity as a cause. Ask your M.D. for a routine heavy metal toxicity test, then use an alternative health practitioner to learn how to detoxify any heavy metals you might have.

❧

FOODS THAT WILL IMPROVE YOUR MEMORY

- Millet, whole oats, whole wheat, bulgur, whole wheat couscous, whole grain pasta
- Navy beans, black beans, pinto beans, lentils
- Cabbage, mushrooms, seaweed, red peppers, sweet potatoes, shiitake mushrooms, dark leafy greens, parsley, broccoli, asparagus, cauliflower, red peppers, bok choy, green peas
- Mangoes, avocados, dried currants, plantains, bananas, cantaloupe, figs
- Almonds, Brazil nuts, walnuts, flax seeds, sunflower seeds
- Oysters, salmon, bluefish, tuna, roe, mackerel, sardines, swordfish, anchovies, chicken, chicken livers, lamb, game, organ meats
- Pickles, blackstrap molasses, rose hips

MENU SUGGESTIONS FOR IMPROVING MEMORY

Here are two days of menus—one vegetarian, one non-vegetarian—designed to get your brain working. Each "day" starts with dinner and proceeds through the next day's breakfast, lunch, and snacks. The menus include "do ahead" tips (like soaking beans at dinner for the next day's lunch) and use leftovers to build new meals.

Vegetarian	*Non-vegetarian*
Dinner: Twice-Cooked Pinto Beans Wrapped in Corn Tortillas; Persimmon Salsa; Chinese Napa and Celery Salad; avocado slices	**Dinner:** Greek Lentil and Garlic Soup; Grilled Fresh Sardines, Portuguese Style; Curried Cauliflower Crown; Mesclun Salad
Dessert: Hearty Oatmeal-Apple Muffins	**Dessert:** Crispy Walnut and Seed Bars; grain coffee substitute with molasses
Breakfast: Twice-Cooked Pinto Beans, scrambled eggs, and corn tortillas	**Breakfast:** Split Pea and Barley Soup with Spices; whole grain crackers
Snack: Beverly's Cantaloupe with Freshly Grated Ginger	**Snack:** Toasted Nuts with Raisins and Apricots
Lunch: avocado sandwich on whole grain roll, with tomato, sprouts, and red pepper slices	**Lunch:** sardine sandwich on whole grain bread with mustard, lettuce, and sprouts
Snack: Hearty Oatmeal-Apple Muffins (*make Crispy Walnut and Seed Bars*)	**Snack:** baked yam and pickles

Mood Swings, Irritability, Depression

Hormonal changes can bring emotions to the surface. It is common to become angry, irritable, have mood swings, and feel depressed. During menopause, the great majority of women don't experience a major depression, but teariness without provocation and a certain moodiness are fairly typical. Lack of sleep, thyroid problems, and adrenal exhaustion can also have an impact on feelings.

The primary causes of "moodiness" during menopause are wild swings in blood sugar, which is determined by what you eat, and fluctuating estrogen levels, which can be modulated by what you eat. In other words, whatever the physical source, being unusually emotional without apparent reason is a sign that better and more frequent meals are needed. Eating well-balanced meals while eliminating refined sugars, processed foods, and caffeine will keep your spirits on a more even keel.

What to Avoid to Stabilize Moods

Vitamin and Mineral Deficiency: The first step in balancing emotions is to eat unrefined foods that still retain their well-rounded complement of nutrients. Having a mild vitamin deficiency can in itself result in nervousness and low spirits. The B vitamins stabilize brain chemistry and nourish the nervous system. A deficiency of thiamin and folic acid can result in irritability, and vitamin B_6 combats depression and stress. Vitamin E is known to reduce anxiety. A deficiency of minerals—potassium, magnesium, calcium, and boron—can also lead to irritability. All of these vitamins and minerals can be found in unprocessed foods, such as **whole grains**, **beans**, **vegetables**, and **fruits**.

Casey's emotions were known to swing from high to low, from euphoria to weepy moments. Her meals mainly consisted of fast food sandwiches on white bread, iceberg lettuce salads with occasional carrots and celery. She ate no beans and infrequent animal protein. Occasionally Casey ate fruit, and daily she consumed cookies and ice cream. To encourage her to eat better, we suggested she start with brown rice and mixed vegetables from a local Chinese restaurant. She then exchanged her white bread for whole grain products, and added a full range of vegetables and fruits. She found chick-pea hummus and whole wheat bread in the grocery store and within a month her day-to-day emotions were more steady.

What You Need to Stabilize Moods

Estrogenic foods: If your mood swings are the result of highs and lows of fluctuating estrogen levels, then focus on the phytohormone-rich foods that modulate these levels—**vegetables**, **fruits** including citrus, **soybeans**, and **buckwheat**. Foods high in bioflavonoids and boron, two estrogenic nutrients, are also good to include in your meals.

The Happy Meal: A meal composed solely of complex carbohydrates will cause your body to produce its own natural tranquilizer. Eating a bowl of brown rice or any other whole grain will raise the level of serotonin, a brain chemical which elevates mood and regulates sleep. The effect works best when the complex carbohydrate is eaten alone, without fat or protein, which interferes with serotonin synthesis. You can also use this "tranquilizer" in the evening if you're having trouble sleeping.

> *Foods to avoid:* refined sugar; caffeine; alcohol; refined grains; processed and refined foods.

FOODS THAT WILL STABILIZE EMOTIONS

- Whole wheat, bulgur, whole wheat couscous, cornmeal, millet, whole barley, whole grain pasta, kasha
- Black beans, pinto beans, white beans (navy, Great Northern, lima, cannellini), kidney beans, split peas, adzuki beans, lentils, soybeans
- Seaweed, Jerusalem artichokes, fresh corn, potatoes, red peppers, green peppers, leeks, alfalfa sprouts, parsley, sweet potatoes
- Avocados, mangoes, peaches, grapes, raisins, kiwi, all citrus, all berries
- Almonds, hazelnuts, Brazil nuts, pine nuts, sunflower seeds, flax seeds, sesame seeds
- Herring, tuna, oysters, swordfish, striped bass, flounder, mackerel, bluefish, chicken livers, chicken, quail, duck, turkey, game, beef liver, beef, organ meats
- Yogurt, miso, tahini, blackstrap molasses

MENU SUGGESTIONS FOR STABILIZING EMOTIONS

Here are two days of menus—one vegetarian, one non-vegetarian—designed to ward off irritability, bad temper, and weepiness. Each "day" starts with dinner and proceeds through the next day's breakfast, lunch, and snacks. The menus include "do ahead" tips (like soaking beans at dinner for the next day's lunch) and use leftovers to build new meals.

Vegetarian	Non-vegetarian
Dinner: Polenta with Wild Mushroom Sauce; Pinto Bean and Swiss Chard Patties; Fast Salad with red and green peppers, alfalfa sprouts, and parsley	**Dinner:** Whole Wheat Linguini with Fresh Tuna; corn on the cob; Steamed Squash Salad
Dessert: bowl of warmed millet with currants and maple syrup	**Dessert:** Banana Refrigerator Cake
Breakfast: Polenta French Toast with Blackberry Syrup; grain coffee substitute	**Breakfast:** Fresh Fruit Salad of mango, peach, grapes, berries, and orange; whole grain crackers with tahini
Snack: almonds and hazelnuts	**Snack:** baked sweet potato
Lunch: pinto bean and swiss chard patty sandwich on whole wheat pita with avocado, tomato, alfalfa sprouts, and mustard *(make Banana Refrigerator Cake)*	**Lunch:** steamed squash, pasta, and tuna salad
Snack: kiwi and berries	**Snack:** Banana Refrigerator Cake

Weight Gain

It's normal to gain some weight at menopause—about five to ten pounds is the average amount—since after menopause, production of estrogen switches from the ovaries to fatty tissue. To adapt to this, nature increases women's proportion of body fat. A woman's rounded belly is her estrogen factory! In other words, a little thickening around the middle at this time of life is natural and has a purpose that you shouldn't try to subvert. Radical dieting is not recommended at any time of life, especially at menopause. It can put great stress on your vitamin and mineral reserves and your body as a whole. Especially now, you need vitamins, minerals, and healthy fats and oils to produce the energy that food provides.

On the other hand, carrying around lots of excess weight is a strain on the body. Excess weight is associated with an increased risk of heart disease and diabetes in post-menopausal women. If you do need to lose some weight during menopause, create meals featuring whole grains, beans, vegetables, and small amounts of animal protein, and your hunger will be satisfied. It is refined foods that leave you with vague hungers, inspiring binges and overeating as your body craves the missing parts—the fiber, vitamins, and minerals—that are removed in processing. With whole foods, you can lose weight without feeling hungry.

Jody always ate low-fat foods, dieter's lunches, and canned tuna packed in water. In her late thirties and early forties she noticed an increase of two to three pounds a year. She was really concerned that by the time she went into menopause she would be very overweight. She came to us, and to help her lose weight we added almonds, extra-virgin olive oil, fresh fish, vegetables, whole grains, beans, and even a little butter. At the same time, we asked her to cut out cottage cheese, fat-free frozen yogurt, and other "diet" foods, and within two months she had lost several pounds. She also reported having more energy than she remembers ever having, and she no longer worries about gaining a lot of weight at menopause.

Significant weight gain may be a sign of an underactive thyroid. For more information, see Hypothyroidism, page 45.

What to Avoid to Minimize Weight Gain:

Sugar: Unwanted weight gain can be caused by eating refined sugars. These simple sugars are absorbed and broken down very quickly; as your body can only use some of the sugar for energy, the rest is converted into fat and stored in this form. Hidden sugars are found in catsup, canned soup, packaged foods, and salad dressing.

Dairy foods: We find that many women avoid weight gain and when dieting lose more weight when they are eating few or no dairy products. (And there are plenty of other ways to get calcium.) The new "healthy" dairy products are no help—choosing low or no-fat dairy products often creates cravings for the fats that are missing in the dairy foods.

Excess fat: Our recipes translate into meals that provide 25 to 30 percent calories from fat. This amount of fat, when supplied by quality fats and oils, will not add pounds. It will allow your body to achieve its natural weight.

What You Need to Maintain a Healthy Weight

Fiber: A normally functioning digestive tract requires fiber to provide bulk. **Whole grains**, **beans**, **vegetables**, and **fruits** add plenty of fiber while helping the body move the digested foods through the intestines and, after the nutrients have been absorbed, assisting in evacuation. A low-fiber diet is associated with obesity; an increase in fiber-containing foods can help with weight loss.

Exercise: Brisk walking or any low-impact aerobic exercise is the best way to reduce body fat and at the same time maintain good muscle tone, and is recommended on a daily basis or a minimum of three times a week for at least twenty minutes each day. The more you exercise the faster your metabolism will burn excess calories, instead of storing food as fat.

Foods to avoid: refined sugars; hydrogenated fats; processed oils; deep-fried and fast foods; fatty meats; dairy products; refined grains; processed and packaged products; sodas and other junk foods.

FOODS THAT WILL ASSIST IN WEIGHT LOSS

- All whole grains, including millet, brown rice, whole wheat, bulgur, wholee wheat couscous, whole grain pasta, whole oats, quinoa
- All beans, including adzuki beans, chick-peas, lentils, black beans, pinto beans, all white beans (Great Northern, navy, lima, cannellini)
- Fresh vegetables, especially dark leafy greens, yams, sweet potatoes, seaweed, broccoli, asparagus, winter squash, carrots, artichokes, bok choy, garlic
- Apples, pears, all berries, all melons
- Flatfish (flounder, sole), salmon, swordfish, sardines, tuna, cod, turkey, chicken, game
- Almonds, chestnuts, walnuts, sunflower seeds, flax seeds
- Rose hips, blackstrap molasses, miso, water

MENU SUGGESTIONS FOR MINIMIZING WEIGHT GAIN

The following page has two days of menus—one vegetarian, one nonvegetarian—designed to help you maintain a healthy weight. Each "day" starts with dinner and proceeds through the next day's breakfast, lunch, and snacks. The menus include "do ahead" tips (like soaking beans at dinner for the next day's lunch) and use leftovers to build new meals.

Vegetarian	*Non-vegetarian*
Dinner: Adzuki Beans with Squash Purée; Bulgur and Walnut Pilaf; Broccoli with Currants; Your Basic Green Salad	**Dinner:** Fresh Chicken Dinner and Soup, Too; Crusty Baked Tomatoes with Sunflower Seeds; Curried Barley with Caramelized Onions; Leafy Greens Vietnamese Style
Dessert: Summer Fresh Fruit Compote	**Dessert:** Fresh Blueberry Cobbler *(bake butternut squash and Butternut Babaganoush)*
Breakfast: bulgur, walnut, and oatmeal hot cereal; Summer Fresh Fruit Compote; Hot Mint Tea	**Breakfast:** 1 or 2 soft-boiled eggs; whole grain English muffin; rose-hip tea
Snack: 10 almonds or roasted chestnuts 2 rice cakes with all-fruit jam	**Snack:** Fresh Carrot-Apple Juice with Parsley
Lunch: Adzuki bean and squash soup with whole grain rolls and Fast Salad of carrots, celery, and tomatoes	**Lunch:** Crusty Baked Tomatoes Topped with Sunflower Seeds; barley salad with carrots, onions, radishes, and chicken chunks
Snack: Vegetable stock with miso, and an apple	**Snack:** Butternut Babaganoush

Sexuality

You'll hear that women's interest in sex tapers off after menopause. However, a Gallup poll showed that only 3 percent of women named sexual problems as their most serious concern, while 55 percent said sexual activity remained the same, 30 percent indicated it decreased, and 7 percent said that their sexual life had increased. We believe that a healthy body is one that has an appetite for sex and a zest for life. When hormonal changes occur, sluggishness, constipation, bloating, and any other uncomfortable symptoms can limit sexual desire. Add to this sleeplessness and a reduction in vaginal moisture, and a once-vital sex life can become dormant. Improving your diet can boost your sexual energy and improve your bodily condition.

If you find some firing-up is needed and your sexuality is a priority to you, start by handling any other persistent complaints. Healthy adrenals are needed for a good sex life and subsisting on coffee, chocolate, and refined foods is a good way to exhaust these glands. Hot flashes, fatigue, and hypothyroidism can interfere with sexual energies. Avoid oral contraceptives and tranquilizers, as they deplete thyroid function.

What You Need to Maintain Sexual Energy

Vitamin E: As the body's supply of estrogen diminishes, vaginal tissue can begin to thin and become less elastic. Vitamin E, found in **nuts** and **whole grains**, preserves tissue elasticity and encourages the growth of cells in the vaginal wall.

Vitamin A: To maintain and repair vaginal tissue, vitamin A is required. This is found in **dark leafy greens** such as **kale**, **collards**, and **turnip greens**.

Collagen: Vitamin C, vitamin B_6, and copper promote the manufacturing of collagen, the substance that brings firmness to tissue, inside and out. **Potatoes**, **tropical fruits**, and **cashews** contain these three nutrients.

Essential oils: For the health of the vaginal tissue, **fish**, **nuts**, and **seeds** are exceptionally good for you.

Whole foods and phytohormones: These enhance hormonal function and can have a significant effect on vaginal health and sexual response as they nourish specific tissues and the body as a whole. General vitality supports healthy sexual functioning and various glands all contribute. (See page 386 for phytohormone foods).

Vaginal lubrication: Barbara thought her marriage would surely end if she did not find a solution to her vaginal dryness. She had always enjoyed a good sex life with her husband before this. She solved her problem by applying vitamin E oil directly to the vaginal tissue and then she found that just inserting a capsule into the vagina at bedtime worked as well. Within several days her vagina became more moist, and after a while she only needed to insert a capsule every few days.

With menopause there is a difference in the amount and consistency of the fluids secreted in response to sexual stimulation. Vitamin E is a standard treatment to increase secretions and, applied directly to the vaginal wall, it's even used as a lubricant itself, as Barbara found out. Niacin, in **fish**, **whole grains**, and **sunflower seeds**, has also been shown to stimulate the formation of vaginal mucus.

Zinc, niacin, and folic acid: Low histamine levels in the blood are correlated with the inability to achieve orgasm, and zinc, niacin, and folic acid increase histamines. **Oysters**, the classic aphrodisiac, have all three and are especially high in zinc—76.4 mg in a serving of six oysters, whereas the RDA is just 15 mg a day!

Foods to avoid: caffeine; chocolate; refined sugar; all refined oils (use unprocessed, unrefined oils instead); refined and processed foods. Also avoid cigarette smoking.

FOODS THAT WILL ASSIST SEXUALITY

- Whole rye, whole barley, whole oats, brown rice, cornmeal, whole wheat, bulgur, whole wheat couscous, whole grain pasta
- Lentils, adzuki beans, white beans (Great Northern, navy, lima, cannellini), soybeans, pinto beans, black beans, chick-peas
- Carrots, cabbage, beets, green beans, green and snow peas, cucumbers, radishes, parsley, onions, dark leafy greens, tomatoes, winter squash, shiitake mushrooms, bok choy, seaweed, shallots, scallions, summer squash, winter squash
- Cherries, all citrus, apples, pomegranates, all berries, all melons, avocados
- Almonds, hazelnuts, Brazil nuts, chestnuts, walnuts, pecans, flax seeds, sesame seeds, sunflower seeds, pumpkin seeds
- Shrimp, oysters, smelts, crab, trout, mussels, shad, mackerel, roe, salmon, tuna, flatfish (sole, flounder), turkey, chicken, game, organ meats, beef liver, rabbit
- Cinnamon, cider, sauerkraut, blackstrap molasses, rose hips, butter, miso

MENU SUGGESTIONS FOR BOOSTING SEXUALITY

Here are two days of menus—one vegetarian, one non-vegetarian—designed to give you more sexual energy and improve tissue elasticity and lubrication. Each "day" starts with dinner and proceeds through the next day's breakfast, lunch, and snacks. The menus include "do ahead" tips (like soaking beans at dinner for the next day's lunch) and use leftovers to build new meals.

Vegetarian

Dinner: Black Beans with Avocado Salsa Cruda; Mexican Rice with Pumpkin Seeds and Cilantro; romaine and orange salad with vinaigrette

Dessert: Broiled Maple Apples (*make Beet and Potato Salad; Breakfast Corn Muffins*)

Breakfast: Black Bean Soup with Orange and Cinnamon; Breakfast Corn Muffins

Snack: Almonds, hazelnuts, and pecans

Lunch: Beet and Potato Salad on leaf lettuce; Mexican Rice with Pumpkin Seeds and Cilantro

Snack: Breakfast Corn Muffins with apple butter (*make Apricot-Date-Pecan Bonbons*)

Non-vegetarian

Dinner: Taramasalata (Greek Caviar) Spread with whole grain pita triangles; Oyster-Pot Stew; Basic Brown Rice; Composed Salad of Oranges, Avocado, and Endive

Dessert: Apricot-Date-Pecan Bonbons

Breakfast: Breakfast Corn Muffins, almond butter, and all-fruit jam

Snack: Sunflower and pumpkin seeds; fresh orange or apple

Lunch: Oyster-Pot Stew; Basic Brown Rice; Fast Salad of cucumbers, radishes, and scallion

Snack: taramasalata with whole wheat pita

Skin Care

Vitamins E, A, C, and B$_6$ and oils that are good for internal skin also nourish your external skin, which can become thinner and drier at menopause.

The kinds of fats you eat can also make a significant difference in the quality of your skin. The predominant oils produced by the glands in the skin are monounsaturates, which are abundant in olives and almonds. The essential fatty acids are also needed. Several teaspoons a day of flax seed oil, which is high in these, can return a freshness to your complexion.

It's also important to avoid hydrogenated and rancid oils. In the body, these can degenerate and cause age spots, the brownish pigment accumulation in the skin that the French poetically term "fleurs de cimetière."

Drinking six to eight glasses of water a day helps cleanse the skin and keep it pliable.

Vaginitis

When the vaginal environment changes from slightly acidic to alkaline, bacterial growth that was normally inhibited is now stimulated. Vaginitis is more likely to occur when this happens.

Treatments include eating plain yogurt with bacteria-active cultures, which reestablish a healthy bacterial population. While live bacteria can do a lot of good, basic changes are needed to remedy the underlying causes of vaginitis. The elimination of refined grains, sugar, and dairy products (other than yogurt) has proven consistently to relieve and eliminate vaginitis.

Hypothyroidism

Hypothyroidism is not a symptom of menopause but is a common coincidental occurrence that is frequently undiagnosed *because the symptoms are similar to the complaints of menopause*. If you frequently lack zest and energy, feel sleepy but are getting plenty of rest, it could be your thyroid gland that's underactive. In hypothyroidism, the thyroid gland either produces abnormally low amounts of thyroid hormones or the hormones that are produced are not properly utilized, as happens in thyroiditis. According to Dr. Serafina Corsello, executive medical director of the Corsello Centers for Nutritional-Complementary Medicine in New York, this condition is seen more and more frequently in female patients. It is evidence of a poorly functioning thyroid in which the immune system attacks the gland and causes an inflammatory condition. Other common symptoms of hypothyroidism often blamed on menopause include painful and excessive menstrual periods, nervousness, depression, unexplained weight gain, low sexual desire, memory loss, dry and scaly skin, and sleeplessness. Hypothyroidism occurs in one out of eight women by the age of fifty.

If you want to find out if you have hypothyroidism, you can ask your doctor to give you the common blood test for this condition, TSH. However the TSH test does not reveal mild cases of this ailment and is not sensitive enough to use for early diagnosis.

Instead, you need to use the basal body temperature test, the most sensitive indicator of thyroid function, and this test you can perform yourself.

Dr. Corsello's basal body temperature test: Collect your first urine of the morning in a styrofoam cup (which will maintain the temperature) in which you have placed a basal temperature thermometer and leave it in the urine for three minutes. For the most reliable results, this procedure needs to be done every morning for a month, with typically the most accurate readings coming the fifth to the seventh day after your period begins. If your temperature is consistently below 98° F, your thyroid might be underactive. Report your observations to your doctor for a final diagnosis. Avoid refined and processed foods, which are low in nutrients, and make a special effort to eat foods that are high in vitamins and especially minerals.

What can you do for an underactive thyroid? Most people know that table salt is iodized because we need iodine for a healthy thyroid, but the story of iodine and how it interacts with chlorine and fluoride to affect the thyroid is a little more complicated.

What to Avoid for Thyroid Health

Chlorine and fluoride: Chlorine and fluoride, widely present in municipal water supplies, block iodine receptors in the thyroid gland, resulting in reduced thyroid hormone production. For this reason, we strongly recommend drinking and cooking with filtered water if your tap water contains these chemicals.

Eat these in moderation: Certain foods when eaten raw block the use of iodine in thyroid hormone production. Cruciferous vegetables—**cabbage**, **cauliflower**, **broccoli**, **brussels sprouts**, **turnips**, as well as **mustard greens**, **spinach**, and **kale**—which are terrific for you in every other way, can block iodine receptors. **Rutabaga**, **soybeans**, **peanuts**, **pine nuts**, **pears**, **peaches**, and **millet** are on this list. There's no reason to avoid these foods; just make sure to get enough iodine along with them. Cooking them usually inactivates the iodine-blocking substance.

Avoid oral contraceptives and tranquilizers, as they deplete thyroid function.

What You Need for Thyroid Health

Iodine: This important nutrient is used by the thyroid and assists in the regulation of the metabolism. Iodine is found in all the foods of the sea—**fish, shellfish,** and **seaweed**—and **sea salt** contains trace amounts of iodine. (Iodized salt contains aluminum, which can interfere with thyroid function, but sea salt contains iodine naturally, is free of aluminum, and contains no additives.) Kelp or kombu is a common seaweed that is an excellent source of iodine, low in sodium, and easily absorbed by the body. Just eat fish twice a week and seaweed several times a month and you'll get a sufficient amount of iodine and many trace minerals. Too much iodine can actually inhibit the thyroid gland, though it would be difficult to consume enough to cause this effect.

Nutrient balance: Thyroid health also depends on having sufficient and balanced quantities of all nutrients, especially thiamine, vitamin A, zinc, manganese, and vitamin E, all of which help in the absorption of iodine. **Whole grains, beans,** and **orange-colored fruits and vegetables** are good sources of these. Certain amino acids which are abundant in animal foods are important too.

Foods to avoid: iodized salt (use sea salt instead); processed and refined foods; raw cruciferous vegetables and other foods listed above. Also avoid chlorine and fluoride.

FOODS THAT WILL ASSIST THE THYROID

- Brown rice, whole wheat, bulgur, whole wheat couscous, whole oats, whole grain pasta
- Chick-peas, black-eyed peas, white beans (Great Northern, navy, lima, cannellini)
- Seaweed, fresh corn, dark leafy greens, mushrooms, sweet potatoes
- Avocados, pineapple, mangoes, papayas, apricots, all berries
- Brazil nuts, almonds, chestnuts, cashews, hazelnuts, pumpkin seeds, sunflower seeds, sesame seeds
- Lobster, oysters, shrimp, tuna, herring, eggs, duck, game, beef liver
- Miso, butter, carob powder

MENU SUGGESTIONS FOR HEALING HYPOTHYROIDISM

Here are two days of menus—one vegetarian, one non-vegetarian—designed to reinvigorate a sluggish thyroid. Each "day" starts with dinner and proceeds through the next day's breakfast, lunch, and snacks. The menus include "do ahead" tips (like soaking beans at dinner for the next day's lunch) and use leftovers to build new meals.

Vegetarian

Dinner: Creamless Mushroom Cream Soup; Black-Eyed Peas with Roasted Vegetables; Spiced Rice with Nuts and Seeds; Your Basic Green Salad

Dessert: Apricot Cashew "Mousse"

Breakfast: Fresh Herb Frittata; whole grain rolls

Snack: freshly roasted chestnuts

Lunch: black-eyed pea with roasted vegetable soup; carrot slices and radishes *(make Walnut Cream (substituting cashews), Carob Cake with Walnuts)*

Snack: mango and papaya slices

Non-vegetarian

Dinner: Venison Shish Kebab; Bulgur, Green Bean, and Walnut Pilaf; Turnips with Tops in Velouté Sauce; Fast Salad of cucumber and tomato

Dessert: blackberries, raspberries, and strawberries with cashew cream

Breakfast: whole grain toast with almond butter; Apricot-Cashew "Mousse"

Snack: Carob Cake with Walnuts

Lunch: Venison Shish Kebab chunks; chicory salad

Snack: Miso soup with nori

❧ 4 ❧

Staying Healthy:
Foods for a Lifetime of Vitality

The diseases associated with women over fifty years of age are osteoporosis, heart disease, and breast cancer. As women enter this time of their lives many are prescribed hormone replacement therapy for long-term health. But often, what they're eating and what that might be contributing to their prognosis is overlooked. We feel that making better food choices is the preferred "therapy," and will often avert the need for any medical intervention. And until all is known about the side effects of these medications, diet is also the safest therapy.

Osteoporosis

Bone is ever changing, constantly remodeling and rebuilding. What you eat day to day affects your bone condition over a lifetime, and what you don't eat is as important as what you do eat. There are foods that have the needed vitamins and minerals for bone health and those that deplete your supply and interfere with bone maintenance. Taking more calcium does not resolve bone problems caused by malnutrition and metabolic imbalance.

The strength of your bones depends on their density and the condition of their crystalline structure. In part, the quality of your bones is determined by your ancestral heritage, but what you've eaten over a lifetime, especially in the bone-building years up to age twenty, is equally important. Many minerals and vitamins are required to build a bone that's strong yet flexible.

The list is long: magnesium, manganese, vitamin K, folic acid, boron, vitamin B$_6$, zinc, strontium, copper, silicon, vitamin C, vitamin D . . . and calcium. Each performs an essential task; calcium alone cannot make bone.

To monitor the condition of your bones, you can have a bone-density test, and this may be important, especially if members of your family have osteoporosis. If your bone density is within an average range for your age, body build, and genetic background, then a health-supportive and nutrient-rich diet along with exercise can be enough to keep your bones healthy. If not, then it is critical to avoid the foods that deplete bone structure—sugar, caffeine, anything high in phosphorous, and too much animal protein—and to eat foods with the full range of vitamins and minerals necessary for bone-building.

What You Need to Maintain Healthy Bones

A balance of magnesium and calcium: Calcium and magnesium work in tandem and need to be present in a certain ratio. Magnesium is necessary for the absorption of calcium; without sufficient magnesium, calcium crystals can form in abnormal sizes and shapes, which is why you need to balance your consumption of the two minerals. The American diet is high in calcium foods, thanks to an abundance of dairy products that contain calcium, yet it is low in foods that contain the much-needed mineral magnesium.

How much of each mineral do you need? The usual recommendation is two parts calcium to one part magnesium, but there is also some consensus that one to one is the best ratio. If you've been eating a high-calcium diet, you'll especially want to increase your magnesium intake. **Whole grains**, **nuts**, and **beans** are good sources of magnesium and can be included in every meal. And if you plan to supplement those two minerals, consider supplementing in a ratio of at least one part magnesium to two parts calcium.

Currently the RDA for women over fifty is 1,500 mg of calcium. We think this is a high dose, since our bodies can adapt to lower amounts, and the more calcium taken at any one time, the less that is absorbed. And even when it is absorbed and circulating in your blood, it can't be used to build bone if its partner nutrients are missing. A further problem is that circulating calcium that doesn't become bone may be deposited elsewhere—in joints where it can cause arthritis, on the bone where it can cause spurs, and in the soft tissues of the arteries, which leads to heart disease.

The amount of calcium an individual requires depends on what she is eating. If you eat a lot of foods like refined sugar that deplete the body of minerals, you'll need additional calcium to compensate. In Asia and Africa, where people depend on unrefined, whole foods, diets are low in calcium, as low as 300 to 500 mg a day, yet osteo-porosis is virtually unknown.

Good calcium sources: Enjoy **fish** with their bones, **almonds**, **dark leafy greens**, **seaweed**, and unhulled **sesame seeds**. Many other foods have small amounts of calcium, and these can all add up to give you a day's worth of calcium while providing you with the other minerals needed to absorb and use this calcium.

Sunshine: As you plan your calcium intake, remember that you also need vitamin D for calcium absorption, which your body makes from sunshine. Include a daily five-minute walk in the sun for the health of your bones.

Foods That Deplete Calcium

Meat: Eating large amounts of animal protein creates an acid state in the body. In order to neutralize this acid state, calcium is drawn from the bones, weakening them in the process. For many Americans, the average protein intake is around 100 grams a day; a more healthful amount is 55 to 65 grams a day, depending on your calorie intake. Converting these grams to animal sources of protein, 65 grams translates into an egg, a 4-ounce hamburger, and a chicken leg, but you won't even need this much from animal sources since your diet will include complex carbohydrates and beans, which also contain protein.

Sugar: Refined sugar also has an acid effect on the system. The more sugar consumed, the more unbalanced the body chemistry can become.

Caffeine: Caffeine is in chocolate, cola sodas, "energy drinks," and some over-the-counter medicines, as well as in coffee and tea, even decaffeinated. Drinking as little as two cups of coffee or four cups of tea a day can result in some calcium loss; consumed daily for years, these beverages can do real damage. Couple this with the intake of other products containing caffeine, and the chances for bone loss are even higher.

High-phosphorous foods: Meat, phosphorous-containing sodas, and phosphate food additives (found in processed cheeses, salad dressings, and baked goods) demineralize bones. These foods upset the natural phosphorous-to-calcium ratio, so calcium is pulled from the bones to correct the imbalance. Worst of all are the high-phosphorous colas, which also contain a lot of sugar and caffeine. These drinks are among the worst foods imaginable for someone trying to prevent osteoporosis. Even the sugar-free varieties do damage.

Other: Smoking is correlated with osteoporosis and is best avoided completely. A lack of impact exercise like energetic walking, running, and weight-lifting is also a risk factor.

Dairy and Osteoporosis

Milk and milk products are high in protein and phosphorus and very low in magnesium. As milk and milk products are produced today, they also contain added hormones and residues of antibiotics. Dairy foods are not an essential for preventing osteoporosis. The countries with the highest rates of osteoporosis—the United States, Great Britain, and Sweden—are also the countries with the highest dairy consumption. There are other sources of calcium that offer better proportions of mineral balance and less protein and it is these sources that we prefer over dairy foods.

If you do crave dairy foods, use them as a condiment. Goat cheese and active-bacteria yogurt are fine in small amounts.

FOODS FOR BONE HEALTH

- Whole wheat, bulgur, whole wheat couscous, brown rice, cornmeal, buckwheat, whole grain pasta
- Adzuki beans, chick-peas, soybeans, white beans (Great Northern, navy, lima, cannellini), lentils, kidney beans
- Dark leafy greens, seaweed, broccoli, beets, asparagus, spinach, watercress, parsley, all mushrooms (including shiitake), potatoes, tomatoes
- Avocados, all berries, papayas, all citrus, figs, all melons, mangoes, bananas, kiwi, plantains
- Brazil nuts, hazelnuts, pistachios, almonds, walnuts, sunflower seeds, sesame seeds, flax seeds, pumpkin seeds
- Sardines with bones, mackerel, shrimp, oysters, mussels, crab, salmon, tuna, eggs
- Blackstrap molasses, tofu, tempeh, tahini, sunshine

To Avoid	To Eat
• Canned, frozen, and packaged, refined and processed foods	• Fresh vegetables, including dark leafy greens
• Large amounts of animal foods	• Protein from vegetable sources, including whole grains and beans
• Large amounts of dairy	• Bacteria-active plain yogurt and other dairy products used as a condiment
• Refined sugar and products made with sugar	• Natural sweeteners in small amounts, including maple syrup, blackstrap molasses, and fruit juices
• Soda, alcohol, caffeinated and decaffeinated coffee, caffeinated tea, baked products containing aluminum baking powder	• Herbal tea, grain coffee substitute

Heart Disease

Eating whole grains and beans along with fresh fruits and vegetables will not only lessen the symptoms of PMS and menopause, but will also reduce the risk of heart disease. Base your meals on vegetarian whole foods, small amounts of animal protein (optional), and use the highest quality fats and oils, which contain the vitamins, minerals, and anti-oxidants you need for heart health.

Hypertension: While high sodium intake can lead to hypertension, deficiencies of potassium and magnesium have also been correlated with high blood pressure. Correcting deficiencies of potassium and magnesium can return blood-pressure levels to normal. We have found that when people with hypertension eat the way we cook, their blood pressure drops. Our recipes contain sea salt and are also full of the very minerals that are missing when eating refined foods and commercial salt. For lowering hypertension, **vegetables**, **fruits**, **whole grains**, **beans**, **nuts**, and **seeds** belong "on the menu."

Fats and heart disease: Our recipes compose into meals that provide 25 to 30 percent of the calories from fat and we cook with only fats and oils of top quality: **extra-virgin olive oil**, **flax seed oil**, **unrefined sesame oil**, and **unsalted butter**. We never use hydrogenated and refined vegetable oils, including margarine and vegetable shortening, that contain transfatty acids. These promote blood clots and raise cholesterol.

Extra-virgin olive oil is one of the staple fats used in the recipes and provides the mono-unsaturates that lower cholesterol. Both extra-virgin olive oil and flax seed oil contain essential fatty acids (EFAs) that lower triglycerides, lessen your risk of blood clots, and break up cholesterol deposited on arterial walls. Unrefined sesame oil is relatively rich in the EFA linoleic acid and, unlike toasted or dark sesame oil, it contains natural preservatives that give it a longer shelf life. Unsalted butter provides some needed saturated fat and is fine to include in your diet when you reduce saturated fat from other sources. A healthy diet includes all of these fats.

Sugar and heart disease: Sugar is being studied for its effect on heart disease. The current average intake of refined sugars is 145 pounds per person per year in the United States. The body converts excess sugar into saturated fat and cholesterol, and sugar raises the level of triglycerides in the blood.

Please note: About 25 percent of all women who use oral contraceptives develop hypertension and hypertension is listed as one of the possible side-effects of hormone replacement therapy.

Cholesterol is made by the liver, which produces as much as the body needs. In a person who is healthy and well nourished, increased cholesterol in the diet naturally leads to the liver making less. To maintain this balance, the body needs a sufficient supply of vitamins and minerals—that is, nutrient deficiencies may be at the root of high cholesterol levels in the blood. Further, it is now thought that only oxidized cholesterol is a risk factor for heart disease. Eating plenty of foods high in antioxidant vitamins and minerals (beta carotene, vitamin C, and selenium, to name some) can prevent this oxidation.

When whole grains and beans are a daily part of your menu and meat and dairy foods are mostly or completely omitted, there is room for cholesterol-containing foods that are extraordinarily nutritious, such as eggs, liver, and shellfish. Three to four eggs a week and liver or shellfish once every two or three weeks can be safely recommended within this context of eating. We do, however, recommend that you have your cholesterol checked once a year, especially if you have a family history of high cholesterol or if you are overweight.

FOODS FOR A HEALTHY HEART

- Whole wheat, bulgur, whole wheat couscous, buckwheat (kasha), cornmeal, quinoa, whole grain pasta
- White beans (navy, Great Northern, lima, cannellini), soybeans, adzuki beans, black beans
- Broccoli, tomatoes, green peppers, winter squash, dark leafy greens, seaweed, onions, scallions, garlic, shallots
- Avocados, all berries, all melons, all citrus, plantains, mangoes
- Almonds, Brazil nuts, hazelnuts, sesame seeds, sunflower seeds
- Salmon, shrimp, mackerel, haddock, oysters, flatfish (flounder, sole), eggs, beef, beef liver, organ meats, lamb
- Blackstrap molasses, rose hips

To Avoid	To Eat
• Canned, frozen, and packaged foods with high sodium content	• Fresh vegetables and fruit
• Large quantities of meat	• Whole grains and beans, fish and shellfish, small portions of meat
• Hydrogenated and refined oils, margarine	• Unrefined oils, nuts, seeds, butter in small amounts
• Refined sugar and products made with sugar	• Natural sweeteners in small amounts, including maple syrup, blackstrap molasses, and fruit juices
• Caffeinated and decaffeinated coffee, caffeinated tea, soda, alcohol	• Herbal tea and grain coffee substitute

Breast Cancer

There are many theories about the importance of diet in preventing breast cancer. Eating plenty of vegetables and fruits for the fiber and cancer-fighting substances they contain, lowering fat intake, maintaining normal weight, and drinking clean water seem to be good advice, but these may be meaningful strategies only in individual cases. Breast cancer develops in many ways and goes through several stages, and when and how various foods affect the development of cancer is still being debated. We may never find a single cause or diet regimen that protects every woman, but while the research continues, there are some foods that do deserve attention.

Healthy fats: We recommend healthy fats in moderate amounts. Advocates of low-fat diets believe that fat intake must drop to at most 20 percent of total calories to make a difference in cancer prevention. Whatever the effective amount, the type of fat eaten is even more important. Diets high in olive oil have been associated with relatively low rates of cancer.

When heated and exposed to oxygen, fats oxidize, creating free radicals. This makes it most important to use unrefined fats and oils which have not been exposed to heat during any point of processing, unlike refined oils and hydrogenated oils which have. The fats we recommend to cook with are extra-virgin olive oil, unrefined sesame oil, and unsalted butter. Butter is included because of its stability when heated. Our recipes keep the fats at safe temperatures.

Essential fatty acids, which are found in fish, flax seed oil, and walnuts, deteriorate quickly and need careful handling. When flax seed oil is used in a recipe, we use it raw and uncooked because of its fragility at high temperatures. As you increase your consumption of foods that contain EFAs, it's important to also increase your intake of free-radical-quenching anti-oxidants.

Anti-oxidants: Free radicals attack cell walls and trigger tumor growth. Anti-oxidants, found in **fruits** and **vegetables**, stop free radicals from doing their damage. The anti-oxidants include vitamin C, vitamin E, beta-carotene, and selenium. Pantothenic acid, copper, manganese, and zinc also play a part. These nutrients are most effective when all are present and able to work together.

Lignans: Flax seeds are the richest source of these anticancer substances, with one hundred times more than whole wheat, which is the next best source. These seeds show up in many of our recipes, as does flax seed oil, which contains small amounts of lignans.

Phytohormones: High estrogen levels are associated with breast cancer. Phytohormones modulate body estrogen, reducing estrogen activity when there is an excess. Soybeans and soy products are especially high in phytohormones, which may be the reason why Japanese women on a traditional diet have lower rates of breast cancer.

Fiber: Fiber reduces estrogen levels by decreasing the amount of circulating estrogen in the blood, and in this way lowers the risk of breast cancer. Less estrogen is reabsorbed and more is excreted. Studies show that people who eat large amounts of fiber have a low risk of cancer. Finland, a country which has the highest consumption of fat in the world, has a low rate of breast cancer, with the Finns eating more than twice as much fiber as Americans.

Iodine: A deficiency of iodine has been linked to breast cancer. This important mineral is only needed in trace amounts and can be found in many foods, including **seaweed**, **saltwater fish**, **shellfish**, **asparagus**, **garlic**, and **lima beans**.

Special foods: Certain foods contain cancer-fighting compounds (phenols, indoles, and others) and we've made a point to include these in the recipes. They are found in **cruciferous vegetables**, **citrus fruits**, **caraway seeds**, **garlic**, **onions**, **leeks**, and **chives**. There's also evidence that **seaweed** is cancer-protective, and it may be beneficial to eat some on a weekly basis.

Organic foods: There is a growing suspicion that the pesticides and other chemicals used by agriculture (and which end up in the water supply as well as in our foods) are associated with breast cancer. The use of these chemicals parallels the modern-day increase in the disease. DDT is part of the group of pesticides known as organochlorides, which stimulate estrogen production and in this way may lead to breast cancer. Although DDT has not been used on American soil for at least a decade, much DDT still enters our food supply on imported fruits and vegetables from foreign countries. Residual DDT may also be in the water supply. The issue of organochlorides makes the strongest case for buying organic foods.

FOODS THAT ARE BREAST CANCER PROTECTIVE

- Whole wheat, bulgur, whole wheat couscous, brown rice, cornmeal, whole rye, whole barley, whole grain pasta
- Chick-peas, adzuki beans, navy beans, soybeans
- Seaweed, shiitake mushrooms, onions, dark leafy greens, carrots, garlic, cucumbers, cabbage, parsley, peas
- All berries, all melons, all citrus, mangoes
- Brazil nuts, almonds, walnuts, flax seeds, sesame seeds, sunflower seeds, pumpkin seeds
- Oysters, clams, mussels, lobster, crab, mackerel, salmon, eggs, chicken livers, chicken, beef liver, game, organ meats
- Sauerkraut, miso, blackstrap molasses

See the following page for a list of foods to eat and to avoid.

To Avoid	To Eat
• Canned, frozen, and commercially prepared fruits and vegetables	• A variety of fresh fruits and vegetables
• Refined flour and baked goods made from this	• High fiber foods including whole grains and beans
• High intake of fat of all kinds, processed and hydrogenated oils	• Unrefined and unprocessed oils including those that contain essential fatty acids
• Produce exposed to higher levels of pesticides (grapes, lettuce, tomatoes), imported fruits and vegetables, commercially raised meats, especially fatty cuts; fish from polluted waters	• Organic produce and lean meats raised without chemicals, deep water ocean fish

❧ 5 ❧

Cooking with Us

Shopping—Learning Some New Steps

Changing the way you eat is going to give you the opportunity to discover some new ways to shop. Supermarkets will still provide many items, including beans, some whole grains, and fresh vegetables and fruits, and new destinations will contribute other ingredients as you increasingly switch to natural and organic foods.

Natural food stores are a source of hundreds of wholesome foods. You can find a large variety of whole grains and beans, as well as sugar-free and preservative-free packaged items. Most natural food stores now sell organic produce and meats, and many will special-order items for you. These stores are a great resource, and the sales staff can help with reading labels and choosing brands as well as assisting with related products, including food and health books, herbs, and supplements.

You may also decide to become involved with a food cooperative, a purchasing group that pools funds to purchase foods and goods at a discount; generally, co-ops have the additional goal of creating a mini-community of like-minded shoppers and eaters. There are co-ops in cities and towns across the United States.

Ethnic and import grocery stores are good sources for condiments and specialty foods from other cuisines, some of which are occasionally included in the recipes. Farmers' markets are a wonderful resource for fresh-picked, seasonal produce, home-made baked goods, as well as organic meats, fish, fresh herbs, and flowers.

Some of the foods we recommend may be new to your pantry, yet there will be plenty of familiar ones, too. As you prepare our recipes, the new ingredients will start accumulating on your shelves and you'll find yourself using them in your old favorites, too. Allow yourself (and your family) to change habits over several months, even years, and in the meantime use up the foods that are no longer "on the menu"—or better yet, give them away. Purchase large enough quantities of ingredients to cook more than one recipe. The dry staples (whole grains, beans, herbs, and spices) stay fresh for months; meat and poultry can be frozen for short periods of time, and most fresh produce lasts at least a week. The only buy-it and eat-it food is fresh fish. Much fish is available flash-frozen and can be stored; just check to see that it's preservative-free.

Whole Foods in the Supermarket

Brown rice, wild rice, barley, and old-fashioned oatmeal are common staples in the average supermarket. We prefer the brands that keep all of the nutrients intact and are not "quick-cooking." There is always a large variety of dried beans which can be interchanged with each other in most recipes.

Purchase whole wheat pita and whole grain breads without preservatives or hydrogenated oil. The ingredient lists of better breads will have whole-wheat flour first and sometimes rye or barley flour. White flour (even unbleached or unbromated) will not be on the ingredient list at all.

In the nut and seed aisle, there are raw varieties, including whole almonds, walnuts, and sunflower seeds. Tahini or sesame butter can be found in the ethnic foods section and extra-virgin olive oil will be available in several brands. All-fruit (no sugar added) jams are now very common, and there are many varieties of caffeine-free herbal teas and grain-coffee substitutes like Caffix or Postum.

The refrigerated areas have unsalted butter and plain yogurt with bacteria-active cultures. There may also be cheeses such as pecorino romano (made from sheep milk) and olives, such as Greek and black oil-cured.

The produce section will often carry dark leafy greens such as collards, dandelion, and kale, romaine, and other green-leaf lettuces. Besides the old standbys like broccoli and cauliflower, you'll find "exotic" produce like portobello mushrooms and daikon radishes. You can try a new vegetable every week. If you don't see the fruit or vegetable you're looking for, ask the produce manager if the store ever carries it. Sometimes it's just out of season.

We've included a "shopping list" of great whole foods that are available in the supermarket. In each category we've left space so you can add more items to this shopping list. Obviously, you won't buy them all every time you shop! Photocopy the following two pages and you can be on your way.

WHOLE FOODS IN YOUR GROCERY STORE

Beans
Black beans
Black-eyed peas
Chick-peas
Great Northern beans
Kidney beans
Lentils
Lima beans
Navy beans
Pink beans
Pinto beans
Split peas
_____
_____
_____
_____

Whole Grains
Barley
Brown rice
Oatmeal
Wild rice
_____
_____
_____
_____

Fruit
Apples
Avocados
Bananas
Berries
Grapefruit
Lemons
Limes
Melons

Vegetables
Artichokes
Asparagus
Beets
Broccoli
Brussels sprouts
Cabbage
Carrots
Cauliflower
Celery
Collards
Corn, fresh
Cucumbers
Dandelion greens
Endive
Garlic
Ginger, fresh
Green beans
Herb, fresh _____
Herb, fresh _____
Kale
Leeks
Lettuce, green leaf
Lettuce, red leaf
Lettuce, romaine
Lettuce, Boston
Lettuce, _____
Mushrooms
Mustard greens
Onions, yellow
Onions, red
Onions, Spanish
Parsnips
Peppers, green
Peppers, red
Potatoes

Dried Fruit & Nuts
Almonds
Cashews
Currants
Dates
Figs
Pecans
Pistachios
Raisins
Walnuts
_____
_____
_____

Condiments
Extra-virgin olive oil
Cider vinegar
Mustard, prepared
Pure vanilla extract
All-fruit jam
Pure maple syrup
_____
_____
_____
_____

Beverages
Herbal teas
_____
_____

Miscellaneous
Butter, unsalted
Whole grain bread
Whole wheat pita

Fruit
Oranges
Pears
Seasonal fruit
Tangerines
_____
_____
_____
_____
_____
_____
_____
_____

Vegetables
Radicchio
Rutabaga
Scallions
Shallots
Summer squash
Swiss Chard
Tomatoes
Turnips
Turnip greens
Watercress
Winter squash
Yams
Zucchini
_____
_____
_____

Miscellaneous
Yogurt
_____
_____
_____

Other
_____
_____
_____
_____
_____
_____
_____
_____

A Guide to the Natural Food Store

Natural food stores are wonderful places to investigate a variety of packaged mixes, breakfast cereals, drinks, and other foods that have never been advertised on television. There may be all sorts of foods and terminology that are new to you, but most stores have an informed staff that can explain what is meant by "stone-ground" flour, "free-range" chickens, and "unsulphured" apricots.

And there is so much more! Here you'll find many common staples, organically grown and free of chemicals, preservatives, and added sugar. Whole grains, beans, sweeteners, dried fruit, and beverages are sold in wider variety than you will ever find in a supermarket. There's a new world of condiments and flavorings like salted plum vinegar (umeboshi), kuzu, brown rice syrup, and unrefined sesame oil waiting for you, plus dozens of tasty whole grain pastas and crunchy chips. Nut and seed butters are available in an astounding variety, such as hazelnut and macadamia, as are conserves made from organically grown fruits. Often organic produce and sometimes organic meats are available.

In spite of their reputation, natural food stores are not necessarily more expensive. Staples are usually sold in bulk at a savings, and other items which appear expensive, such as nut butters and flax seed oil, are actually cost-effective since they are potent nutritionally and eaten in small quantities. With unrefined foods, you're getting much more nutrient value for the dollar.

In the Appendix we list brand names of some of the staples that we find to be the best quality, as well as brand names of some of the whole-food versions of convenience foods, such as instant soup, packaged pilaf, and cake mixes. There's also a list of mail-order resources.

Here's a shopping list for you to take to the natural food store. We've included many items from our recipes and added lines so you can customize the list. Make several copies and keep them handy to fill out before you head to the store.

A GUIDE TO YOUR NATURAL FOOD STORE
(You'll find a lot of these foods organically grown.)

Beans
Adzuki beans
Black beans
Black-eyed peas
Chick-peas
Great Northern beans
Kidney beans
Lentils
Lima beans
Navy beans
Pinto beans
Red lentils
Split peas
Tempeh
Tofu
_____
_____
_____

Whole Grains
Amaranth
Barley, pearled
Couscous, whole
   wheat

Vegetables (seasonal)
Beets
Broccoli
Burdock
Buttercup squash
Cabbage
Carrots
Celery
Cucumbers
Garlic
Ginger, fresh
Green beans
Herbs, fresh_____
Leafy greens
Lettuce
Onions
Potatoes
Watercress
Yams
Zucchini
_____
_____
_____
_____

Beverages
Herbal teas
Coffee substitutes
Organic coffee
Apple juice
Juice_____
Iced tea
Milk, rice
Milk, _____
_____

Grain Products
Cereal, brown rice
Cereal, dry _____
Cereal, oatmeal
Crackers
Granola, maple
Pancake mix
Rice cakes
Sourdough bread
Whole grain bread
Whole grain
   muffins & pita
_____

Whole Grains
Barley, whole
Brown rice, basmati
Brown rice, long
Brown rice, short
Brown rice, medium
Bulgur
Kasha
Millet
Oatmeal
Pasta, buckwheat
Pasta, corn
Pasta, whole wheat
Pasta, _____
Quinoa
Wild rice
_____
_____
_____

Whole Grain Flour
Cornmeal
Whole wheat
Whole wheat pastry
_____
_____
_____
_____
_____
_____
_____
_____

Fruit (seasonal)
Apples
Bananas
Berries
Citrus
_____

Dried Fruit (unsulphured only)
Apples
Apricots
Currants
Dates, Medjool
Dates, pitted
Figs, black/white
Mixed fruit
Peaches
Prunes
Raisins

Nuts & Seeds
Almonds, whole
Brazil nuts
Cashews
Nut butter _____
Pumpkin seeds
Sesame seeds
Sunflower seeds
Walnuts
_____
_____
_____
_____
_____
_____

Condiments
Arrowroot powder
Brown rice vinegar
Butter, unsalted
Extra-virgin olive oil
Flax seed oil
Herbs & spices,
   non-irradiated
Kuzu
Miso, chick-pea
Sea salt, plain
Sea salt, herbal
Shoyu soy sauce
Umeboshi paste
Umeboshi vinegar
Unrefined sesame oil
_____
_____
_____

Dried Vegetables
Agar-agar
Arame
Kombu
Nori
Shiitake
_____
_____
_____
_____
_____
_____

Shopping Tips

- Farmer's market produce often has been grown with fewer pesticides and other chemicals.
- Imported fruits and vegetables can have higher amounts of pesticides and chemicals than domestic produce.
- Foods that are in season are often less expensive.
- Whole grains, beans, and dried vegetables and fruits such as mushrooms, tomatoes, apricots, and figs can be purchased in volume since they store for at least six months.

RECIPES FOR A HEALTHY MENOPAUSE

About the Recipes

The recipes have been written with the foods and nutrients in the quantities that are needed to maintain great health. The most important ingredients that women need show up more frequently. Walnuts, fish, citrus fruit, and dark leafy greens are included in many recipes; foods that are of lesser importance are used less often. Beans are used often in salads, soups, and meat dishes for the magnesium they contain, a mineral to eat in quantity along with calcium found in dark leafy greens, meat-bone stocks, and seaweed. The recipes give the best balance of nutrients to preserve and restore every system of the body.

We cook with some ingredients that may be new to you, but when possible we also include the more familiar and standard counterparts of unusual items, such as cider vinegar instead of brown rice vinegar, arrowroot for kuzu, lemon juice plus salt rather than salted plum vinegar. The idea is to keep introducing new flavors and ingredients without making the recipes seem unfamiliar. If an ingredient is missing from your shelf, just use something else that is similar. We encourage you to be flexible with all the ingredients, adding or leaving out a vegetable or changing a seasoning. Make notes on the recipes so that you can duplicate your results next time.

The dishes we've created have a range of flavors, an international mix contributed by the wholesome traditional foods that many cultures have used for centuries. You'll find a description of the more unusual ingredients in the Appendix (page 366). Often the ingredient lists are short, and the recipes steer away from fancy chopping or difficult techniques. These are recipes for everyday living.

At the end of the recipes are suggested accompaniments. Names of dishes capitalized are recipes in the book; lowercase suggestions are foods that can be assembled easily. The nutritional stars show you the nutrients each dish contains. The most plentiful are marked with three stars (★★★) and the remaining important nutrients are listed next to a single star (★).

Cooking Day by Day

Now, how to have these wonderful dishes on hand when you want them? The key is to always have something happening—some beans soaking, grains steaming, an organic chicken defrosting—while you're attending to something else. There are many time-savers such as recipes like Fresh Chicken Dinner and Soup, Too. And when we're boiling potatoes, we piggyback hard-cooking some eggs in the same pot. This way you'll produce the maximum amount of cooked food, while spending a minimum amount of time in the kitchen.

Many of the recipes are designed to provide leftovers to use in a later meal, so Black Bean Loaf can be used as a sandwich filler, or a grain pilaf as the base of a tossed salad with vinaigrette. We rarely cook all the dishes in a meal from scratch—especially grains and beans, which are usually from a previous cooking session. Here are some quick tips.

TIPS TO FASTER MEAL PREPARATION

- Keep vegetables that store well on hand for future use: carrots, potatoes, beets, onions, celery, ginger, garlic, winter squash, parsnips, and turnips.
- Soak beans in the evening and put them to cook in the morning as you get ready for work. Turn the beans off and let them sit in the pot covered all day. The beans will be ready for seasoning when you return for dinner.
- While cleaning up from dinner, cook a pot of grain, roast a chicken, soak or cook beans, simmer a compote, or start a stock.
- Wash lettuce, then wrap in a cotton cloth or paper toweling and store in a plastic bag to have quick and easy, already clean salad greens on hand.
- Cooked grains and beans can be seasoned quickly with the addition of caramelized onions and garlic, herbs (basil, oregano, thyme), and spices (chili powder, curry powder).
- Already cooked vegetables, grains, or beans can become a soup with the addition of stock or water plus seasoning.
- Leftover beans can be puréed into a dip or loaf or made into a stew.
- Leftover grain can become the base of a salad, soup, or stir-fry.

Getting Support

If cooking seems overwhelming right now, consider finding someone to help you. It doesn't have to cost a lot and you may be able to trade talents with someone. You might find someone to do weekly cooking through a natural food store—look at the bulletin board or post your own note. Perhaps your housekeeper cooks; you can provide produce and a chicken to be made into several meals, or it may be helpful to have your shopping done for you. Many large supermarkets and specialty stores offer telephone shopping and delivery services.

Eating with Us

We invite you to start eating the way we do; begin today to enjoy all the foods that are "on the menu." Take a look through the recipes and find something special to your tastes. In a short time you can be savoring the natural and fresh flavors of the foods we recommend. These ingredients will give you dependable energy while keeping you well, just like they do for us. It's easy to shift to eating foods that are better for you. From your first bite you'll be on your way.

❧ 6 ❧

Soups and Stocks

SOUPS

Greek Lentil and Garlic Soup

Spring Greens Potage with Asparagus

Butternut Squash and Yam Bisque with Toasted Pumpkin Seeds

Tuscan Bread Soup with Basil Infusion

Creamless Mushroom Cream Soup

Seafood Bisque with Chives

Turkey Soup with Barley-Rice

Black Bean Soup with Orange and Cinnamon

Escarole and Kidney Bean Soup

Garlic Soup with Bruschetta

Split Pea and Barley Soup with Spices

STOCKS

Calcium-Rich Fish Stock

Vegetable Trimmings Stock with Lentils

Soups

A warm and soothing bowl of soup can be full of good-for-you ingredients—just what you need to ease tension and lift your spirits. Most soups are easy to make and successfully take additional ingredients. Sample the soup as it is cooking and let your tastes inspire you, using our recipes as a base. We've created several formats made with beans, leafy greens, grains, and vegetables, and in a variety of textures such as creamy, chunky, and chewy.

Stocks

Making a stock to use in a recipe may sound complicated and time-consuming, but the procedure really only takes a couple of minutes and very little effort. Once it's made, you'll have a quick way of increasing the vitamins and minerals in any dish you're cooking.

When making a stock from vegetables or their trimmings, we prefer organic vegetables because their skins are sweeter and they've been spared chemical sprays and waxing. Stay away from cabbage, cauliflower, and other cruciferous vegetables since they have a strong sulphur taste which will overpower the broth.

To make stock richer in flavor and nutrients, use organic beef or chicken bones, plus a little vinegar to draw out the calcium in the bones. Rich-tasting vegetarian stocks with depth of flavor are made by adding lentils, miso, or herbal sea salt. (Remember to reduce the salt in a soup recipe if you've used miso or herbal salt in the stock.) For fish stock, use the bones, head, and tail (and vinegar) or the flesh from a light meat fish. Fish stock is best used only for fish recipes.

Cook a vegetable stock about 15 to 20 minutes, a beef or poultry stock 30 minutes, and a fish stock 20 minutes. Strain it, then simmer the liquid uncovered to concentrate the flavors and reduce the quantity. You can also take a tip from chefs and add a flavor spark—a squeeze of lemon, a splash of vinegar, or a few chopped tomatoes.

This broth can be frozen for many months. When you need stock, just slip some into a pot and cover with a lid. Heated on a low flame, it melts quickly. Keep several kinds in your freezer.

❧ Greek Lentil and Garlic Soup ❧

Yield: 2 quarts   (*4 generous servings plus extra*)

We've created a variation on this Greek specialty, a standard family classic in many kitchens, and included flax seed oil to give you the essential fatty acids you need. EFAs are components of many tissues and organs that are stressed and undergoing changes at menopause, including the adrenal and sex glands, brain cells, and skin tissue. For some additional taste and texture, garnish each bowl with a few Mediterranean olives.

 2 cups green or brown lentils, washed
 8 cups vegetable or chicken stock (see index) or filtered water
10 cloves garlic, peeled
 1 bay leaf
 2 onions, diced
 2 carrots, diced
 3 stalks celery, diced
 2 potatoes, peeled and diced
 2 teaspoons oregano
 2 teaspoons sea salt
¼ teaspoon freshly ground black pepper
  Juice of 1 lemon or 2 tablespoons cider vinegar
 1 bunch watercress, spinach, or scallions, chopped coarsely (about 2 cups)
 4 teaspoons flax seed oil or extra-virgin olive oil
 8 to 12 Greek or black oil-cured olives (optional)

1. In a medium stockpot, place lentils and stock or water over a high flame. Add whole cloves of garlic and bay leaf, and bring to a boil, covered. Lower flame and simmer for 10 to 15 minutes.

2. Add onions, carrots, celery, potatoes, and oregano. Return soup to a boil, reduce heat to a simmer, and cook, covered, 30 minutes.

3. Add salt, pepper, and lemon juice. Remove bay leaf. (For a creamier texture, purée part of soup in a blender.)

4. Ladle soup into deep bowls, place a generous pinch of greens on top (about 2 to 4 tablespoons), and drizzle ½ teaspoon flax seed or olive oil on each. Add 2 or 3 olives to each bowl.

VARIATIONS: Other diced vegetables can be added in step 2, such as green peppers, parsnips, potatoes, parsley root, rutabaga, or butternut squash.

SUGGESTED ACCOMPANIMENTS: Pilaf with Brown, Wehani, and Wild Rices; Your Basic Green Salad; Classic Candied Yams Revised; and Fresh Blueberry Cobbler.

★★★   OMEGA-3 FATTY ACIDS, FOLIC ACID

★   VITAMIN K, VITAMIN C, IRON, VITAMIN B_6

❧ Spring Greens Potage with Asparagus ❧

Yield: 2 quarts   (4 generous servings plus extra)

Maintaining the strength of your bones depends in part on whether or not you have sufficient vitamin K in your system. This soup is good insurance, with asparagus, spinach, potatoes, and peas all contributing this important vitamin. Asparagus also contains some vitamin E, called the "menopause vitamin" because it assists in alleviating so many of the signs of menopause.

2 tablespoons unsalted butter
2 potatoes, peeled and diced
1 leek or 1 bunch scallions, sliced and washed (see page 80)
4 cups chicken stock (see index), (organic preferred) or filtered water
1 pound young asparagus (see Note)

½ cup fresh peas or handful stringbeans, broken into thirds
2 teaspoons herbal sea salt
Freshly ground white pepper
1 tablespoon lemon juice
12 leaves spinach, shredded (about 1 cup)

1. In a medium stockpot, heat butter and add potatoes and leeks. Sauté over medium heat for 3 to 4 minutes.

2. Add stock, bring to a boil, and turn down flame to a simmer; cook, covered, 4 to 5 minutes, until potatoes are softened.

3. Break tips off asparagus and set aside. Cut stalks into four or five pieces, about 1 to 1½-inch lengths. Add stalks and peas, and cook, uncovered, 1 minute, until bright green. Add herbal salt, a few grinds of pepper, and lemon juice. Drop in spinach and asparagus tips and serve.

NOTE: Young asparagus have very thin stalks. If these are not available, use regular asparagus and scrape the stalks with a peeler, removing the more woody part.

SUGGESTED ACCOMPANIMENTS: Chicken Salad, Tomatoes Stuffed with Couscous, and Broiled Maple Bananas.

★★★   VITAMIN K, VITAMIN C, FOLIC ACID
  ★   VITAMIN B$_6$, VITAMIN E, COPPER, THIAMIN, VITAMIN A

❧ Butternut Squash and Yam Bisque ❧ with Toasted Pumpkin Seeds

Yield: 2½ quarts   (4 generous servings plus extra)

This soup is full of vitamin A, which is needed at all times in a woman's life. Vitamin A, in the yam, butternut squash, and butter, encourages skin growth and repair. And our garnish of pumpkin seeds and arame provides magnesium, good for irregular heartbeats that can sometimes occur during menopause.

SOUP:

2 tablespoons unsalted butter or stock
1 onion, diced
1 butternut, long-neck, buttercup, or Hubbard squash, about 1 to 1½ pounds, peeled, seeded, and cubed
1 yam, peeled and diced
1 teaspoon sea salt
¾ teaspoon cinnamon or 1 cinnamon stick
½ teaspoon ground ginger or 4 slices fresh ginger
6 cups vegetable stock (see recipe) or filtered water

¼ cup arame
1 cup filtered water
3 tablespoons salted plum vinegar (umeboshi) or 3 tablespoons lemon juice and ¼ teaspoon sea salt
1 teaspoon herbal sea salt
¼ teaspoon freshly ground white pepper
2 teaspoons fresh ginger juice (see recipe)
½ cup pumpkin seeds, toasted

ROUX:

¼ cup unsalted butter or extra-virgin olive oil

½ cup whole wheat or oat flour

1. In a medium pot, heat butter and onion. Cook on a medium flame for 2 minutes.
2. Add squash, yam, salt, cinnamon, and ginger to onion. Stir and let cook 2 to 3 minutes, uncovered.
3. Add stock, cover, and bring to a boil. Lower heat to a simmer and cook until the vegetables are soft, about 20 to 30 minutes.
4. Soak arame in 1 cup filtered water to soften, about 15 minutes.
5. Prepare roux by heating butter and flour in a heavy frying pan, such as cast iron. Stir constantly until fragrant, golden, and nutty-smelling, about 4 or 5 minutes. Be careful that the roux doesn't smoke or burn.

6. Add a few tablespoons of broth from the soup to the roux. Continue to stir, adding half ladles of broth until the roux has the consistency of gravy. Turn off heat.

7. Remove cinnamon stick and ginger slices, if used, from squash and yams. Purée soup and roux in blender or processor until smooth. (Be careful not to fill blender more than halfway, and cover with lid before turning on. For extra precaution, place a cloth over the lid to keep any hot liquid from splattering out.) While blender is still running, add several ladles of squash and broth. Cover and continue blending until smooth, then pour soup into a separate pot or bowl; repeat with remaining until the entire soup is puréed.

8. Heat soup over a low flame, cooking for 5 minutes while seasoning to taste with the plum vinegar, herbal salt, pepper, and ginger juice.

9. Ladle soup into bowls and garnish with a few strands of soaked arame and 1 tablespoon pumpkin seeds.

VARIATION: Try this soup made with all yams.

SUGGESTED ACCOMPANIMENTS: Black Beans with Avocado Salsa Cruda, Collard Greens with White Onions, and Old-Fashioned Oatmeal Raisin Cookies.

★★★ VITAMIN A
  ★ MAGNESIUM, VITAMIN C, MANGANESE, LINOLEIC ACID, IRON

❧

Vitamin A is essential for health, but among Americans, vitamin A deficiencies are common. To assure yourself a good supply, do a color check on your meals and make sure you regularly serve orange foods that contain beta-carotene, which converts to vitamin A.

Here's your orange-foods list, with your foods ranked in richness of beta carotene:

yams	winter squash:	pumpkin
sweet potatoes	butternut	cantaloupe
carrots	acorn	mangoes
	buttercup	apricots
	Hubbard	persimmons
	long-neck	papayas

❧

❧ Tuscan Bread Soup with Basil Infusion ❧

Yield: 2½ to 3 quarts   (4 generous servings plus extra)

Enjoy the flavors of Tuscany with this classic bread soup that has its own special nutritional wisdom. When you combine this hearty, rich broth with whole grain bread, you'll be supplying yourself with manganese and the B vitamins which work together to nourish the brain and fortify the nerves.

2 tablespoons extra-virgin olive oil
1 tablespoon flax seed oil
8 fresh basil leaves, minced
2 tablespoons unsalted butter
1 onion, chopped
8 cloves garlic, peeled
2 leeks, cleaned (see page 80) or
  2 additional onions

6 cups vegetable stock (see recipe)
1 teaspoon sea salt
½ pound whole wheat bread
  (stale or fresh sourdough, Italian, or
  other hearty whole grain bread)
  Freshly ground black pepper

1. Make infusion by mixing olive oil and flax seed oil together in a small bowl and adding minced basil. Set aside.

2. In a large stockpot, place butter, onion, and whole garlic cloves. Sauté over medium heat for 5 to 7 minutes.

3. Add leeks to onion mixture and cook another 3 to 4 minutes. In a blender or processor, purée onion mixture with 1 cup stock and salt.

4. Return purée to pot, add 5 cups stock, cover and bring to a boil. Lower heat and simmer 10 minutes.

5. With a serrated knife, cut bread into 1-inch cubes.

6. Add bread cubes and black pepper to stockpot. Stir, reduce flame to low, and let cook 10 to 15 minutes, covered.

7. Ladle soup into individual bowls and garnish with 2 teaspoons of oil and basil infusion.

SUGGESTED ACCOMPANIMENTS: Butternut Babaganoush, Pinto Bean and Swiss Chard Patties, and Strawberry Tart with Walnut Crust.

★★★   OMEGA-3 FATTY ACIDS
  ★   MANGANESE, SELENIUM, FOLIC ACID, MAGNESIUM, THIAMIN

Two Ways to Clean Leeks

1. Leave roots on leek and cut it in half lengthwise from white part through greens, without separating leek into two pieces. Under running water, hold leek upside down, allowing water to cascade down interior part of each leaf while using your thumb and forefinger to encourage any dirt to dislodge. After cleaning is complete, shake any excess water out of leek, and place on cutting board to remove roots. Complete the cut, separating leek into two separate pieces and chop in 1/4-inch pieces, removing any tough outer green leaves.

2. Slice white part of leeks into 1/4-inch rounds. Remove any tough outer green leaves, and slice inner and more tender green leaves into 1/4-inch slices. Place with leek rings in large bowl of water. Separate rings to allow sand to rinse out and drop to bottom of bowl. Remove cleaned leeks from bowl with your fingers or a slotted spoon.

In either case, save tough outer green leaves and roots for stock.

Extra virgin means oil that is from the first pressing and is not refined or heated. Virgin is from the second pressing and has had heat used in processing, and pure olive oil is from the third pressing with heat and chemicals added to further extract any oil from the olives. We only recommend extra-virgin olive oil since this is the finest of the olive oils and the only grade that has not been heated.

❧ Creamless Mushroom Cream Soup ❧

Yield: 2 quarts   (4 generous servings plus extra)

Here's a comforting food that's smooth and soothing for those times you're feeling stressed—a nondairy soup that tastes and feels creamy. The oatmeal lends richness and a velvety texture when blended, but without the calories of heavy cream. Oats also contribute some phytohormones as a bonus. This soup is good for your bones because of the vitamin D in the mushrooms.

2 10- to 12-ounce boxes mushrooms
1 onion, diced
2 cloves garlic, chopped
4 cups vegetable stock (see recipe) or filtered water

¼ cup rolled oats
1 tablespoon herbal sea salt
¼ teaspoon freshly ground white pepper
2 scallions, chopped

1. In a medium stockpot, put mushrooms, onion, garlic, stock, and oats. Bring to a boil, lower heat, and cook, covered, 15 minutes.

2. Purée entire contents of pot in a blender or processor, in batches. Place each blenderful in a bowl.

3. Return purée to pot and season with herbal salt and pepper, cooking for another 2 or 3 minutes.

4. Serve in bowls and garnish with several teaspoons of scallions. Serve hot.

SUGGESTED ACCOMPANIMENTS: Warm Lima Beans with Basil, Tomato, and Chèvre; Savory Corn Muffins with Onion and Poppy Seeds; and Beverly's Cantaloupe with Freshly Grated Ginger.

★★★ VITAMIN D, NIACIN, PANTOTHENIC ACID, RIBOFLAVIN, COPPER, SELENIUM
★ VITAMIN K, FOLIC ACID, THIAMIN, VITAMIN C, IRON

Cream soup can be made with almost any vegetable. Try carrots, yams, potatoes, leeks, onions, butternut squash, zucchini, parsnips, cauliflower, celery, and asparagus. Vegetables like celery and asparagus will need straining to remove the fibrous parts. After puréeing the soup, add asparagus tips, broccoli florets, or fresh peas for added texture and crunch.

❧

While we can't claim that this soup is a miracle cure for gray hair, it does contain vitamins and minerals that are needed for hair color. Deficiencies of pantothenic acid, folic acid, copper, and iron have been known to manifest as silver threads among the gold, and this soup can increase your stores of these nutrients.

❧

❧ Seafood Bisque with Chives ❧

Yield: 2½ quarts   (4 generous servings plus extra)

Throughout life, and especially at menopause, we need a steady supply of omega-3 essential fatty acids. Fish is high in these wonderful oils. Here is a delicious way to enjoy a healthful dose.

2 onions, chopped
3 tablespoons unsalted butter
4 cups fish or shrimp stock
   (see index)
2 potatoes, peeled and chopped
1 stalk celery, chopped
1 clove garlic, chopped
2 tablespoons whole wheat pastry flour
1 bay leaf
   Pinch saffron

1½ teaspoons herbal sea salt
½ pound shrimp, shelled and deveined
½ pound bay scallops or lobster pieces
½ pound cod, cut into chunks
   Freshly ground white pepper
1 teaspoon lemon juice or salted plum vinegar (umeboshi)
½ bunch chives, cut in half

1. In a medium pot, sauté onions in butter for 2 minutes. Add 2 cups stock, potatoes, celery, garlic, flour, bay leaf, saffron, and herbal salt and bring to a boil, covered. Reduce heat to a simmer and cook covered until vegetables are soft, about 15 minutes.

2. Remove bay leaf and, using a blender or processor, purée ingredients.

3. Return purée to pot, add remaining 2 cups stock, shrimp, scallops, and cod. Bring to a boil and simmer until shrimp turn pink, and scallops and cod become opaque, about 3 minutes. Season with white pepper and lemon juice. Serve in bowls with several chive strands fanned out, floating on top of soup.

SUGGESTED ACCOMPANIMENTS: Broccoli Rabe with Tomato and Spirals, Swordfish Steaks Marinated in Curry Powder Rub, and cucumber and tomato slices.

★★★   VITAMIN B_{12}, OMEGA-3 FATTY ACIDS
★   SELENIUM, COPPER, VITAMIN C, VITAMIN D, VITAMIN B_6

Vitamin B_{12} leaches into cooking water and is lost if fish broth is discarded. Cook fish in its own stock, and you'll insure that this vitamin, which nourishes the nervous system, makes it to the table.

❧ Turkey Soup with Barley-Rice ❧

Yield: 2½ quarts (4 generous servings plus extra)

This soup provides you with an assortment of anti-oxidants, those anti-aging nutrients that work cell by cell to keep your body youthful. There's beta-carotene in the carrots, vitamin C in the parsley, and selenium in the brown rice.

STOCK: (see Notes)

1 turkey carcass, neck, gizzard, and heart (organic preferred)
3 quarts filtered water
1 tablespoon brown rice vinegar or cider vinegar
½ bunch parsley or carrot tops

SOUP:

¼ cup barley, washed (see Notes)
¼ cup brown rice, washed (see Notes)
8 cups turkey stock (from above)
2 onions, diced
2 carrots, diced
3 stalks celery, diced
1 parsnip, diced
½ rutabaga, diced (optional)
2 teaspoons basil
1 tablespoon marjoram
2 to 3 cups leftover cooked turkey, cut into pieces
2 teaspoons herbal sea salt
Freshly ground black pepper
½ bunch parsley, leaves only
1 lemon, cut into wedges, organic preferred (optional)

STOCK:

1. In a large stockpot, place carcass, neck, gizzard, heart, water, vinegar, and parsley (stems and leaves). Bring to a boil, covered. Skim off any foam that comes to the top. Turn flame to medium, leave uncovered, and let cook 30 minutes.

2. Using tongs, remove carcass and discard.

3. Using a large bowl with a colander sitting in it, strain turkey parts and parsley. Set stock aside.

SOUP:

1. In a large stockpot, put barley and rice into 4 cups stock. Bring to a boil, covered, lower flame, and let cook 30 minutes.

2. Add 4 cups stock, onions, carrots, celery, parsnip, and rutabaga to cooking rice and barley. Bring to a boil, covered, reduce flame to a simmer, and cook 15 minutes.

3. Add basil, marjoram, turkey pieces, herbal salt, and pepper. If desired, cut gizzards and heart into pieces, remove any meat from neck, and add these.

4. Serve in large bowls, each garnished with parsley leaves and a lemon wedge.

NOTES: **1.** If you already have stock made, start with soup directions.

2. Already-cooked grain can be used and will shorten the cooking time by half.

SUGGESTED ACCOMPANIMENTS: Asparagus Mimosa with Lemon and Flax Seed Oil, Butternut Squash and Yam Purée, and Fresh Blueberry Cobbler.

VARIATION: The hard rinds of Parmesan or pecorino romano cheese can be added to flavor soups such as this one. Just add the rinds (with the wax removed) and allow them to simmer slowly while the other ingredients are cooking.

★★★ VITAMIN A, VITAMIN B$_{12}$
★ VITAMIN K, SELENIUM, VITAMIN C, FOLIC ACID, IRON

Soup is marvelous to have on hand when you are not in the mood to cook, but after a few days in the refrigerator, it may need some reviving. Here's a trick we use: Add something fresh that you've just chopped, such as several cloves of garlic, an onion, or some freshly grated ginger, and stir it into the soup while it's heating. You'll be adding some fresh flavor and new energy.

❧ Black Bean Soup with Orange and Cinnamon ❧

Yield: 2 quarts   (4 generous servings plus extra)

Here's one of those traditional dishes we like so much, a soup from South America that includes many ingredients that are on a woman's menu. The black beans are a great source of folic acid, which keeps the brain functioning; the orange contains bioflavonoids, which lessen hot flashes; and cinnamon is used medicinally to lessen the cramps that can occur in perimenopause.

Before you begin, have on hand 1 cup dried black beans that have been sorted, washed, and soaked 6 to 8 hours or overnight.

2 to 2½ cups soaked black beans
(from 1 cup dried)

4 cups filtered water or vegetable stock
(see recipe)

¼ eating orange, organic preferred,
seeded (see Note)

1 cinnamon stick

1 onion, minced

1 yam, peeled and diced

1 ripe plantain, peeled and sliced

2 to 3 teaspoons herbal sea salt

½ bunch cilantro or parsley, chopped

1. Lift beans from soaking water with your hand or a slotted spoon and place them in a large stockpot, with the water, orange, and cinnamon. Bring to a boil, lower flame, and simmer 45 minutes. Discard the soaking water.

2. Add onion, yam, and plantain, and continue cooking until yam and beans are soft, about 20 minutes.

3. Remove cinnamon stick and discard. In a blender or processor, purée cooked orange (with rind) with 1 or 2 ladlefuls of beans and broth. Return to pot and season with herbal salt. Serve with several teaspoons of cilantro or parsley.

NOTE: If the orange is not organic, please remove the skin before cooking.

SUGGESTED ACCOMPANIMENTS: Mexican Rice with Pumpkin Seeds and Cilantro, romaine and red onion salad, and Light Lemon Pudding Parfait with Kiwi Slices.

★★★   FOLIC ACID
 ★   VITAMIN K, VITAMIN C, THIAMIN, MAGNESIUM

Fruits that contain bioflavonoids, ranked in order of foods with the greatest concentration of this nutrient:

oranges	dried currants	apricots
lemons	grapes	blackberries
limes	plums	papayas
grapefruit	cherries	cantaloupe

❧ Escarole and Kidney Bean Soup ❧

Yield: 2½ quarts   *(4 generous servings plus extra)*

Both dark leafy greens and beans are staples for bone health, so we combined them into this soup. You can use collards, kale, or endive in place of the escarole, and any beans can replace the kidney beans. Serve it with whole grain bread or bruschetta on the side and you will feel really nurtured and pleasantly full.

Before you begin, have on hand 1 cup dried kidney beans that have been sorted, washed, and soaked 6 to 8 hours or overnight.

2 to 2½ cups soaked kidney beans (from 1 cup dried)

6 cups filtered water or vegetable stock (see recipe)

2 bay leaves

2 sprigs fresh rosemary or 2 teaspoons dried rosemary

5 cloves garlic, peeled

½ head escarole, chopped into bite-sized pieces

½ teaspoon freshly ground white pepper

1 teaspoon sea salt

1 teaspoon hot sauce

1 tablespoon brown rice vinegar or cider vinegar

Olive oil

1. Lift beans from soaking water with your hand or a slotted spoon and put them in a large pot, with the water, bay leaves, rosemary, and whole garlic. Bring to a boil, covered, reduce to a simmer, and cook 50 minutes. Discard soaking water. (See Note.)

2. Add escarole, white pepper, salt, hot sauce, and vinegar. Cook uncovered over medium heat for 5 minutes, until the greens have wilted.

3. If desired, a small portion can be blended for a thicker broth.

4. Ladle into bowls and drizzle with olive oil. Serve while hot.

NOTE: If using cooked beans, cook beans and herbs only 10 minutes in step 1.

SUGGESTED ACCOMPANIMENTS: Slice of whole wheat bread and a baked yam.

★★★ VITAMIN K; FOLIC ACID

★ IRON, VITAMIN C, MANGANESE, COPPER, THIAMIN, MAGNESIUM

❧ Garlic Soup with Bruschetta ❧

Yield: 2½ quarts   (4 generous servings plus extra)

Having food already prepared and waiting allows you to heat up some nourishment quickly anytime fatigue overtakes you. Because this soup is made with garlic, it digests very easily and it also gives a boost to your immune system, which may need some help if you're feeling worn out. Settle into a comfortable chair and sip some of this gently fortifying broth.

SOUP:

- 2 tablespoons extra-virgin olive oil
- 2 leeks, sliced thin (about 2 to 3 cups; see box, page 80)
- 15 to 20 cloves garlic, peeled
- 6 cups filtered water or vegetable stock (see recipe)
- 4 potatoes, peeled and quartered
- ½ teaspoon sea salt
- 1 tablespoon lemon juice
- 2 teaspoons herbal sea salt
- ¼ teaspoon freshly ground white pepper

BRUSCHETTA:

- ½ loaf whole wheat Italian bread or 4 slices hearty whole grain bread
- 1 clove garlic, peeled
- 2 tablespoons extra-virgin olive oil
- ¼ bunch parsley, minced

SOUP:

1. In a medium stockpot, heat olive oil with leeks and whole garlic. Cook until vegetables begin to soften, about 3 to 5 minutes.

2. Add water or stock, potatoes, and salt. Bring to a boil, cover, and reduce heat, cooking gently for 30 minutes.

3. Meanwhile, make bruschetta. Cut the bread into thin slices, and quarter or halve if slices are large. Toast in the oven until golden and crisp. Remove toast and rub each slice with garlic. (The toast will act like a grater and the garlic flavor will be imparted.) Drizzle olive oil over the toast and sprinkle with parsley.

4. When the soup is cooked, purée half or all of the vegetables in a blender or processor, adding lemon juice, herbal salt, and pepper. Stir well.

5. Ladle into bowls, placing 1 or 2 slices of bruschetta in each, or serve alongside.

VARIATION: For a heartier soup add broccoli florets, pieces of cooked chicken, tofu, rice, millet, or pasta, or give it a protein boost and do what the Mexicans do—

drop a raw egg right into your bowl of hot soup (it will cook in the hot broth)—and add several squeezes of fresh lemon.

SUGGESTED ACCOMPANIMENTS: Tuscan White Beans with Tuna and Lemon, Your Basic Green Salad, and Italian Almond Cake.

★★★   VITAMIN C
　★   VITAMIN B$_6$, VITAMIN K, POTASSIUM, THIAMIN, MANGANESE, COPPER, IRON

You can easily make a sauce from this soup by cooking it over medium heat, uncovered, until reduced to half the volume, about 15 to 20 minutes. Or add diluted arrowroot or kuzu and cook until clear.

❧ Split Pea and Barley Soup with Spices ❧

Yield: 2 quarts   (4 generous servings plus extra)

By stabilizing blood sugar, this soup helps to prevent hot flashes and mood swings. It pairs a grain and a legume which, when combined, provides you with both complex carbohydrates and protein for a steady supply of energy. Try a bowlful and notice that your energy supply lasts longer.

1 cup green or yellow split peas, washed	3 stalks celery, diced
¼ cup barley, washed	1 parsnip, diced
1 6-inch strip kombu or kelp seaweed (optional)	1 teaspoon caraway or cumin seeds
6 cups filtered water	1½ teaspoons herbal sea salt
2 onions, diced	½ teaspoon black pepper
2 carrots, diced	1 tablespoon flax seed oil or extra-virgin olive oil
	½ bunch scallions, chopped

1. In a large stockpot place split peas, barley, kombu, and water. Bring to a boil, covered. Lower flame and simmer for 30 minutes.

2. Add onions, carrots, celery, parsnip, and caraway seeds. Return to a boil, reduce flame, and simmer until split peas fall apart and barley is soft, about 45 minutes.

3. Add herbal salt and pepper, and cook for 1 or 2 minutes. If kombu has not dissolved, remove with tongs and chop or slice and return to soup. Turn off flame and add flax seed or olive oil, stirring well.

4. Serve in individual bowls, garnished with scallions.

SUGGESTED ACCOMPANIMENTS: Greek Cucumber and Yogurt Dip; Composed Salad of Oranges, Avocado, and Endive; baked yams; and Fresh Blueberry Cobbler.

★★★ VITAMIN A, OMEGA-3 FATTY ACIDS
★ FOLIC ACID, VITAMIN K, THIAMIN, MANGANESE, MAGNESIUM

Seaweed can be incorporated into many dishes without changing their flavor and it adds considerable nutrients. The kombu we tucked into this pea-soup recipe adds iron, potassium, and iodine. Iodine is needed for thyroid health, and a deficiency of iodine has been linked to breast cancer.

❧ Calcium-Rich Fish Stock ❧

Yield: 4 quarts

Stocks are a traditional way to easily acquire the calcium and other minerals that are stored in animal bones. The secret to releasing the minerals is to add a little vinegar. Its flavor will dissipate as the stock cooks.

4 quarts filtered water
1 pound fishbones with head and tail, washed in cold water (see Note)
2 bay leaves
3 to 4 white or black whole peppercorns

2 tablespoons cider vinegar or brown rice vinegar
1 onion, peeled and quartered
1 carrot, cut in half
4 cloves garlic, unpeeled and mashed
2 stalks celery, cut in half

1. In a large stockpot, place water, fishbones, head, and tail. Add bay leaves, peppercorns, and vinegar. Bring to a boil, covered.

2. Add onion, carrot, garlic, and celery. Lower heat and simmer uncovered 30 minutes. Allow to cool about 10 to 15 minutes.

3. Place a colander in a large bowl or pot and pour the soup into the colander. Discard the bones and vegetables. Allow the stock to sit 5 minutes to settle any particles.

4. Without disturbing the stock, gently pour all of the stock, except what is in the bottom inch of the pot, into storage containers. (The bottom inch will contain inedible particles.)

NOTE: Some common varieties of fish to use are red snapper, flounder, sole, catfish, cod, scrod, or any light-tasting white-meat fish.

SUGGESTED USES: Use stock in any grain, bean, soup, or sauce recipe, which will make the flavor more full-bodied.

★★★ VITAMIN A, VITAMIN B$_{12}$, SELENIUM, CALCIUM
★ VITAMIN D, VITAMIN B$_6$, NIACIN, POTASSIUM, VITAMIN C, FOLIC ACID

Miso Soup

A fish stock like the one we give here makes a good base for miso soup. Use 1 to 2 teaspoons miso paste per cup of hot stock or water. Be sure to treat the miso as the living substance it is, rich in micro-organisms, and add the miso only during the last minute of cooking or directly into your bowl. (This keeps the miso from reaching a high temperature.) The miso paste is easier to add if it is first mixed with a small amount of broth or water.

❧ Vegetable Trimmings Stock with Lentils ❧

Yield: 2 quarts

When you use this stock made with an assortment of trimmings, you give yourself a significant amount of ten or more different nutrients, the variety you need because they all work together. A deficiency in one disables another. In vegetables, vitamins and minerals are often concentrated just below the skin, and this recipe gives you a way to benefit from these nutritious scraps.

2 quarts filtered water ¼ cup lentils, washed
6 to 8 cups vegetable trimmings
(see Note)

1. In a large stockpot, put water, vegetable trimmings, and lentils. Bring to a boil, covered. Lower heat to medium and simmer for 30 to 45 minutes.
2. Remove pot from heat and allow stock and vegetables to cool about 10 minutes. Prepare a large bowl with a colander in it. Drain stock through colander. When cool, discard vegetable trimmings and lentils.
3. Let stock settle, then gently pour into storage containers, being careful not to disturb the bottom inch of the bowl, where there may be sand and small particles. After pouring, discard this.

NOTE: Use the peels from carrots, potatoes, and parsnips; onion and garlic skins; leek trimmings; the stems of mushrooms and parsley; corncobs; and butternut-squash seeds.

★★★ VITAMIN A, VITAMIN K, VITAMIN C, FOLIC ACID
★ IRON, VITAMIN B₆, POTASSIUM, COPPER, MANGANESE, MAGNESIUM

❧

Lentils give this stock a deep, rich, and meaty flavor, while adding a little protein. To make a still richer stock, add beef or chicken bones with a little vinegar to draw out their abundant calcium.

❧

7

Salads and Dressings

SALADS

Your Basic Green Salad
Fast Salad
Composed Salad of Oranges, Avocado, and Endive
Carrot and Cabbage Slaw with Fresh Fennel
Three-Bean Salad
Mesclun Salad with Organic Liver and Rosemary
Classic Potato Salad Revisited
Grated Beet and Hijiki Medley
Bowl of Antipasto
Chinese Napa Cabbage and Celery Salad
Steamed Summer Squash Salad
Bulgur Wheat Salad
Marinated Arame Salad with Horseradish
Leafy Greens Vietnamese Style
Beet and Potato Salad
Cold Seafood Salad
California Waldorf Salad

DRESSINGS

Your Basic Easy Dressing
Mustard Vinaigrette
Lime-Cilantro and Red Onion Vinaigrette
Creamy Plum Dressing
Tahini-Garlic Dressing
Creamy Yogurt Dressing
Sweet Almond-Butter Dressing

Salads

Salads are great food for menopause since they can be made with so many different ingredients. They can be quick and easy to prepare, whether they are made with fresh ingredients or are a way to use already cooked foods.

Traditional salad ingredients provide fiber, raw vegetables add crunch, and everything adds useful vitamins and minerals. Start with colorful vegetables, add some fish or nuts and a savory salad dressing, and you'll have a variety of flavors and textures. Serve this with a slice of whole grain bread and you'll quickly have more than a salad—you'll have a mini-meal!

Dressings

When seasoning salads with dressing, use just enough for flavoring and your salad will remain a low-calorie dish. (Any oil label that reads "lite" refers to the color and taste, not the calories. All oils have 9 calories per gram.) We start with the best quality oils—extra-virgin olive oil, flax seed oil, or unrefined sesame oil. Added to this is an acid for tang, such as lemon juice or vinegars like brown rice, cider, or salted plum. For additional flavoring sometimes mustard, herbs, spices, garlic, ginger, miso, or scallions are added. Salt is good for bringing out the flavors of the dressing, yet when using salted plum vinegar or miso, it is not usually necessary to use any additional salt since they already contain enough.

Washing Greens

Fill a large bowl or the sink with plenty of fresh water, preferably filtered, so that there is lots of room for the sand and particles to free themselves from the greens and drop to the bottom of the container. Cut ¼ inch off the ends of the greens so that the leaves can detach, and submerge the greens several times in the water. Remove the greens from the water with your hands, and repeat this procedure, first emptying the bowl of water and sand, then refilling it with fresh water. Wash the greens until there is no sediment left in the bowl.

We do not recommend putting salt or vinegar in the water to help in cleaning as they leach out the vitamins and minerals.

❧ Your Basic Green Salad ❧

Yield: Any amount

Everyone knows how to make a salad—iceberg lettuce, waxed cucumbers, and hothouse tomatoes with bottled ranch dressing. Not anymore! Here's a reminder of the variety of vegetables to choose from to make a nutrient-packed, colorful, tasty, and textured salad. Go wild!

Mild-Flavored Greens

romaine
spinach
Boston lettuce
bibb lettuce
red-leaf or ruby lettuce
green-leaf lettuce
oak-leaf lettuce
corn salad

Tangy-Flavored Greens

escarole
chicory
watercress
arugula
purslane
sorrel
Belgian endive
radicchio
cabbage—green, savoy, red

Fresh Herbs

parsley—Italian, curly
basil
dill
oregano
rosemary

Sprouts

alfalfa
mung bean
lentil
radish
cabbage

Onions

Vidalia
red
yellow
shallots
scallions
chives

1. Choose one or several lettuces. Wash (page 94) and spin dry.
2. Tear greens into bite-size pieces (about 1 cup per person) and place in a serving bowl. If you like, add the leaves of fresh herbs, sprouts, and chopped onions.
3. Add your dressing of choice and for crunch and variation add some salad crunchies. Toss and munch.

Salad Crunchies

green or red peppers
red or white radishes
carrots
cucumbers

sunflower seeds
pumpkin seeds
walnuts
almonds

❧ Fast Salad ❧

Yield: Serves 1

With a minute or two of slicing, you'll have a tasty salad. Use its quick crunch and flavor for a vegetable snack or part of a meal.

1 **kirby cucumber**
1 **plum tomato**
2 **radishes or 1 scallion (optional)**

1 **or 2 tablespoons Paul Newman's Own: Olive Oil and Vinegar Dressing (or a homemade version)**

Chop vegetables; add dressing.

★★★ CHROMIUM, VITAMIN C
★ POTASSIUM, FOLIC ACID, VITAMIN A, PANTOTHENIC ACID

❧ Composed Salad of Oranges, ❧ Avocado, and Endive

Yield: 1½ quarts   (4 generous servings)

Avocados do contain a lot of fat—California avocados can contain as much as 30 grams—but two-thirds of that fat is the beneficial mono-unsaturated kind that lowers the LDL cholesterol (the kind you don't want) and increases HDL (the kind that's healthy). So please don't be fat-phobic and enjoy avocados when in season.

2 **endive**
2 **navel oranges, peeled and sliced into rounds**
1 **avocado, pitted and cut into 12 slices (see Note)**

8 **red radishes, trimmed and chopped**
Lime-Cilantro and Red Onion Vinaigrette (see recipe)

1. On an individual salad plate, arrange four endive leaves in a fan. Join them in the middle of the plate and let the slim ends point outward.
2. Cover the base of the fan with three orange slices (which should leave about half of the plate still empty).
3. Take three slices of avocado and arrange these so they mirror the fan of the endive.
4. Sprinkle radishes over oranges. Drizzle dressing over arrangement.

NOTE: To seed avocado, cut avocado in half lengthwise, and twist one half away from pit, then remove pit from other half. Holding each half in the palm of your hand, cut the flesh into 6 slices. Run the knife between the outer shell and the flesh to remove the slices.

SUGGESTED ACCOMPANIMENTS: Great Northern Ragout Provençal, Savory Oatmeal Muffins with Sunflower Seeds, and Light Lemon Pudding Parfait with Kiwi Slices.

★★★   VITAMIN K, VITAMIN C
★   FOLIC ACID, PANTOTHENIC ACID, COPPER, VITAMIN B$_6$, POTASSIUM, MAGNESIUM

Vitamin C

An elegant glass carafe of freshly squeezed orange juice may look beautiful sitting on the patio table you've prepared for a Sunday brunch, but it's losing its vitamin C every minute—as much as 50 percent in the first half hour! Vitamin C also disappears quickly from orange slices.

⚜ Carrot and Cabbage Slaw with Fresh Fennel ⚜

Yield: About 2 quarts   (4 generous servings plus extra)

Here's a combination that includes three phytohormone vegetables—celery, parsley, and fennel—plus currants which contain bioflavonoids, all estrogenic compounds that quell hot flashes and stabilize mood swings. Keep a batch of this slaw on hand; it's a good way to have vegetables without cooking some for every meal.

2 carrots, peeled
¼ head green cabbage, core removed
  and shredded
1 stalk celery
½ red onion
1 fennel bulb
1 teaspoon sea salt
½ bunch parsley, chopped coarsely

3 scallions, chopped
¼ cup currants (optional)
1 recipe Creamy Plum Dressing
  (see recipe)
1 endive, separated into individual
  leaves
½ head red-leaf lettuce, about 8 leaves

1. Grate carrots, cabbage, celery, and onion, and place in a medium bowl.
2. Remove any damaged outer stalks from fennel. Cut feathery leaves and tough

stalks from top of fennel, leaving only the bulb. Cut in quarters, remove core, mince or grate and add to bowl.

3. Toss grated vegetables with salt and stir. Let sit 10 minutes

4. Put a colander in the sink, and pour salted vegetables into it, allowing any liquid from salting process to be drained and discarded. Rinse with filtered water and shake to drain.

5. Place drained vegetables in a mixing bowl. Add parsley, scallions, and currants. Pour dressing over and toss. If time permits, allow slaw to sit at least 20 minutes.

6. Place a spoonful of slaw in each endive leaf, arrange on a lettuce-lined platter, and serve.

VARIATIONS: Try celeriac or jicama instead of fennel.

SUGGESTED ACCOMPANIMENTS: Creamless Mushroom Cream Soup, Black-Eyed Peas with Roasted Vegetables, Savory Corn Muffins with Onion and Poppy Seeds.

★★★   VITAMIN A, VITAMIN K, VITAMIN C, FOLIC ACID
★   MANGANESE, IRON, THIAMIN, VITAMIN B_6

To peel or not to peel: Since more nutrients in fruits and vegetables lie just under the skin, it's better not to peel your vegetables if you don't have to. To decide whether or not that beautiful-looking carrot needs to shed its skin, peel off one strip. Taste it. If it is tasty, don't peel; if the peel is bitter, then peel the carrots.

❧ Three-Bean Salad ❧

Yield: 1 quart   (4 generous servings plus extra)

The three-bean salad sold at the delicatessen is usually so sweet you could serve it for dessert. Our version of this American classic is made without sugar and lets the taste of the sweet onions and richly flavored beans come through. Beans are a staple for women because they are a good source of protein and fiber, and bean salads are another way to include them regularly in your menus.

Before you begin, have on hand ½ cup dried kidney or pinto beans and ½ cup dried black-eyed peas that have been sorted, washed, and soaked in separate containers.

1 **cup soaked kidney or pinto beans (from ½ cup dried)**
1 **cup soaked black-eyed peas (from ½ cup dried)**
  Filtered water
1 **teaspoon sea salt**
½ **pound green beans or 1 cup shucked fresh peas**

1 **recipe Your Basic Easy Dressing (see recipe)**
2 **stalks celery, diced**
½ **red onion, minced**
1 **carrot, minced or grated**

1. Remove beans from soaking water with hands or a slotted spoon and place in separate pots. Pour enough water over the beans to cover by at least 1 inch. Bring to a boil, covered, lower flame, and simmer kidney beans 40 to 45 minutes and black-eyed peas 35 to 40 minutes. After 20 minutes add ½ teaspoon salt to both pots and continue cooking (see below). Discard soaking water.

2. Pick through green beans and break off the vine tip. Wash. Break or cut into thirds or quarters. In a small pot, bring ½ cup water to a boil. Add green beans and steam 3 to 4 minutes, until bright green. Remove with a slotted spoon and place in a serving bowl.

3. Drain beans (save cooking liquid for soup) and add with green beans. Pour dressing over while hot and toss well. Add celery, onion, and carrot.

4. Marinate in the refrigerator for at least 30 minutes. This salad tastes better and better as the days pass, but after a day or two, some additional seasoning may be needed.

VARIATIONS: Try other bean combinations such as chick-peas and black beans, navy beans and lima beans, or cannellini and kidney beans. The addition of fresh corn kernels, red pepper, or sun-dried tomatoes adds a lovely color and texture.

SUGGESTED ACCOMPANIMENTS: Greek Cucumber and Yogurt Dip, Kasha and Red Pepper Timbales, and Old-Fashioned Oatmeal Raisin Cookies.

★★★ FOLIC ACID, OMEGA-3 FATTY ACIDS
  ★ VITAMIN A, VITAMIN K, IRON, MANGANESE, MAGNESIUM, VITAMIN C

Adding salt halfway through the cooking time keeps beans from falling apart and getting too mushy. It doesn't matter if you're making soup, but for a salad this technique produces beans that look their best.

❧ Mesclun Salad with ❧ Organic Liver and Rosemary

Yield: About 2 quarts (4 servings)

Mesclun is a European salad mix of tasty and tender leaves of baby lettuces, such as chicory, frisée, and radicchio, plus culinary herbs, and it's starting to become available in the supermarket. If gardening is your hobby, in mild-weather months you can grow your own. Young plants are especially full of nutrients and enzymes—premium fuel for a woman at any stage of her life.

2 tablespoons filtered water
1 tablespoon unsalted butter or extra-virgin olive oil
4 or 5 chicken livers, organic only, or 2 turkey livers, organic only (see Note page 257)
2 teaspoons rosemary

¼ teaspoon sea salt
    Freshly ground black pepper
2 quarts loosely packed mesclun salad (see Note)
½ cup Mustard Vinaigrette or Tahini-Garlic Dressing (see recipe)

1. In a small sauté pan, heat water and butter. Add chicken livers, rosemary, and salt. Cook over medium heat 3 to 5 minutes, turning once or twice. The livers should still be tender and not hard. Be careful not to overcook.

2. Turn off heat and dust the livers with pepper.

3. Divide salad into four or five portions and place on large salad plates. Pour several teaspoons of dressing over each salad. Arrange cooked livers in center of each salad. Serve immediately, with extra dressing in a bowl on the side.

NOTE: Mesclun can be used for the base of any leafy salad, without the organic liver and rosemary. If mesclun is not available, use a mix of escarole, chicory, watercress, and arugula.

SUGGESTED ACCOMPANIMENTS: Black Bean Soup with Orange and Cinnamon, and whole grain sourdough bread.

★★★   VITAMIN A, VITAMIN K, VITAMIN B$_{12}$, FOLIC ACID, OMEGA-3 FATTY ACIDS
  ★   VITAMIN C, RIBOFLAVIN, IRON, MANGANESE

❧ Classic Potato Salad Revisited ❧

Yield: 2½ quarts   (4 generous servings plus extra)

Potatoes are high in potassium, a mineral you need. Stress can deplete your supply of potassium, and it can also be lost in the perspiration of a hot flash. Instead of mayonnaise, use one of our dressings made with healthy oils and convert this favorite into a menopause food.

6 red Bliss, Yukon Gold, or eastern potatoes	3 stalks celery, minced
1 quart filtered water	1 carrot, grated
2 eggs, organic and free-range preferred (optional)	½ bunch parsley, chopped coarsely
½ red onion, diced	1 recipe Your Basic Easy Dressing or Creamy Plum Dressing (see recipe)
	1 teaspoon prepared mustard

1. In a medium stockpot, put potatoes in water with eggs. Cover, bring to a boil, reduce flame, and simmer 5 minutes. Remove eggs with a slotted spoon. Keep cooking the potatoes until soft when pierced with a fork, about 10 to 15 minutes more.

2. Run cold water over eggs to cool. Peel and dice fine.

3. In a medium bowl place chopped eggs, onion, celery, carrot, parsley, dressing, and mustard.

4. Remove potatoes from cooking water with slotted spoon and place in bowl of cold water. Allow potatoes to sit in water until cool enough to touch, about 5 minutes. Peel potatoes by holding under water and slipping the skins off with your hands or a paring knife.

5. Cut potatoes into cubes or slices. Add to vegetables and dressing and toss. Cover and marinate in refrigerator at least 30 minutes. Of course, as the salad marinates over several days, it gets better!

VARIATIONS: Add chopped dill pickles, scallions, cucumbers, and/or capers.

SUGGESTED ACCOMPANIMENTS: Great Meatloaf with Tomato Sauce, corn on the cob, Sautéed Mushrooms with Garlic, Old-Fashioned Oatmeal Raisin Cookies.

★★★   OMEGA-3 FATTY ACIDS
 ★   VITAMIN C, VITAMIN K, VITAMIN A, VITAMIN B_6, POTASSIUM, COPPER, FOLIC ACID

Mayonnaise not only has a high fat content, it is usually made from fats that have been deodorized and bleached with chemicals, which make them tasteless, and many also contain preservatives and sugar. Our alternative to this is to use a dressing that is made from unrefined sesame or flax seed oil and to mix or blend these oils with mustard, which will emulsify the oil with the vinegar or lemon juice. Though the fat content will be just as high, you can certainly make homemade mayonnaise with extra-virgin olive oil, if you like the taste.

Dr. Serafina Corsello, executive medical director of the Corsello Centers for Nutritional-Complementary Medicine in New York, has created an oil mixture that's ideal for menopause. It combines 8 ounces each of premium extra-virgin olive and flax seed oils with the oil from three capsules of vitamin E, which acts as a natural preservative. To this—for flavor and improving circulation and other health benefits—she adds 2 to 3 cloves of garlic cut in half. Dr. Corsello advises women to use 1 tablespoon daily to begin and increase to several tablespoons daily within a month. (This allows the body time to adjust its metabolism to good-quality fats.) It can be used as a base for salad dressing, or drizzled over hot vegetables. Keep it refrigerated.

❧ Grated Beet and Hijiki Medley ❧

Yield: 2 cups (4 servings plus extra)

If you don't already eat seaweed, find out what you've been missing and prepare this delicious gourmet salad. First there's the color—the deep magenta of the beets, mixed with the black hijiki—then there's the velvety texture. And check out those nutritional stars!

¼ **cup hijiki**
Filtered water
1 **large beet**
1 **cup unfiltered apple juice**
3 **slices fresh ginger**
½ **navel orange, cut into quarters (see Note)**

1 **tablespoon brown rice vinegar or cider vinegar**
1 **tablespoon lemon juice**
¼ **teaspoon sea salt**

1. In a small bowl, place hijiki in 3 to 4 inches of water. Let soak for 20 minutes.
2. Place beet in a small saucepan and cover with water. Bring to a boil, covered, reduce heat, and simmer 20 to 30 minutes, until soft when pierced with a fork.
3. Lift the hijiki from the soaking water with your hands or a slotted spoon and place in a small pot. Discard soaking water. Add apple juice, ginger, and orange to hijiki. Bring to a boil and cook, covered, 15 minutes.
4. Remove orange pieces and discard. Remove hijiki to a bowl, season with vinegar, lemon juice, and salt. Stir well.
5. Remove beet from pot and place in a bowl. Cover with cold water and, when cool enough, slip off skin under water. Remove beet from water and grate. Add to hijiki, stir, and serve.

NOTE: Use the skin only if the orange is organic. If only commercial oranges are available, then peel.

SUGGESTED ACCOMPANIMENTS: Turkey Soup with Barley-Rice; Tempeh, Green Beans, and Carrots with Mustard Sauce; Broiled Dates Stuffed with Almonds.

★★★ CALCIUM, FOLIC ACID
★ MANGANESE, IRON, MAGNESIUM, VITAMIN C, VITAMIN A, POTASSIUM, THIAMIN, RIBOFLAVIN, PANTOTHENIC ACID, COPPER, VITAMIN B_6

⚜ Bowl of Antipasto ⚜

Yield: 4 generous servings plus extra

This antipasto is a spectacular way to increase your count of vegetable servings each day—you need three to five. Arrange a showy display on a large platter or in an oversized salad bowl and serve this grand salad to company. Everyone will find something that they like and the next day you can graze on the leftovers. Snacking will help steady both your blood sugar and emotions between meals.

1 quart filtered water or more as needed
2 stalks broccoli, cut into spears
2 carrots, cut into sticks
1 cauliflower, cut into florets
1 zucchini, cut diagonally into ¼-inch pieces
1 yellow summer squash, cut diagonally into ¼-inch pieces
½ head escarole or ½ bag prepared chopped lettuce
1 green pepper, sliced into ½-inch pieces

1 red pepper, sliced into ½-inch pieces
1 10-ounce carton mushrooms
1 pint cherry tomatoes
4 scallions
20 kalamata or Greek olives
½ bunch parsley or dill, chopped coarsely
1 recipe Your Basic Easy Dressing (see recipe)
1 recipe Taramasalata (see recipe) or White Bean Spread (see recipe)

1. In a large stockpot, covered, bring water to a boil.
2. Blanch broccoli by immersing in boiling water. Leave pot uncovered and return to a boil, cooking about 4 minutes. Broccoli should be bright green and tender, but not soft.
3. With a slotted spoon, remove broccoli from water and place in a bowl of cold water to stop the cooking process. Leave in the water for several minutes, until cooled. Pour water and broccoli into a colander and drain for several minutes.
4. Return water to a boil and repeat procedure for the carrots, cauliflower, zucchini, and summer squash, blanching and cooling each individually. Place cooked vegetables on a tray while waiting for all to be blanched.
5. On a large, shallow platter, arrange lettuce leaves to cover the entire surface. Organize vegetables in mounds around the platter, alternating colors and including the peppers, mushrooms, tomatoes, scallions, and olives. Leave room for two small serving bowls that will contain dressing and dip.
6. Scatter parsley or dill over vegetables, pour dressing and dip into bowls, and place on platter. Serve with toothpicks or forks and small plates.

VARIATIONS: Add a few chunks of imported goat or sheep-milk cheese, such as feta or ricotta salata; roasted peppers; Easy Onion and Pepper Slices (see recipe); skewered and then grilled steamed vegetables; eggplant salad, and so on. Create a feast!

SUGGESTED ACCOMPANIMENTS: Whole wheat Italian bread, Asparagus Fusilli, Soft-Shell Crabs, and Italian Almond Cake.

★★★   VITAMIN A, VITAMIN K, VITAMIN C, FOLIC ACID, PANTOTHENIC ACID
  ★   VITAMIN B$_6$, RIBOFLAVIN, NIACIN, POTASSIUM, OMEGA-3 FATTY ACIDS, IRON, MANGANESE, MAGNESIUM, SELENIUM

When blanching, to test if vegetables are cooked enough, lift a piece with a slotted spoon and pierce with a fork. There should be a slight resistance.

To rehydrate yourself after a day of hot flashes, eat juicy vegetables, such as summer squash, zucchini, and cucumbers. Watery foods help replenish your supply of liquid. Think of water as a nutrient, along with vitamins and minerals.

❧ Chinese Napa Cabbage and Celery Salad ❧

Yield: 1½ quarts *(4 generous servings plus extra)*

Napa cabbage matches common cabbage in most nutrients but towers over it in vitamin A content. We need this nutrient for eyesight, which can begin to weaken as we age. We've combined the napa cabbage with celery, a source of phytohormones.

1 small head or ½ head Chinese napa cabbage, or red, green, or savoy cabbage, shredded
3 stalks celery, chopped
1 carrot, grated

4 inches daikon radish or 6 white radishes, grated or chopped
1 recipe Creamy Yogurt Dressing (see recipe)
Sea salt and pepper, as needed

1. In a medium bowl, put cabbage, celery, carrot, and radish. Stir in creamy yogurt dressing.

2. If time permits, let salad marinate in the refrigerator for 30 minutes or overnight. Before serving, taste and add a pinch or two of salt, if needed. Grind fresh pepper on top.

SUGGESTED ACCOMPANIMENTS: Calcium-Rich Fish Stock with miso and scallions, Bluefish Marinated in Plum Vinegar, and Spicy Almond Udon with Wilted Spinach.

★★★ VITAMIN A, VITAMIN C, FOLIC ACID, OMEGA-3 FATTY ACIDS
★ VITAMIN B$_6$, POTASSIUM, VITAMIN K, IRON, MANGANESE

❧ Steamed Summer Squash Salad ❧

Yield: 1 quart *(4 generous servings plus extra)*

A salad can be made with ingredients other than lettuce. Cooked vegetables that might usually be served hot can be an innovative change from a raw salad. Try broccoli, zucchini, spinach, green, purple, or wax beans, and even dark leafy greens. Cooked salads last all week long, travel well, and are an easy way to add vegetables to lunch—or any meal.

½ cup filtered water
1 pound yellow squash
1 recipe Your Basic Easy Dressing
  (see recipe)

2 cloves garlic, peeled and sliced
Sea salt and black pepper,
  as needed

1. In a medium saucepan, covered, bring water to a boil.
2. Cut ends off squash, slice in half lengthwise, and cut into ¼-inch slices.
3. Put slices in boiling water, lower heat, and simmer until tender, about 4 minutes. Do not overcook.
4. Remove from pot and place in a serving bowl. While squash is still hot, dress with Your Basic Easy Dressing, and toss with garlic. Add salt and pepper to taste.
5. Serve salad hot, room temperature, or cold.

SUGGESTED ACCOMPANIMENTS: Chicken with Garlic and Vinegar, Baked White and Orange French Fries.

★★★ VITAMIN B_6, VITAMIN C
★ MANGANESE, FOLIC ACID, SELENIUM, MAGNESIUM, THIAMIN, COPPER, VITAMIN K, OMEGA-3 FATTY ACIDS

❧ Bulgur Wheat Salad ❧

Yield: 4 cups   *(4 generous servings plus extra)*

Also known as tabouleh to some, versions of this salad are classic to Middle Eastern cooking. It's easy to prepare—while the wheat is cooking there's time to chop the vegetables and mix the dressing. The bulgur provides a complex carbohydrate to give you an even supply of energy.

1 teaspoon sea salt
2 cups filtered water, boiling
1 cup bulgur wheat
½ cup lemon juice or ⅓ cup vinegar
¼ cup extra-virgin olive oil
2 tablespoons flax seed oil

2 ripe tomatoes, chopped
2 stalks celery, minced
1 bunch parsley or ½ bunch mint,
  chopped
½ cup sunflower seeds

1. In a small pot heat water to boil with salt. Add bulgur, cover, and return to a boil. Lower heat to a simmer and cook 5 minutes. Turn off heat and let bulgur remain covered in the pot for 10 to 15 minutes.

2. Pour into a bowl and add lemon juice, olive and flax seed oils. Stir well and let cool 10 minutes.

3. Add tomatoes, celery, parsley, and sunflower seeds. Stir well. Serve at room temperature or chilled.

Suggested accompaniments: Chick-pea Hummus on a bed of chicory, Oven-Fried Chicken with Herbs, and Fresh Blueberry Cobbler.

Variations: Add chopped garlic, scallions, or red onion.

★★★   omega-3 fatty acids, vitamin k, linolenic acid, vitamin c
   ★   magnesium, manganese, thiamin, folic acid, pantothenic acid

❧ Marinated Arame Salad with Horseradish ❧

Yield: ½ cup   *(4 servings plus extra)*

Horseradish has long been used by some cultures for its medicinal properties. It stimulates digestion and circulation and has antibiotic properties as well. This spicy-tasting root is used as a naturopathic treatment for urinary tract infections, which some women are more prone to during and after menopause. Arame is a variety of seaweed.

¼ cup arame
Filtered water
1½ inches fresh ginger, grated
   (about 2 to 3 teaspoons)
1 tablespoon unrefined sesame oil
1 tablespoon brown rice vinegar or
   cider vinegar
1 teaspoon shoyu soy sauce
1 teaspoon prepared horseradish,
   white or red

½ teaspoon extra-virgin olive oil
¼ teaspoon unsulphured blackstrap
   molasses
¼ teaspoon maple syrup
Pinch sea salt
4 to 6 green lettuce leaves
3 scallions, chopped

1. Place arame in a medium bowl and cover with 3 to 4 inches of water. Let soak for 10 to 15 minutes.

2. Lift the arame from the soaking water with your hand or a slotted spoon and place in another bowl. Discard soaking water.

3. Add ginger, sesame oil, vinegar, soy sauce, horseradish, olive oil, molasses, maple syrup, and salt. Stir well and let stand at least 30 minutes before serving.

4. Arrange lettuce on a platter and place marinated arame on top. Top with scallions and serve.

SUGGESTED ACCOMPANIMENTS: Kale with Capers and Black Olives; Bulgur, Green Bean, and Walnut Pilaf; Frozen Banana Maple-Walnut Whip.

★★★ CALCIUM, IODINE, LINOLEIC ACID
★ VITAMIN E, FOLIC ACID, MAGNESIUM

❧ Leafy Greens Vietnamese Style ❧

Yield: 4 generous servings

Here's a traditional Vietnamese salad that you assemble yourself and eat with your hands—which can be a lot of fun if you share a platter with family and friends. We use greens that are high in vitamins A, K, and C, good for immunity and bone health, and add a bonus in the sunflower seeds to give you essential fatty acids. These oils are components of cell walls throughout your body, and are important for good health.

½ head romaine lettuce, about 8 to 10 whole leaves
1 bunch watercress
1 cup alfalfa sprouts or other variety
10 to 12 sprigs parsley
10 to 12 sprigs cilantro
1 recipe Lime-Cilantro and Red Onion Vinaigrette (see recipe)
4 scallions, sliced thin
¼ cup sunflower seeds

1. Place romaine on a large serving platter. Arrange mounds of watercress, sprouts, parsley, and cilantro with romaine.

2. Make dressing and pour into a decorative bowl. Stir scallions and seeds into dressing and serve with a spoon.

3. To eat: Take a romaine leaf onto your plate. Cover it with one or two sprigs of watercress, a pinch of sprouts, and some of the parsley and cilantro. Place 2 or 3 teaspoons of dressing on greens. Roll up the leaf from narrow end, hold, and eat over a plate. (Pieces will fall out—that's part of the fun!)

VARIATIONS: Add cooked chicken or turkey slices, avocado, beans, or other greens to make your fantasy salad roll.

SUGGESTED ACCOMPANIMENTS: Chinese Steamed Whitefish with Fresh Coriander, Millet-Rice with Green Beans and Tomatoes, and Banana Refrigerator Cake.

★★★ VITAMIN A, VITAMIN K, VITAMIN C, FOLIC ACID, LINOLEIC ACID

⚜ Beet and Potato Salad ⚜

Yield: 2 quarts   (4 generous servings plus extra)

Instead of eating a fast-food or deli lunch, plan ahead and brown-bag your own. Here's a hearty root salad that travels well, made with oil and vinegar rather than mayonnaise, which can spoil. The beets are a source of iron which you may be lacking, a problem for some women in perimenopause. Your body will thank you for this special care.

1 bunch beets with beet greens, if available

3 potatoes

2 quarts filtered water

1 white or yellow onion, sliced (see Note)

1 teaspoon herbal sea salt or more as needed

3 tablespoons cider vinegar

2 tablespoons extra-virgin olive oil

1 tablespoon flax seed oil

1. Remove beet greens, leaving 1 inch of stem on beets. Wash beets and greens separately; set greens aside. Place beets with potatoes in a medium pot. Cover with water. Bring to a boil, covered, lower flame and simmer until soft when pierced with a fork, 30 to 40 minutes. (Potatoes may be done before beets and can be removed.)

2. Using tongs, remove potatoes and beets to a bowl. Leave cooking water in pot. Pour cold water over vegetables and, when cool enough to handle, holding vegetables under the water, slip off skins. Place in a bowl.

3. Place beet greens, if using, into cooking water from beets and potatoes. Cover and simmer 7 to 10 minutes until wilted and soft. With tongs, remove greens to a

colander (do not pour water out on top of greens, since there may be sand in the bottom of the pot.) Let cool and chop.

4. Cut beets and potatoes into bite-size chunks. Add beet greens, onion, herbal salt, vinegar, olive oil, and flax seed oil. Toss well and let marinate for at least 30 minutes at room temperature.

NOTE: For a less spicy onion taste, steam onions in a small amount of water before adding to potatoes and beets.

VARIATIONS: Add hard-boiled eggs, scallions, olives, or cooked carrots or turnips.

SUGGESTED ACCOMPANIMENTS: Chicken with Garlic and Vinegar, Greens Four Calcium, and Broiled Maple Apples.

★★★ FOLIC ACID, OMEGA-3 FATTY ACIDS
  ★ VITAMIN C, VITAMIN B$_6$, POTASSIUM, MANGANESE, COPPER

Unless you've been diagnosed with iron-deficiency anemia, it's best not to supplement with iron, which can be toxic in high amounts. If you're not menstruating, you're no longer losing iron each month, and iron from foods should be sufficient. A recent study (with only male subjects) showed that excess iron might lead to increased risk of heart disease and cancer.

❧ Cold Seafood Salad ❧

Yield: 4 generous servings

Relish the sensual pleasure of chewy calamari (squid), succulent shrimp, and velvety scallops. These treasures of the sea contain selenium and essential fatty acids, and the calamari contains copper, which is good for your bones.

½ cup filtered water or fish stock
  (see recipe)
½ pound cleaned calamari, cut into
  rings
½ pound shrimp, shelled and deveined
½ pound bay scallops
2 stalks celery, minced
½ red onion, minced

3 tablespoons extra-virgin olive oil
1 tablespoon flax seed oil
1 tablespoon prepared mustard
¼ bunch parsley, minced
Juice of 2 lemons
½ teaspoon herbal sea salt
Freshly ground black pepper
1 head Boston or Bibb lettuce

1. In a medium saucepan, bring water to a boil. Add calamari, cover, and cook for 1 minute. Remove with a slotted spoon to a baking pan or wide bowl, allowing it to cool. Repeat procedure with shrimp and scallops, cooking each for 1 minute. Remove to pan to cool.

2. In a medium bowl, add celery, onion, olive and flax seed oils, mustard, parsley, lemon juice, salt, and pepper. Stir well. Add semi-cooled shellfish, stir well, cover and refrigerate at least 1 hour, stirring several times.

3. Taste salad and adjust seasoning. (As the salad absorbs the flavoring it may need additional seasoning.) Set aside four Boston lettuce cups, and shred the remaining lettuce. Place the shredded lettuce on four salad plates. Spoon the seafood salad into the lettuce cups and place on the shredded lettuce to serve.

VARIATIONS: Add pine nuts and raisins or black currants.

SUGGESTED ACCOMPANIMENTS: Large chunks of whole wheat bread, Pasta e Fagioli, Broccoli with Currants, Savory and Spicy Cocktail Mix.

★★★   VITAMIN B$_{12}$, OMEGA-3 FATTY ACIDS
  ★   COPPER, SELENIUM, VITAMIN K, VITAMIN C (AND MANY MORE NUTRIENTS)

❧ California Waldorf Salad ❧

Yield: 6 cups   (4 generous servings plus extra)

Here's our updated version of this tea-room salad from the fifties, a perfect brunch dish. This dish is filled with foods for menopause—apples and pears have boron, black currants and apricots contain bioflavonoids, figs have calcium, and the garnish of pomegranate is an estrogenic fruit.

2 Golden Delicious apples, diced
2 d'Anjou or green pears, diced
  Juice of ½ lemon
6 unsulphured dried white figs, chopped (about 1 cup; see Note)
½ cup unsulphured dried apricots, chopped
½ cup almonds, chopped coarsely

¼ cup dried currants
¼ cup sunflower seeds
1 recipe Sweet Almond-Butter Dressing (see recipe)
½ head green- or red-leaf lettuce (about 8–10 leaves)
1 pomegranate, cut into 6 to 8 wedges

1. Place diced apples and pears in a medium bowl and sprinkle with lemon juice. Toss fruit to coat.

2. Add figs, apricots, almonds, currants, and sunflower seeds to fruit. Toss well.

3. Push fruit to the sides of the bowl to make a well in the center, where the juices will drain. Pour the dressing into this well and stir in the juices that accumulate. Then mix through the entire salad. (If there is not enough liquid at the bottom of the bowl, add some more fruit juice.)

4. Serve on a bed of leafy lettuce. Garnish with pomegranate wedges.

NOTE: If dried fruit is very dry and hard, pour 1 cup boiling water over uncut fruit and cover for 5 to 10 minutes to soften. Remove with a slotted spoon, and save the liquid for cooking hot cereal. Fresh figs can be used when in season.

SUGGESTED ACCOMPANIMENTS: Whole Grain Crackers with Four Seeds, and Zen Punch.

★★★ VITAMIN K, VITAMIN C, FOLIC ACID, LINOLEIC ACID, VITAMIN E, MAGNESIUM, MANGANESE, COPPER

Here's an easy way to juice a lemon so that some of the membrane part is included in the juice (country-style lemon juice!). Take half a lemon and, using a fork, remove any visible seeds. Insert the fork into the center of the lemon and cup the lemon in your other hand. Over a bowl, squeeze the lemon around the fork, while moving the fork back and forth inside the lemon. Twist the lemon around the fork several times, then discard the lemon rind and use the fork to remove any remaining seeds from the squeezed juice.

The preservative sulphur dioxide is known to produce side-effects—nausea, diarrhea, asthma attacks, and hives—in some people, and it is banned on fresh fruits. Some dried fruits are sulphured to retain their moisture and bright color. Organically grown dried fruits are unsulphured and can be found in natural food stores.

❧ Your Basic Easy Dressing ❧

Yield: ¼ cup

2 tablespoons extra-virgin olive oil	⅛ teaspoon sea salt
2 tablespoons flax seed oil	½ teaspoon oregano (optional)
4 tablespoons lemon juice or vinegar	

In a small bowl mix together olive and flax seed oils, lemon juice, salt, and oregano. Pour over lettuce greens or cooked vegetables.

❧ Mustard Vinaigrette ❧

Yield: ¾ Cup

¼ cup brown rice vinegar or cider
   vinegar
3 tablespoons prepared grainy mustard
3 tablespoons flax seed oil

2 tablespoons filtered water
1 tablespoon chick-pea or light miso
   Pinch of sea salt
⅛ teaspoon freshly ground black pepper

In a blender mix together vinegar, mustard, flax seed oil, water, miso, salt, and pepper. Purée until smooth.

VARIATIONS: Add garlic, onion, or scallions.

❧ Lime-Cilantro and Red Onion Vinaigrette ❧

Yield: 1 cup

3 tablespoons flax seed oil
3 tablespoons extra-virgin olive oil
   juice of 3 limes (about ¼ cup)
2 tablespoons brown rice vinegar or
   cider vinegar

2 cloves garlic, peeled
½ teaspoon sea salt
¼ bunch cilantro, leaves only
¼ red onion, minced or grated

In the blender mix flax seed and olive oils, lime juice, vinegar, garlic, and salt, blending until smooth. Add cilantro and blend very briefly to chop coarsely. Pour into a bowl and add onion.

❧ **Creamy Plum Dressing** ❧

Yield: ¾ cup

¼ cup brown-rice vinegar or cider
  vinegar
2 tablespoons unrefined sesame oil or
  extra-virgin olive oil
2 tablespoons flax seed oil
2 tablespoons salted plum paste
  (umeboshi)

1 tablespoon dulse granules or flakes
  or 2 salt-cured anchovies
1 tablespoon prepared mustard
  Sea salt
  Freshly ground pepper

In a blender, mix together vinegar, olive and flax seed oils, plum paste, dulse granules, and mustard. Taste, using a lettuce leaf, and add salt and pepper.

❧ **Tahini-Garlic Dressing** ❧

Yield: ½ cup

¼ cup filtered water
3 tablespoons sesame tahini
3 tablespoons cider vinegar or brown
  rice vinegar

1 clove garlic, mashed
½ teaspoon salt

In a blender, mix together water, tahini, vinegar, garlic, and salt. Blend until smooth.

❧ Creamy Yogurt Dressing ❧

Yield: ½ cup

¼ cup plain bacteria-active yogurt
2 tablespoons brown rice vinegar or
  cider vinegar
2 tablespoons salted plum vinegar
  (umeboshi) or 2 tablespoons lemon
  juice and ½ teaspoon sea salt

1 tablespoon flax seed oil
½ teaspoon oregano
Pinch sea salt
Black pepper

In a small bowl mix together yogurt, vinegars, flax seed oil, oregano, salt, and pepper. Pour over salad and toss.

VARIATIONS: Add minced garlic, chopped parsley or dill, or scallions.

❧ Sweet Almond-Butter Dressing ❧

Yield: ½ cup

2 tablespoons almond or cashew butter
2 tablespoons brown rice vinegar or
  cider vinegar
¼ teaspoon prepared mustard

¼ teaspoon sea salt
2 tablespoons filtered water or apple
  juice, more as needed

In a small bowl, mix together almond butter, vinegar, mustard, and salt. Whisk together. Thin with water to make a thick yet pourable dressing.

8

Beans

Tofu Teriyaki with Vegetables
Overnight Baked Beans
Black-Eyed Peas with Roasted Vegetables
Persian-Style Peppers Stuffed with Lentils and Bulgur
Adzuki Beans with Squash Purée
Black Beans with Avocado Salsa Cruda
Tempeh, Green Beans, and Carrots with Mustard Sauce
Pinto Bean and Swiss Chard Patties
Chick-pea Hummus
Tuscan White Beans with Tuna and Lemon
Black Bean Loaf
Colombian Lima Bean and Corn Stew
Cannellini and Kidney Beans with Rosemary
Twice-Cooked Beans Wrapped in Corn Tortillas
Adzuki Bean Chili with Avocado Cream
Great Northern Ragout Provençal
Warm Lima Beans with Basil, Tomato, and Chèvre
Red Lentil Dhal
Tempeh Slices for Sandwiches

❧

Beans are "on the menu" for women—before, during, and after menopause. They are satisfying when you want some simple food, and make great partners with many other ingredients, producing richly flavored dishes. And beans provide top nutritional value, pound for pound costing the least of any food in the market.

Beans are a source of protein—7 grams in a half cup—giving you a way to have a plant-based diet and still get the protein you need. It's been found that large amounts of protein from animal sources draws calcium from the bones, while protein from plant foods doesn't have as much of an effect. Full of nutrients, the vitamins and minerals in beans nourish the adrenals, soothe irritability, and carry oxygen to the brain. Beans are a source of zinc, which is essential for functions throughout your body, and they can help protect your bones. Beans also contain calcium and its counterpart, magnesium.

One cup of cooked beans has only 250 calories. (The only exception is soybeans, which are high in unsaturated fat.) And beans are high in fiber, the kind that lowers cholesterol.

Buy a variety and keep them on hand. Stored at room temperature in a covered container, they keep for at least a year.

Bean Basics

For a truly healthful lifetime of eating, make beans part of your daily meals. While preparing them may seem time-consuming, beans are actually a great convenience food and preparing them is simple, once you learn the basics.

1. **To sort beans:** Most beans need to be sorted first, especially chick-peas, adzuki, and kidney beans. Measure the amount to be used and pour a single layer on a dinner plate (preferably unpatterned). Remove any broken beans and nonbean objects (stones, chaff, and string). Put the sorted beans in a saucepan or bowl and do the same with the remaining beans.

2. **To wash beans:** Pour plenty of fresh water over the beans (at least 4 to 5 cups of filtered water per cup of beans) and swirl the beans with your hand, loosening dirt and particles. Allow the beans to settle for a few seconds, and then carefully pour off most of

the water without losing any beans. Repeat this process at least one more time, or until the water is clear. After the last wash, pour the beans into a strainer and drain off as much water as possible.

3. To soak beans: Almost all beans need to be soaked to help make them more digestible. (Red lentils, green lentils, green and yellow split peas, and adzuki beans can be cooked successfully without soaking. If they are soaked, their cooking time will be reduced by about half.) There are three basic methods for soaking beans:

a. *Countertop soak:* After sorting the beans, place them in a bowl and cover with 3 or 4 inches of filtered water. Let the soaking beans sit in a cool area, uncovered, for 6 to 8 hours or overnight. When soaking is complete, with your hands or a slotted spoon lift the beans out of the water into a pot. Pour fresh filtered water over the beans and proceed with your recipe.

b. *Hot soak:* After sorting and washing beans, place them in a saucepan and cover with 3 or 4 inches of filtered water. Bring the beans to a boil, cover pot, lower heat, and simmer for 5 minutes. Turn off beans and let them sit, covered, in hot water for 2 hours. Remove beans with a slotted spoon, add desired amount of fresh, filtered water, and proceed with your recipe.

c. *Refrigerator soak:* Prepare beans as in countertop soak, cover with a plate or plastic wrap with several air vents poked into it, and refrigerate. This method is preferable to the Countertop Soak during the hot summer months, when heat can cause beans to ferment more quickly.

Once beans are soaked, they will generally increase by two to two and a half times their original volume. They will keep, uncooked, in the refrigerator for two to three days. Whichever method of soaking you use *always* discard the soaking water.

4. To cook beans: For soup, add 1 cup soaked beans to 6 cups of water. If they will be used in stew or salad, be twice cooked, or served plain, use 1 cup soaked beans to 4 cups water. After cooking, remove the beans with a slotted spoon. Reserve any excess bean liquid for soup stock.

5. To season beans: Always add salt *after* the beans have reached their desired texture, and then cook beans an additional 5 minutes to dissolve salt properly. (Add other acid-containing ingredients, such as tomatoes, vinegar, or lemon juice toward the end of cooking or the beans will be tough.) When making bean salad, add salt midway to assist the beans in retaining their skins and shape to avoid a mushy bean salad. Add herbs, spices, and vegetables while the beans are cooking; these will help flavor the beans and the cooking liquid.

6. Cooking times: Here is a quick reference chart for cooking beans. We have included pressure-cooking times only on those beans that are safe to cook in the pressure cooker (some beans lose their skins and can clog the valve).

Beans That Do Not Need Soaking Before Cooking

Bean Type	Cooking Time	Pressure-Cooker Time
Red lentils	20 minutes	Don't use
Green lentils	45 minutes	Don't use
Split peas	1¼–1½ hours	Don't use
Adzuki beans	1½ hours	40 minutes

Beans That Do Need Soaking Before Cooking

Chick-peas	1½–3 hours	50–60 minutes
Black beans	1½ hours	45 minutes
Kidney beans	50–60 minutes	30 minutes
Pinto beans	45 minutes	25 minutes
Anasazi beans	45 minutes	25 minutes
Large lima beans	1 hour	30 minutes
Small lima beans	45 minutes	20 minutes
Great Northern beans	45 minutes	25 minutes
Navy beans	40 minutes	25 minutes
Black-eyed peas	35 minutes	15 minutes
Pink beans	40 minutes	20 minutes
Cannellini beans	1 hour	25 minutes
Fava beans (broad beans)*	3 hours	45 minutes

*Soak a minimum of 12 hours or overnight.

The Trouble with Beans, or the Missing Enzyme

Beans are on many people's list of foods-to-avoid because they can cause gas. The reason is a missing enzyme, alpha-galactosidase, which humans do not have, and which breaks down raffinose sugars. It's the undigested raffinose and other undigested sugars in our stomachs that cause gas. But there are many things you can do to avoid this problem:

- Eat beans more often. People who eat beans on a regular basis have less difficulty digesting them.

- Change the bean-soaking water two to three times to remove more of the complex sugars from the beans and leave them uncovered while soaking.
- Never cook the soaking liquid—it's full of those tough-to-digest complex sugars.
- Rinse beans after soaking to remove any remaining sugars.
- After soaking, cook beans with a 6-inch strip of kombu seaweed, 1 or 2 bay leaves, 2 slices of fresh ginger, or 1 teaspoon thyme or cardamom, all of which are helpful in the digestion of beans.
- Cook beans slowly, at a low simmer rather than a rapid boil, and cook beans thoroughly.
- Reduce or eliminate intake of dairy products, since beans seem to be more gaseous when eaten with dairy foods.
- Finally, there's always Beano. It's a liquid alpha-galactosidase, that missing enzyme. (For a free sample, see the Appendix.)

❧ Tofu Teriyaki with Vegetables ❧

Yield: 1 quart   (4 generous servings)

Tofu is made from soybeans, which contain high amounts of phytohormones. The infrequency of hot flashes in Japanese menopausal women has been linked to their high consumption of this food. Enjoy its custardlike texture.

1 pound firm tofu
3 tablespoons unrefined sesame oil
1 onion, sliced
1 carrot, sliced diagonally
1 green or red pepper, seeded and sliced

1 recipe Teriyaki Marinade, including thickener (see recipe)
1 teaspoon prepared mustard
1 teaspoon dark sesame oil

1. Remove tofu from package and cut into ½-inch-thick slices. Lay out on two sheets of paper toweling, and then cover with two more sheets. Press toweling down on top of tofu to squeeze out water. Let sit for 5 minutes.

2. In a medium sauté pan, heat 1 tablespoon unrefined sesame oil and tofu slices. Cook until golden brown, about 5 to 6 minutes. Turn slices over, adding 1 more table-

spoon sesame oil to pan, and cook until golden. Remove to a brown bag to drain off any excess fat.

3. Heat remaining 1 tablespoon sesame oil and add onion, cooking over medium-high heat for 1 minute. Add carrot and then pepper, cooking 1 minute after each addition.

4. Add mustard and dark sesame oil to teriyaki marinade and mix well.

5. Return tofu to sauté pan, placing on top of vegetables. Pour teriyaki sauce over tofu and vegetables. Cover and let cook on low heat for about 7 to 10 minutes.

6. Serve hot.

SUGGESTED ACCOMPANIMENTS: Calcium-Rich Fish Stock with miso, Spicy Almond Udon with Wilted Spinach, and Strawberry Tart with Walnut Crust.

★★★   LINOLEIC ACID, IRON, OMEGA-3 FATTY ACIDS, VITAMIN A
★   MANGANESE, MAGNESIUM, VITAMIN C, CALCIUM

> If the food you've sautéed has absorbed too much fat, place it on a brown paper bag to soak up the extra oil. Paper towels do not work as well; after the initial absorption, the food tends to reabsorb the fat from the toweling.

Tofu was first made in China about 164 B.C. from soybeans and nigari, a calcium-rich liquid taken from sea water. Today tofu is made with refined calcium sulfate and it is still an excellent source of calcium—100 mg in a 3.5-ounce serving.

Tofu comes in several textures. Soft tofu contains more water and is good for making dips and sauces. Firm tofu is preferable for slicing, cubing, and cooking with other ingredients; it can be used for dips and sauces when more liquid is added.

❧ Overnight Baked Beans ❧

Yield: 6 cups   (4 generous servings plus extra)

When beans appear on American menus, they are often in this form, baked with seasonings and sugar. As a nutritional bonus, we've used unsulphured blackstrap molasses instead of brown sugar and corn syrup. Refined sugars contain no vitamins or minerals, while blackstrap molasses contains vitamins B_6, E, and K, plus calcium, copper, iron, magnesium, and selenium. Cook these beans overnight, while you sleep.

5 cups filtered water
2 cups dried kidney or pinto beans, sorted and washed
5 cloves garlic, peeled
1 or 2 onions, cut into cubes
¼ cup unsulphured blackstrap molasses

1 tablespoon mustard
⅛ teaspoon cayenne
1 or 2 teaspoons sea salt, to taste
2 teaspoons flax seed oil

Preheat oven to 325°.

1. In a medium ovenproof pot, put the water, beans, whole cloves of garlic, onion, molasses, mustard, and cayenne. Stir well.

2. Cover pot and place in 325° oven for 8 hours or overnight.

3. Stir in salt and cook another 5 minutes.

4. Just before serving, stir in flax seed oil.

VARIATIONS: Add a ripe plantain for a Caribbean zest.

SUGGESTED ACCOMPANIMENTS: Baked chicken brushed with Quick Barbecue Sauce, Steamed Yellow Squash Salad, Savory Corn Muffins with Onion and Poppy Seeds, and Fresh Summer Fruit Compote with sunflower seed cream (see Walnut Cream).

★★★   FOLIC ACID, OMEGA-3 FATTY ACIDS
  ★   IRON, MAGNESIUM, COPPER, PHOSPHORUS, VITAMIN B_6, CALCIUM, THIAMIN

❧ Black-Eyed Peas with Roasted Vegetables ❧

Yield: About 10 cups   (4 generous servings)

Life can leave you feeling exhausted and in no mood to cook, especially if you've been experiencing PMS or menopause symptoms. Here's a two-in-one dish that cuts back on time and effort in the kitchen. Roast the vegetables and cook the beans; then add vinaigrette to make a salad, or water to make a richly flavored soup, and eat these on different days. This dish is even good to eat just like it is!

Before you begin, sort, wash, and soak 1 cup dried black-eyed peas 6 to 8 hours or overnight.

ROASTED VEGETABLES:

2 potatoes, peeled and diced
2 carrots, peeled and diced
1 onion, diced
1 parsnip, peeled and diced
1 parsley root, peeled and diced
   (optional)

½ rutabaga, peeled and diced
2 tablespoons extra-virgin olive oil or
   unsalted butter
1 teaspoon oregano
½ teaspoon black pepper
½ teaspoon sea salt

PEAS:

2 to 2½ cups soaked black-eyed peas
   (from 1 cup dried)

4 cups filtered water

Preheat oven to 375°.

1. In a medium baking dish, put potatoes, carrots, onion, parsnip, parsley root, and rutabaga. Sprinkle with olive oil, oregano, pepper, and salt. Put into 375° oven and bake for 45 minutes, turning several times.

2. Remove beans from soaking water with your hands or a slotted spoon and put in a medium pot with water. Bring to a boil, covered, lower heat, and simmer for 30 minutes.

3. Drain water from peas and add roasted vegetables.

THE SOUP

Yield: 2 quarts   *(4 generous servings plus extra)*

½ recipe cooked Black-Eyed Peas with Roasted Vegetables (about 4 cups)
4 cups vegetable stock or filtered water (see recipe)

½ teaspoon herbal sea salt
1 bay leaf
1 tablespoon salted plum vinegar (umeboshi) or red miso

1. Place cooked peas with roasted vegetables in a medium-size pot. Add stock, herbal salt, and bay leaf. Bring to a boil, covered, lower heat, and cook 15 minutes.
2. Using a potato masher, mash some of the peas and vegetables. Remove bay leaf and discard. Add salted plum vinegar and serve hot.

SUGGESTED ACCOMPANIMENTS: Serve with whole grain pita bread, broiled fish, and watercress salad.

★★★   VITAMIN A, VITAMIN C, FOLIC ACID
★   MANGANESE, COPPER, MAGNESIUM, POTASSIUM, THIAMIN

THE SALAD

Yield: 1½ quarts   *(4 generous servings plus extra)*

½ recipe cooked Black-Eyed Peas with Roasted Vegetables (about 4 cups)
2 stalks celery, diced
½ red or white onion, diced
½ bunch parsley, chopped coarsely

2 cloves garlic, pressed
3 tablespoons flax seed oil
3 tablespoons cider vinegar
1½ tablespoons prepared mustard
½ teaspoon sea salt

1. Place peas and roasted vegetables in a medium bowl.
2. Add celery, onion, and parsley.
3. In a small bowl, mix together garlic, flax seed oil, vinegar, mustard, and salt. Pour over beans and vegetables, stir well. Let marinate at least 30 minutes. This salad gets better as the days go on.

SUGGESTED ACCOMPANIMENTS: Serve with slices of whole grain bread and lettuce leaves for a perfect lunch.

★★★   VITAMIN K
★   VITAMIN A, VITAMIN C, VITAMIN E, FOLIC ACID, POTASSIUM, LINOLEIC ACID

❧ Persian-Style Peppers Stuffed ❧ with Lentils and Bulgur

Yields: 6 stuffed peppers (4 generous servings plus extra)

Eating grains and beans together gives you a low-fat, high-fiber source of protein. Here's a favorite Middle Eastern dish that does this in a particularly savory way. Dried currants provide sweetness as well as estrogenic bioflavonoids, and cinnamon, used medicinally to ease cramps which you may have in the perimenopause years, rounds out the flavors.

3 cups filtered water
1 cup green or brown lentils, washed
1 cup bulgur wheat
1½ teaspoons sea salt
4 tablespoons extra-virgin olive oil
1 onion, diced
4 plum tomatoes, chopped
¼ cup dried currants
¼ bunch parsley, chopped
2 tablespoons chopped fresh mint or 4 teaspoons dried

1 tablespoon chopped fresh tarragon or 2 teaspoons dried
2 scallions, chopped (optional)
¼ teaspoon freshly ground black pepper
1 teaspoon cinnamon
Juice of 1 lemon or ¼ cup vinegar
6 well-shaped green peppers with stems

1. In a medium pot, put water with lentils, bulgur, and ½ teaspoon salt. Bring to a boil, covered, lower heat, and simmer 30 minutes. Turn off heat and let sit 10 minutes.

2. Preheat oven to 350°.

3. In a medium sauté pan, heat two tablespoons oil and add onion, cooking until golden.

4. In a large bowl, place cooked lentils and bulgur, onion, tomatoes, currants, parsley, mint, tarragon, scallions, pepper, cinnamon, lemon juice, 1 teaspoon salt, and 2 remaining tablespoons oil. Mix well.

5. Slice tops off peppers, leaving ¼ inch of top attached to stem to make a "lid." Clean out seeds. Spoon stuffing into peppers and replace cap. Place in a baking pan at least 2 inches deep. Pour ½ inch filtered water into pan. Cover with parchment paper and foil and bake 30 minutes, until peppers are soft. Uncover peppers and cook another 10 to 15 minutes, until the peppers start to brown.

VARIATIONS: This stuffing can be used to fill red peppers, tomatoes, onions, zucchini, pattypan squash, cabbage leaves, grape leaves, or poultry.

SUGGESTED ACCOMPANIMENTS: Napa Cabbage and Celery Salad, beet slices with Creamy Yogurt Dressing, and Apricot-Date-Pecan Bonbons.

★★★ VITAMIN C, FOLIC ACID, VITAMIN K
★ MANGANESE, MAGNESIUM, IRON, VITAMIN B$_6$

❧ Adzuki Beans with Squash Purée ❧

Yield: 6 cups   (*4 generous servings plus extra*)

We invite you to try this intriguing combination—a substantial texture coupled with a delicate taste. This dish is food for your thyroid gland, which can especially begin to slow down as you enter menopause. It contains the essential amino acid phenylalanine and also iodine, two nutrients your thyroid needs for proper functioning.

BEANS:

1½ cups adzuki beans, sorted and washed
4½ cups filtered water
    6-inch strip kombu or kelp sea vegetable

    2-inch piece fresh ginger, grated (about 1½ tablespoons)
¼ teaspoon sea salt

SQUASH PURÉE:

1 butternut or other winter squash, peeled, seeded, and cut into cubes, about 4 to 6 cups
½ cup filtered water
½ cup apple juice or more as needed
3 tablespoons unsalted butter

2 teaspoons ginger juice (see Notes)
1 teaspoon sea salt
   Maple syrup to taste (optional)
2 teaspoons flax seed oil
½ bunch fresh parsley or scallions, chopped

BEANS:

1. In a medium pot, place beans, water, and kombu. Bring to a boil, covered, lower heat, and cook over medium-low heat 1½ hours (pressure cook 45 minutes).

2. Add grated ginger and salt, and stir thoroughly, breaking up kombu (or remove it, chop fine, then return to pot). Cook 5 more minutes, covered.

SQUASH PURÉE: (see Notes)

1. In a medium pot, put squash and water. Bring to a boil, covered, reduce heat to medium-low and cook 20 to 30 minutes, until squash is soft when a fork is inserted.

2. In a blender or processor, purée cooked squash in batches with some cooking liquid and apple juice, until all squash has been puréed. Add butter, ginger juice, and salt. Stir squash purée well.

3. Taste purée; if it is not sweet enough, add a few drops of maple syrup at a time until desired flavor is achieved.

TO SERVE:

With a slotted spoon, place beans in individual bowls. Pour ½ teaspoon flax seed oil over each. Top with several generous tablespoons of purée. Garnish with parsley or scallions.

NOTES: 1. For ginger juice, press as many slices of ginger in clean garlic press as necessary to achieve 2 teaspoons.

2. The squash can be baked instead of steamed. When puréeing, some stock or filtered water will need to be added.

VARIATION: For a time saver, just toss squash chunks on top of beans in their last half hour of cooking.

SUGGESTED ACCOMPANIMENTS: Basic Brown Rice, Broccoli with Black Currants, and Baked Apples Stuffed with Raisin-Ginger Chutney.

★★★   VITAMIN A, FOLIC ACID, OMEGA-3 FATTY ACIDS
  ★   VITAMIN C, VITAMIN K, IRON, MAGNESIUM, MANGANESE, COPPER

❧

Whenever you can, slip a little seaweed into your cooking. The vegetables from the sea—kombu, kelp, nori, wakame, hijiki, and arame—contain 10 to 20 times the minerals of land vegetables. It's a particularly good idea to have some seaweed before and after any kind of X-ray, including mammograms, since seaweeds contain sodium alginate, known to protect against the effects of radiation.

❧

❧ Black Beans with Avocado Salsa Cruda ❧

Yield: 1½ quarts   (4 generous servings plus extra)

Many of our bean recipes are high in folic acid, but this one gives you a double dose because the avocado also contains this important B vitamin. Folic acid is critical to brain function and can bolster your ability to remember what you've just said, sometimes a problem in menopause.

Before you begin, sort, wash, and soak 1 cup dried black beans 6 to 8 hours or overnight.

BEANS:

2 to 2½ cups soaked beans
   (from 1 cup dried)
3 cups filtered water or stock
2 cloves garlic, peeled and mashed
2 bay leaves

1 tablespoon oregano
1 teaspoon cumin seeds or ½ teaspoon
   ground cumin
1 teaspoon sea salt

SALSA CRUDA:

2 cloves garlic, peeled
1 onion, minced
1 avocado, peeled, seeded, and
   chopped (see Note)
2 teaspoons lemon juice

½ bunch parsley, minced
2 tablespoons extra-virgin olive oil
1 tablespoon flax seed oil
   Several pinches paprika (optional)

1. Remove beans from soaking water with your hands or a slotted spoon and place in a medium pot. Add water, garlic, bay leaves, oregano, and cumin seeds. Bring to a boil, lower heat, and simmer, covered, 1 hour. Discard soaking water.

2. Stir in salt and continue cooking 5 minutes, uncovered.

3. Mince 2 cloves garlic. Place in a small bowl with onion, avocado, lemon juice, parsley, olive oil, and flax seed oil. Mix well and place avocado pit in bowl.

4. Serve beans in bowls; they will be a little soupy. Place several tablespoons of avocado mixture on each. If you like, dust with paprika.

NOTE: To seed avocado, cut in half lengthwise around pit. Remove pit and, using a spoon, scoop flesh out of the skin. Keep the pit and place it in the center of the salsa cruda when serving and storing—it keeps the avocado from turning black.

SUGGESTED ACCOMPANIMENTS: Mexican Rice with Pumpkin Seeds and Cilantro, Butternut Squash and Yam Purée, Your Basic Green Salad, and fresh orange, pear, and apple slices.

★★★   FOLIC ACID, VITAMIN A, VITAMIN K
   ★   THIAMIN, MAGNESIUM, COPPER, VITAMIN C

❧ Tempeh, Green Beans, and Carrots ❧ with Mustard Sauce

Yield: 2 quarts   (4 generous servings plus extra)

Tempeh, which originates from Indonesia, is a fermented soybean patty. It is a whole food and, unlike tofu which has been processed, contains all of soy's nutrients and fiber. Tempeh is on the favored-foods list because of the estrogenic properties of soybeans.

TEMPEH:

2 8-ounce packages tempeh
¼ cup shoyu soy sauce
2 cups filtered water
6 cloves garlic
3 slices fresh ginger
1 tablespoon curry powder

1 tablespoon unrefined sesame oil
2 onions, sliced
2 carrots, sliced diagonally
2 teaspoons basil
¼ pound green beans, cut in half

SAUCE:

½ prepared cup grainy mustard
1 cup filtered water or vegetable stock
   (see recipe)

2 tablespoons unfiltered apple juice
4 tablespoons arrowroot or
   2 tablespoons kuzu

1. Remove tempeh from packages. Cut each block lengthwise into four equal strips.

2. In a medium saucepan, place tempeh, soy sauce, water, garlic, ginger, and curry powder. Bring to a boil, covered, lower to a simmer, and cook 20 minutes.

3. In a medium sauté pan, heat 1 tablespoon sesame oil and add onions. Sauté over medium heat until they begin to turn translucent.

4. Add carrots and basil, cover, and cook 5 minutes. Turn off heat and let sit until tempeh is ready.

5. Place a colander in a bowl and pour tempeh and its marinade into it (marinade can be reserved for soup flavoring and stock); allow tempeh to cool.

6. Brush tempeh with oil on both sides. Broil until golden, turning once, about 5 minutes per side.

7. Cut tempeh into triangles. Add to vegetables with green beans, cover, and heat over medium heat 10 minutes.

8. In a small bowl, mix mustard, water, apple juice, and arrowroot, stirring well. Pour over tempeh and vegetables, stir until sauce thickens and clears, then cook another 30 seconds. Serve immediately.

Suggested accompaniments: Bulgur, Green Bean, and Walnut Pilaf; Your Basic Green Salad; and Broiled Maple Apples.

★★★ VITAMIN A, LINOLEIC ACID, MANGANESE, OMEGA-3 FATTY ACIDS, VITAMIN B$_{12}$, SODIUM

★ COPPER, MAGNESIUM, FOLIC ACID, NIACIN

Tempeh naturally contains cottony spores, which are safe to eat when they are white, gray, or black. The darker the color, the stronger the taste of the tempeh. If the spores turn yellow or red, read this as a stop sign—proceed no further—and throw the tempeh away.

❧ Pinto Bean and Swiss Chard Patties ❧

Yield: 12 patties   (4 servings plus extra)

Both Swiss chard and spinach contain oxalic acid, which can combine with calcium, keeping you from absorbing this mineral. In this recipe we steam these vegetables with just the liquid that clings to their leaves after washing. The minimal water forces the leaves to release additional liquid, and in the process they also release some of their oxalic acid. Don't drink or cook this liquid, which is full of oxalates. Throw it out.

Before you begin, sort, wash, and soak 2 cups dried pinto or kidney beans 6 to 8 hours or overnight.

4 to 5 cups soaked pinto or kidney beans (from 2 cups dried)
5 cups filtered water
1 bunch Swiss chard or spinach (about 10 ounces), washed
2 tablespoons extra-virgin olive oil
2 cloves garlic, minced
1 medium onion, minced

1 bunch scallions, chopped
1 teaspoon sea salt
½ teaspoon ground black pepper
¼ teaspoon ground nutmeg or allspice
¼ to ½ cup whole wheat bread crumbs
2 tablespoons unsalted butter or extra-virgin olive oil

1. Remove beans from soaking water with your hands or a slotted spoon, put into a medium pot, and add water. Bring to a boil, covered, lower heat, and simmer until beans are soft, about 45 minutes. Discard soaking water.

2. Put washed, wet greens into a medium pot. Over medium-high heat, bring greens to steaming, lower heat, and cook until wilted, about 5 minutes.

3. Remove beans from cooking liquid with a slotted spoon. (Reserve water for stock or other use.) Place beans in a bowl and allow to cool.

4. Drain greens in a colander, discarding the liquid. Let cool briefly, then place on a cutting board and chop coarsely.

5. In a medium sauté pan, heat olive oil, and add garlic, onion, and scallions. Cook until softened, about 2 or 3 minutes. Add the greens, cook another 2 minutes stirring well, and turn off flame.

6. Preheat the oven to 350°.

7. In a processor or with a potato masher, purée the beans. Remove beans to a medium bowl and mix with the greens mixture, salt, pepper, nutmeg, and bread crumbs, stirring well.

8. Oil a baking sheet or line with parchment paper. Using wet hands, form 12 patties and place them close together on baking sheet. Bake at 350° for 25 minutes. Serve hot or cold.

SUGGESTED ACCOMPANIMENTS: Butternut and Yam Purée; Pilaf with Brown, Wehani, and Wild Rices; Fast Salad of cucumber, radishes, and scallions; and Beverly's Cantaloupe with Freshly Grated Ginger.

SUGGESTIONS FOR USE: Place warmed patties on sliced whole wheat bread with mustard, lettuce, tomato, and a pickle on the side for a satisfying lunch.

★★★ VITAMIN K, FOLIC ACID

  ★ MAGNESIUM, IRON, VITAMIN A, MANGANESE, THIAMIN

❧ Chick-pea Hummus ❧

Yield: 2 cups

Hummus is a Middle Eastern dish, traditionally made with fava beans or chick-peas. The cooked beans are puréed with tahini, a sesame-seed butter high in essential fatty acids. Treat yourself to some scooped up on pita-bread triangles and eaten with salt-cured olives.

Before you begin, sort, wash, soak, and cook 1 cup dried chick-peas.

2 cups cooked chick-peas, with cooking liquid reserved (see Note)
Juice of 2 lemons
2 cloves garlic
1 tablespoon extra-virgin olive oil, plus additional for serving (optional)

2 tablespoons sesame tahini
½ to 1 teaspoon sea salt
Paprika
10 Greek or black olives

1. In a blender or processor, combine chick-peas, lemon juice, garlic, olive oil, tahini, and ½ teaspoon sea salt. Purée, adding a small amount of bean liquid at a time, if needed, to allow machine to run smoothly. Taste and add more salt, if needed.

2. Pour hummus onto a dinner plate. Shake plate to spread hummus in a thin layer. Sprinkle with paprika and place olives along the rim. (Traditionally, several teaspoons of olive oil are drizzled on top of hummus before sprinkling with paprika.)

VARIATIONS: Instead of lemon juice, use cider vinegar or brown rice vinegar. Try making this purée with other beans, such as kidney, navy, or black beans.

NOTE: Use only as much cooking liquid as needed to make a spreadable consistency. Use remaining liquid for a soup stock or discard.

SUGGESTED ACCOMPANIMENTS: Serve with whole grain crackers or pita bread, or vegetable sticks.

★★★ FOLIC ACID, LINOLENIC ACID, MANGANESE, THIAMIN, MAGNESIUM
★ VITAMIN C, IRON, COPPER

While sesame seeds are a good source of calcium, tahini does not supply significant amounts of this mineral because, when the hull of the seed is removed to make the seed paste, most of the calcium is also removed.

❧ Tuscan White Beans with Tuna and Lemon ❧

Yield: 6 cups   (4 generous servings plus extra)

Here's our version of this simple traditional dish, a meal cooked in one pot. It uses extra-virgin olive oil, which is the only unrefined oil sold mass market. This oil is the product of the first pressing of the olives and still contains phytosterols, chlorophyll, magnesium, vitamin E, and beta-carotene, all important to a woman's health.

Before you begin, sort, wash, and soak 2 cups dried white beans 6 to 8 hours or overnight.

4 or 5 cups soaked navy or Great Northern beans (from 2 cups dried)	2 ripe tomatoes, seeded and chopped
4 tablespoons extra-virgin olive oil	½ pound fresh tuna fillet
½ teaspoon sage	1 teaspoon herbal sea salt
2 cloves garlic, sliced	1 teaspoon pepper
4 cups filtered water	2 lemons, organic preferred
	1 teaspoon sea salt

1. In a medium casserole, put beans with 2 tablespoons of the olive oil, sage, garlic, water, and tomatoes. Bring to a boil, covered, lower heat, and simmer until beans are tender, about 45 minutes.

2. Wash tuna in cold water and cut into pieces. Place in a container with a cover and sprinkle with herbal salt, ½ teaspoon pepper, and juice of 1 lemon. Cover and place in refrigerator, about 30 minutes.

3. Add the halves from the juiced lemon to the casserole.

4. Add tuna chunks, salt, remaining ½ teaspoon pepper and remaining 2 tablespoons olive oil. Stir, cover, and continue cooking 5 more minutes.

5. Slice remaining lemon into wedges. Serve beans and tuna in wide bowls and place 1 or 2 lemon wedges on top.

SUGGESTED ACCOMPANIMENTS: Garlic bruschetta (see Garlic Soup with Bruschetta), Asparagus Mimosa with Lemon and Flax Seed Oil, and Poached Pears in Ginger-Kuzu Sauce.

★★★ VITAMIN B$_{12}$, FOLIC ACID, OMEGA-3 FATTY ACIDS
★ SELENIUM, THIAMIN, MAGNESIUM, IRON, PHOSPHORUS

❧ Black Bean Loaf ❧

Yield: 1 loaf (4 generous servings plus extra)

Beans are an important part of a woman's menu because they contain needed vitamins, minerals, and fiber. This recipe puts beans into a versatile loaf form so that you can use slices as you would a meatloaf, in sandwiches, or for a snack. Black beans contain thiamin and manganese, which nourish the nervous system and dampen menopausal irritability.

Before you begin, sort, wash, and soak 2 cups dried black beans 6 to 8 hours or overnight.

4 to 5 cups soaked black beans (from 2 cups dried)	2 onions, minced
4 cups filtered water	6 cloves garlic, chopped coarsely
2 bay leaves	1 tablespoon oregano
1 carrot, cut in half	2 teaspoons sea salt
2 inner stalks celery with light green leaves, cut in half	¼ teaspoon cayenne powder
2 tablespoons extra-virgin olive oil	¼ cup red miso or 2 teaspoons sea salt
	1 cup whole wheat bread crumbs

1. Remove beans from soaking water with your hands or a slotted spoon and put into medium saucepan with water, bay leaves, carrot, and celery. Cover and bring to a boil over high heat, then reduce heat to low and simmer 1 hour, until beans are soft. Discard soaking water.

2. Heat oil in a large skillet and cook onions over medium-high heat. (See Note.)

3. Add garlic to onions with oregano, salt, and cayenne. Stir well. Reduce heat, cover, and cook 10 to 15 minutes, until onions are very soft.

4. Drain beans (save bean liquid for soup stock). Remove and discard bay leaves.

5. Add beans, carrot, and celery pieces to skillet and stir well to absorb the cooking juices from the onions. Turn off heat.

6. Preheat oven to 350°.

7. In batches, purée bean mixture in processor or blender. (If using a blender you may need some additional bean liquid; also add an additional ¼ cup of bread crumbs.) Add miso to one of the batches. Put into another bowl or pot. When all of the bean mixture has been puréed, stir in ¾ cup of bread crumbs (1 cup if puréed in blender) and stir the mixture together well.

8. Oil or butter a 4-cup loaf pan, then cover bottom and sides with remaining ¼ cup bread crumbs, shaking them back and forth until no more will stick. Pour the extra crumbs that do not stick to the pan into a small container. Spoon the pâté into the loaf pan, pat with the back of a wet spoon, and sprinkle the top with the remaining crumbs.

9. Bake in 350° oven for 30 minutes until the loaf starts to pull away from the sides of the pan.

10. Let cool at least 20 minutes before removing from pan to slice.

11. To remove from loaf pan, slip a knife around the perimeter, place a plate on top of the loaf and, holding both the plate and the loaf pan, quickly flip it over. Remove pan, cut loaf into slices, and serve for dinner.

VARIATIONS: Bean loaves can be served as a pâté with whole wheat pita triangles, toast points, or crackers.

NOTE: To save time, add the vegetables to the beans while cooking them. After the beans have softened, add flavorings, salt, and oil. Proceed with step 7.

SUGGESTED ACCOMPANIMENTS: Millet-Rice with Peas and Tomatoes, Cilantro Salsa, Mesclun Salad with Organic Liver and Rosemary, and Light Lemon Pudding Parfait with Kiwi Slices.

★★★   FOLIC ACID, THIAMIN, MANGANESE, MAGNESIUM
  ★   LINOLEIC ACID, OMEGA-3 FATTY ACIDS, VITAMIN A, COPPER

Beans are food for the brain. They have lecithin, which contains choline from which acetylcholine is made, and this chemical is the brain's major messenger for transmitting thoughts. Lecithin is found in many other foods, ranked here in order of concentration:

egg yolks	brewer's yeast	cabbage
peanuts	green leafy vegetables	cheese
liver	cauliflower	beans

❧ Colombian Lima Bean and Corn Stew ❧

Yield: 2 to 3 quarts   (4 generous servings plus extra)

This recipe is a vegetarian version of the traditional dish sancocho, which is usually made with sausages, meat, and chicken. Gabriel Vasquez, chef-owner of Bachué, a New York restaurant, created the original adaptation. Our version of this recipe includes beans, plus some more unusual foods—plantains, yucca, and taro—giving you a delicious way to widely vary your diet, a fundamental for good health.

Before you begin, sort, wash, and soak 1 cup large dried lima beans 6 to 8 hours or overnight.

2 to 2½ cups soaked lima beans (from 1 cup dried)
8 cups filtered water
4 cloves garlic, peeled
2 bay leaves
2 tablespoons extra-virgin olive oil
2 large onions, diced
2 carrots, diced
1 green plantain, peeled and sliced (see Note)

1 yucca or 2 taro (yautia), peeled and sliced
2 potatoes, peeled and diced
3 ears of corn, shucked and cut into rounds
1 large pinch saffron
2 teaspoons sea salt
½ teaspoon herbal sea salt
½ bunch cilantro, chopped coarsely
½ bunch scallions, chopped coarsely

1. Remove beans from soaking water with your hands or a slotted spoon, put into a large Dutch oven, and add 6 cups fresh water. Bring to a boil with whole garlic and bay leaves, lower heat, and simmer 30 to 40 minutes. Discard soaking water.

2. In a large sauté pan, heat olive oil and add onions, carrots, plantain, yucca, and potatoes, stirring after each addition.

3. Add onion mixture to lima beans along with corn and saffron. Add remaining 2 cups of water to sauté pan, heating and stirring until the bottom of the pan is clean and the flavors from the onions and other vegetables have colored the water. Add to the Dutch oven, bring to a boil, covered, lower heat, and simmer until the beans are soft, about 30 minutes.

4. Add salt, cook another 5 minutes. This is a thick and soupy stew. Serve in roomy bowls garnished with several tablespoons of cilantro and scallions.

NOTE: Green plantains are an unripe, larger relative of the common banana. In their green state, they have a high carbohydrate content, and are cooked as a starchy vegetable would be. To peel, cut off the ends and score it down the side lengthwise. Pry open the skin and remove the plantain.

Yucca is a type of starchy tuber that can be substituted with taro, battata, Jerusalem artichokes, or any other tuber. Always peel them.

VARIATIONS: Add celery, yams, or butternut squash, and use fresh fava beans or peas instead of lima beans.

SUGGESTED ACCOMPANIMENTS: Mexican Rice with Pumpkin Seeds and Cilantro, Collard Greens with White Onions, and Broiled Maple Apples.

★★★   VITAMIN A, VITAMIN K, FOLIC ACID, VITAMIN C
★   MAGNESIUM, IRON, MANGANESE, THIAMIN

❧ Cannellini and Kidney Beans ❧ with Rosemary

Yield: 1 quart   (4 generous servings plus extra)

Rosemary is a woman's herb, useful in many ways. It is prescribed medicinally to counteract depression, improve circulation, strengthen fragile blood vessels that begin to weaken, and ease painful periods. It is also a good accompaniment for beans because rosemary reduces flatulence and stimulates digestion.

Before you begin, sort, wash, and soak ½ cup dried cannellini beans and ½ cup dried kidney beans in separate bowls 6 to 8 hours or overnight.

1 **cup soaked cannellini beans (from ½ cup dried)**	2 **stalks celery, minced**
1 **cup soaked kidney beans (from ½ cup dried)**	1 **carrot, minced**
	½ **red onion, minced**
4 **cups filtered water**	1½ **tablespoons minced fresh rosemary**
4 **cloves garlic, minced**	2 **tablespoons extra-virgin olive oil**
	Sea salt and fresh pepper

Preheat oven to 375°.

1. Remove beans from soaking water with your hands or a slotted spoon and put into an ovenproof casserole. Discard soaking water.
2. Add water, cover, place in preheated oven, and bake 20 minutes.
3. Add garlic, celery, carrot, onion, and rosemary to the beans. Cook until beans are soft, about another 20 minutes, stirring two or three times.
4. Season with olive oil, salt, and pepper, stirring well. Cook another 5 minutes.
5. Remove casserole and cool for 10 minutes before serving.

SUGGESTED ACCOMPANIMENTS: Hungarian Pasta with Cabbage, steamed carrots, Your Basic Green Salad with Creamy Plum Dressing, and Banana Refrigerator Cake.

★★★   FOLIC ACID, VITAMIN K
 ★   VITAMIN A, IRON, MAGNESIUM, CALCIUM, COPPER

❧ Twice-Cooked Beans Wrapped in ❧ Corn Tortillas

Yield: 1½ quarts   (4 generous servings plus extra)

Here's a delicious way to give yourself calcium, which is found in both the pinto beans and the corn tortillas. These long-cooked beans can be made soupy and turned into a sauce, or cooked down to a pastier consistency that works for spreading. The generous cooking time makes the beans easier to digest. Try some for breakfast.

Before you begin, sort, wash, and soak 1 cup dried pinto or kidney beans 6 to 8 hours or overnight.

2 to 2½ cups soaked pinto beans
    (from 1 cup dried)
4 cups filtered water
4 cloves garlic, peeled
1 bay leaf
3 tablespoons extra-virgin olive oil
1 teaspoon chili powder
1 onion, chopped
1 green pepper, seeded and minced

6 scallions, chopped
2 plum tomatoes, seeded and
    chopped
2 teaspoons herbal sea salt
¼ teaspoon white pepper
8 corn tortillas
4 leaves romaine lettuce, shredded
1 recipe Cilantro Salsa (see recipe)

   1. Remove beans from soaking water with your hands or a slotted spoon, put in a medium pot, and add water, garlic, and bay leaf. Bring to a boil, lower heat, and simmer until beans are soft, about 40 minutes. Discard soaking water.
   2. In a large sauté pan, heat olive oil and chili powder just until the spice bubbles, about 30 seconds. Add onion, pepper, scallions, and tomatoes. Stir and cook over medium-high heat, uncovered, about 5 minutes.
   3. Using a slotted spoon, remove beans from cooking water, reserving water, and put into sauté pan. Cook beans and vegetables over medium-high heat, uncovered, about 20 minutes. As the beans start sticking to the pan, add ½ cup of the bean cooking liquid at a time, stirring well after each addition. This will make a thick, gravylike sauce that can be left thick or thinned, as desired.
   4. Add herbal salt and white pepper, stir well, and cook another 2 minutes.
   5. To warm tortillas, heat a dry cast-iron pan and put in one or two tortillas at a time, turning once after 30 seconds. If they bubble up in places, press down with a spatula. Place the warm tortillas on a clean cloth and wrap to keep softened and warm.

6. Place a tortilla on a plate and put several tablespoons of beans on it. Add some shredded lettuce and salsa. Roll up and serve.

VARIATIONS: If preferred as a soup, add enough additional water and herbal sea salt to create desired consistency, serving tortillas on the side. As a sauce, use over rice or on pasta.

SUGGESTED ACCOMPANIMENTS: Creamless Mushroom Cream Soup, Basic Brown Rice, steamed zucchini, and Broiled Dates Stuffed with Almonds.

★★★   VITAMIN K, FOLIC ACID, VITAMIN C
  ★   MAGNESIUM, IRON, THIAMIN, CALCIUM, MANGANESE

Beans that contain calcium, ranked in order of concentration of this nutrient:

soybeans	kidney
lima	pinto
navy	chick-peas
Great Northern	

❧ **Adzuki Bean Chili with Avocado Cream** ❧

Yield: 2 quarts   *(4 generous servings plus extra)*

If you've only recently begun to eat beans, you'll like adzuki beans because they are easy to digest. Until you can eat beans comfortably, eat small portions and see our other tips for digestion in the bean introduction on pages 122–23.

1½ cups adzuki beans, sorted and washed
4 cups filtered water
2 tablespoons extra-virgin olive oil
1 teaspoon chili powder
½ teaspoon cumin
½ teaspoon oregano
¼ teaspoon cayenne (optional)
2 onions, chopped
2 cloves garlic, minced
1 green pepper, chopped
2 jalapeño chilies, minced

4 ripe tomatoes, seeded and chopped, or 1 cup prepared salsa and ½ cup filtered water
1 teaspoon sea salt
Freshly ground black pepper, if desired
1 ripe avocado, seeded
½ cup plain bacteria-active yogurt
¼ teaspoon herbal salt
Juice of 1 lime
3 scallions, chopped

1. In a medium pot, put washed adzuki beans and water. Bring to a boil and simmer, covered, 1 hour.

2. A few minutes before beans are cooked, prepare the spices. In a small sauté pan, heat olive oil and add chili powder, cumin, oregano, and cayenne. Heat until bubbly, about 30 seconds over medium heat, and immediately add onion. Stir well and add garlic, green pepper, and jalapeño.

3. Pour onion mixture into pot with beans. Add tomatoes. Cook, uncovered, over medium-low heat for about 30 minutes, stirring occasionally. (If more liquid is needed, add water or stock.)

4. Add salt and pepper, stir, and cook another 1 or 2 minutes.

5. Scoop avocado out of shell. Place in a blender with yogurt, herbal salt, and lime juice. Purée until smooth.

6. Serve chili in a deep bowl with several tablespoons of avocado cream. Top with scallions.

VARIATIONS: To add meat, use ½ to 1 pound chopped ground round, ground sirloin, or leftover steak chunks (organic preferred). Sauté in a frying pan to partially cook and drain excess fat. Add to beans with spices and vegetables. Avocado cream can also be made by omitting the yogurt and substituting ¼ cup filtered water and 1 tablespoon flax seed oil.

SUGGESTED ACCOMPANIMENTS: Savory Corn Muffins with Onion and Poppy Seeds, Cilantro Salsa, and orange slices with lime juice, paprika, salt, and pepper.

★★★ FOLIC ACID, VITAMIN C
  ★ VITAMIN K, COPPER, MAGNESIUM, MANGANESE, IRON, ZINC, PANTOTHENIC ACID

❧ Great Northern Ragout Provençal ❧

Yield: 2½ quarts (4 generous servings plus extra)

This bean dish, inspired by the French cassoulet, features three B vitamins: folic acid, which helps prevent fatigue; thiamin, which nourishes the nervous system; and vitamin B_6 (pyridoxine), which combats depression and stress. Keep this dish vegetarian or develop it further, adding some chicken, lamb, rabbit, or game.

Before you begin, sort, wash, and soak 1½ cups dried Great Northern beans 6 to 8 hours or overnight.

2 to 4 tablespoons extra-virgin olive oil
3 onions, sliced
4 cloves garlic, minced
3 ripe tomatoes, seeded and chopped
3 cups soaked Great Northern beans (from 1½ cups dried)
1 teaspoon thyme
1 bay leaf

3 cups vegetable or chicken stock (see index)
1 red pepper, seeded and diced
1 teaspoon sea salt
1 teaspoon freshly ground pepper
1 bunch parsley, leaves only
3 or 4 anchovies, preserved in brine, rinsed, and chopped (optional)

1. In a medium saucepan, heat 2 tablespoons of the olive oil over moderate heat. Add onions and garlic and sauté for 2 or 3 minutes.

2. Add tomatoes and cook, stirring frequently, 5 minutes. Remove beans from soaking water with your hands or a slotted spoon and add with thyme, bay leaf, and stock to saucepan, bring to a boil, lower heat and simmer, covered, until the beans are tender, about 45 minutes, stirring occasionally. Discard soaking water.

3. Add red pepper, salt, and pepper. Stir well, cover, and continue cooking over low heat 15 minutes.

4. Add parsley leaves and anchovies, cover, and cook 5 more minutes.

5. If desired, drizzle another 2 tablespoons olive oil into ragout before serving for additional flavor.

SUGGESTED ACCOMPANIMENTS: Quinoa Risotto, Collard Greens with White Onions, and Peach Crumble with Walnut Cream.

★★★   FOLIC ACID, VITAMIN K, VITAMIN C
★   OMEGA-3 FATTY ACIDS, THIAMIN, MAGNESIUM, IRON, COPPER, VITAMIN B$_6$

❧ Warm Lima Beans with Basil, ❧ Tomato, and Chèvre

Yield: 5 cups   (4 generous servings plus extra)

A little chèvre goes a long way, giving the flavor of cheese without adding a lot of fat. We prefer dairy products made from goat's milk rather than cow because goat's milk has a higher proportion of magnesium to calcium, closer to what our bodies really need. And most brands are produced on small-scale farms. Support your local goat herd!

Before you begin, sort, wash, and soak 1 cup dried lima beans 6 to 8 hours or overnight.

2 to 2½ cups soaked lima beans
    (from 1 cup dried)
4 cups filtered water
1 bay leaf
4 cloves garlic
3 tablespoons extra-virgin olive oil
    Juice of 1 lemon
    Freshly ground black pepper
6 plum tomatoes, seeded and chopped
    coarsely

½ bunch fresh basil, leaves only, or
    1 tablespoon dried
¼ pound chèvre, crumbled or cubed
    (see Note)
    Sea salt (optional)
8 lettuce leaves, such as romaine,
    escarole, or green leaf

1. Lift beans from soaking water with your hands or a slotted spoon and put in a medium saucepan with water, bay leaf, and 3 cloves of garlic. Bring to a boil, covered. Lower flame to a simmer and cook until beans are soft, about 35 minutes. Discard soaking water.

2. Remove bay leaf and discard. Using a slotted spoon, remove beans and garlic to a bowl. Toss with olive oil, lemon, and pepper.

3. Mince remaining clove of garlic and add to beans with tomatoes, whole basil leaves, and chèvre. Toss well. Taste and add salt, if needed.

4. Serve on lettuce leaves while still warm.

NOTE: Chèvre is goat's-milk cheese, and can be substituted with imported feta (made from sheep or goat's milk), ricotta salata, or gorgonzola (blue cheese). The saltiness of cheeses differ, so add salt according to taste.

VARIATIONS: Large lima beans give this dish an elegant appearance, although any type of bean will work well. To use the next day as a salad, allow the beans to return to room temperature or heat slightly.

SUGGESTED ACCOMPANIMENTS: Broccoli Rabe with Tomato and Spirals; Fast Salad of black olives and cucumber and carrot sticks; and Frozen Banana Maple-Walnut Whip.

★★★ VITAMIN K, FOLIC ACID, VITAMIN A, VITAMIN C
★ MAGNESIUM, IRON, OMEGA-3 FATTY ACIDS

❧ Red Lentil Dhal ❧

Yield: 1½ quarts   (*4 generous servings plus extra*)

Lentils contain copper, which is necessary for the formation of collagen, which gives your skin the structure and lift of youth. Lentils also contain boron, which can help you make the best of your own body's estrogen.

4 cups filtered water
2 cups red lentils, sorted and washed
2 teaspoons curry powder (see recipe)
½ teaspoon sea salt

Freshly ground white pepper
2 tablespoons extra-virgin olive oil or
  unsalted butter (optional)

1. In a medium saucepan, put water, beans, and curry powder. Bring to a boil, reduce flame, and simmer 20 minutes.

2. Stir in salt and pepper and, if desired, olive oil or butter.

SUGGESTED ACCOMPANIMENTS: Curried Barley with Caramelized Onions, Indian Chicken with Lemon Slices and Onions, Steamed Spinach, Raisin-Ginger Chutney, and Frothy Mango Lassi.

★★★   FOLIC ACID
  ★   IRON, VITAMIN K, COPPER, MANGANESE, MAGNESIUM, THIAMIN, BORON

Red lentils need to be sorted carefully since they can contain little stones. Wash them quickly so they do not lose too much of their starch (the water will be whitish). After cooking, the beans will fall apart, lose their red color, and turn a yellow ocher. Some store brands may be dyed, and are not recommended. (See Appendix for brand recommendation.)

ꙮ Tempeh Slices for Sandwiches ꙮ

Yield: 16 slices   (4 sandwiches plus extra tempeh)

Tempeh contains manganese, which assists your body in making hormones. It comes plain and preseasoned, ready for heating or to use for a quick and easy mini-meal, between two pieces of whole grain bread spread with mustard or drizzled with one of our sauces.

2 8-ounce packages tempeh
1 cup filtered water
¼ cup shoyu soy sauce

3 slices fresh ginger root
2 teaspoons curry or chili powder
¼ cup unrefined sesame oil

SANDWICH STUFF:

4 whole wheat pitas
4 romaine lettuce leaves
   Prepared mustard

1 ripe tomato, sliced
½ package alfalfa sprouts
   Herbal vinaigrette (optional)

1. Remove tempeh from packages and cut into four equal blocks. Cut each block in half by width, so that thin slabs are formed.

2. In a medium saucepan, place tempeh, water, soy sauce, ginger, and curry. Bring to a boil, covered, then reduce heat to a simmer and cook 20 minutes.

3. Use a colander to drain liquid (which can be reserved for soup), and allow tempeh to cool.

4. Heat 2 tablespoons oil in a large sauté pan, and cook slabs until golden on each side, turning once. Add additional oil to pan as needed. (Tempeh will absorb oil quickly, so do not put in more before turning, and add only a small amount at a time. You may not use all of the oil.) Remove to brown paper to drain.

5. To build a sandwich, warm pita, cut one third off, and stuff it inside pita. Fold lettuce in half and stuff into pita. Spread mustard on tempeh slabs and put three or four slices on top of the lettuce, then add one or two tomato slices and stuff with sprouts. If you like, add several teaspoons of an herbal vinaigrette dressing.

SUGGESTED ACCOMPANIMENTS: Grated Beet and Hijiki Medley and iced herbal tea.

★★★ OMEGA-3 FATTY ACIDS, MANGANESE, FOLIC ACID, MAGNESIUM, SELENIUM, LINOLEIC ACID

★ VITAMIN B$_{12}$, VITAMIN E, THIAMIN

9

Whole Grains and Whole Grain Pasta

WHOLE GRAINS

Basic Brown Rice
Pilaf with Brown, Wehani, and Wild Rices
Spiced Rice with Pistachios and Flax Seeds
Chewy Wheat Berries and Barley with Rosemary
Curried Barley with Caramelized Onions
Bulgur, Green Bean, and Walnut Pilaf
Millet-Rice with Peas and Tomatoes
Indian Millet with Currants and Sunflower Seeds
Kasha Loaf with Yam
Quinoa Risotto
Mexican Rice with Pumpkin Seeds and Cilantro
Roasted Pecans and Wild Rice
Polenta with Wild Mushroom Sauce
Kasha and Red Pepper Timbales
Wild Rice Ring

WHOLE GRAIN PASTA

Whole Wheat Linguini with Fresh Tuna
Spicy Almond Udon with Wilted Spinach
Broccoli Rabe with Tomato and Spirals
Vongole and Linguini (Clams and Pasta)
Pasta e Fagioli
Hearty Rigatoni with Sausages, Garlic, and Broccoli
Hungarian Pasta with Cabbage
Asparagus Fusilli
Tomatoes Stuffed with Couscous
Sesame Salad with Buckwheat Noodles and Fresh Coriander

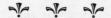

Whole Grains

Grains are normally part of so many of our meals—morning cereal, sandwich bread at lunch, and pasta dishes for dinner—that you have lots of opportunities to eat them in their complete and unrefined form. Whole grains have far more vitamins and minerals than refined grains, and switching to these nutritious foods is one of the best steps you can take to supply yourself with the nutrients you need. Upgrade the refined grains in your diet and you'll also be adding interesting flavors and textures to your meals.

Whole grains, with their bran and germ intact, are a source of B-complex vitamins, which work together to stabilize brain chemistry and convert food into energy. The stress of menopause and PMS can deplete these. Whole grains are also high in magnesium, which strengthens the bone; manganese, which nourishes the thyroid; and copper, which helps form collagen, the structural substance of skin that keeps it firm. During menopause, whole grains are especially useful because they digest and assimilate slowly, giving you a long, steady supply of energy. They stabilize blood sugar, preventing sugar-related mood swings and fatigue.

Natural food stores carry whole grains that are made into flour and flakes. Whole grains are available as pancake mixes and ready-made products, such as pretzels, bagels, waffles, and English muffins. Brown rice, in short and long varieties, is available plain or made into rice cakes, pasta, and pilaf mixes. There are other kinds of rice as well, such as wehani, wild, red rose, Christmas, and brown basmati, each having a unique flavor. Whole wheat is most often sold as flour, available for pastry and breadmaking, and it's available in ready-to-make mixes for cakes, quick breads, and muffins. It is also what pasta and whole wheat couscous are made from. Cracked wheat and bulgur are also made from whole wheat kernels. Oatmeal, the old-fashioned variety, is available in both regular and thick cut, and there is also steel-cut oatmeal and oat flakes. Barley is obtainable whole or pearled, which cooks a little quicker, and is used in flour and breads. There is also rye, cornmeal, buckwheat (kasha), millet, and several grains new on the market—quinoa, amaranth, spelt, and kamut, all available whole and as ready-to-use products.

Whole Grain Pasta

There are a variety of grain pastas on the market—whole wheat, brown rice, buckwheat, spelt, corn, and noodles made from wild yam. They are in a different class from standard white-flour pastas, and rather than compare the two, enjoy the whole grain pastas for their own unique flavors and textures. See Appendix for listing of whole grain pasta brands.

A whole grain contains all of its parts—bran, germ, and endosperm. When a grain or grain product contains these three, it is called a complex carbohydrate. If it is missing any part, it is called a refined grain or just a carbohydrate. Removal of the bran, called hulling or polishing, eliminates the tough outer layer of the kernel, most of the fiber, and many nutrients. Degerminating removes the germ, which carries the essential oils and fat-soluble vitamins E and K. The more a grain is refined, the lower its nutritional value. White flour consists of the endosperm of the wheat only, which is the starchy part of the kernel, without the nutritious bran or germ.

Storage

Store your whole grains and cereal products in glass containers with screw-on lids in a cool and dry place. Kept this way they can stay fresh for a year.

Whole grain flours, flakes, meal, and mixes keep best when refrigerated or frozen. They contain oil, which can go rancid, and once rancid, the oil is toxic to your arteries, tissues, and cells. Stone-ground flours are preferred to steel-rolled milling because grinding the grain into flour with stones keeps the germ from being heated and retains the freshness of the oil in the germ. Once a whole grain is milled, this product will last about four months in the refrigerator and one year in the freezer.

Grain Basics

1. *To wash grains:* Place a measured amount of grain into a saucepan. (It is preferable to use a heavy-bottomed saucepan with a tight-fitting lid.) Pour water on the grain—at least four or five times the amount of water as grain. (We use filtered water.) Swirl the grains with your hand, rubbing them with your fingers, which will loosen dirt, chaff, and other particles. Pour the excess water out without using a strainer. Stop pouring when the grains begin to reach the brim. Repeat the process at least one more time until the washing water seems clear. After the last wash, pour the grain into a strainer and let as much water as possible drain out. Place the grain back in the pot and proceed with the cooking instructions.

Grains that require no washing include bulgur, couscous, any meal, cracked or rolled grains, and kasha.

2. *To soak grains:* Most grains require no soaking, including those that are minimally processed. These grains come as flakes, pearled, rolled, cracked, or as meal or flour. Grains that need soaking are the whole grains—barley (not pearled), wheat, rye, oats, spelt, and kamut. Wash, then soak 1 cup of these in 3 cups of water for 6 to 8 hours or overnight. These grains can be cooked in their soaking liquid and will be done in 1 to 1¼ hours. (The grains that need soaking are much more chewy than other whole grains and their minimally processed relatives.)

3. *To cook grains:* Add a measured amount of filtered water (see chart) and a pinch of sea salt per cup of grain. (This will not make them salty at all, and many recipes will call for larger amounts of salt for taste.) Bring the pot to a boil, covered, reduce the heat to as low as possible, and place a heat diffuser between the pot and the heat. Do this especially if the pot is thin-bottomed or the stove is difficult to adjust to a very low temperature, often true of an electric stove. To make the grain softer for easier digestion or to accommodate someone who is not used to chewing, additional water can be added, about ½ cup more per cup of dry grain.

4. *Cooking times:* Use the cooking time in the recipe or in our grain-cooking chart. Grain-cooking time starts the moment the water has come to a boil. Do not stir whole grains except when preparing the grain in risotto, polenta, or hot cereal style. It is important to cook whole grains thoroughly. At the end of the cooking time, let them stand covered for 5 minutes or more before serving to allow the remaining steam to distribute evenly throughout the grains.

5. *After cooking:* Loosen and fluff the cooked grain with a fork. This will help to separate the grains.

6. *To bake grains:* Start the cooking on the stove top in an ovenproof pot, and then place the covered pot in an oven preheated to 350°.

7. *To pressure-cook grains:* This produces a softer texture than stove-top cooking, and if you prefer a texture closer to steamed grains, just reduce the water by ½ cup or 20 percent. We have included pressure-cooking times only on those grains that are safe to cook in the pressure cooker.

Whole Grain Cooking Times

Grain Type	Liquid	Cooking Time	Pressure-Cooker Time
Amaranth	1¾ cups	20 minutes	5 minutes
Barley, pearl	2 cups	1 hour	40 minutes
Brown rice, long grain	1½ cups	55 minutes	40 minutes
Brown rice, short grain	2 cups	55 minutes	40 minutes
Bulgur	1½ cups, boiling	Bring to boil, turn off flame, and let sit ½ hour	Don't use
Cornmeal	4–5 cups, cold	45 minutes	Don't use
Couscous	1½ cups, boiling	Add liquid, cover, turn off flame, and let sit 10 minutes	Don't use
Cracked grain	2 cups	30 minutes	Don't use
Flaked grain	2 cups	35 minutes	Don't use
Job's tears	2½ cups	55–60 minutes	20 minutes
Kamut	2 cups	60 minutes	35 minutes
Kasha	2 cups, boiling	10 minutes	Don't use
Millet	1¾–2 cups	35 minutes	15 minutes
Oatmeal, creamy texture	2 cups, cold	15 minutes, uncovered	Don't use
Oatmeal, chewy texture	2 cups, boiling	15 minutes, uncovered	Don't use
Oats, steel cut	2 cups	30 minutes	Don't use
Oats, whole	2 cups	55–60 minutes	30 minutes
Quinoa	2 cups	12–15 minutes	Don't use
Rye berries	2 cups	55–60 minutes	30 minutes
Spelt	2 cups	60 minutes	35 minutes
Wheat Berries	2 cups	55–60 minutes	35 minutes

Liquid measurements are for 1 cup of grain.

Tips for cooking whole grain pasta:

1. Cook whole grain pasta longer than you would white-flour pasta (see package directions for cooking time). Undercooked whole grain pasta is tough and more difficult to digest.

2. Use strong flavors in the sauce and the rich flavor of whole grain pasta will have met its match. Try a mix of salty anchovies and mellow sautéed onions, or the full flavors of lemon peel and garlic.

3. When making pasta, add 2 teaspoons sea salt to the cooking water, unless you're cooking Japanese noodles such as soba or udon. These noodles are made with salt and don't need additional in the water.

❧ Basic Brown Rice ❧

Yield: About 2 cups   (4 generous servings)

For the symptoms of perimenopause eat brown rice. It's high in B vitamins that help the liver do its work. The liver metabolizes estrogen and converts it to a weaker form, which may help put you at lower risk for breast cancer. Brown rice also contains good amounts of magnesium which helps lessen the symptoms of PMS.

1 cup short-grain brown rice, washed   **Pinch sea salt**
2 cups filtered water (see Note)

1. In a heavy-bottomed, medium saucepan, put rice, water, and salt. Bring to a boil over high heat, covered. Reduce flame to low and simmer 55 minutes. (Use a heat diffuser if cooking on an electric stove or using a thin-bottomed pot.)

2. Turn off heat and allow cooked rice to sit covered for 5 minutes.

3. With a fork, fluff to separate grains.

NOTE: For long-grain brown rice, reduce water to 1½ cups.

SUGGESTED USES: Use in stuffing, salad, soup, and pudding.

★★★   MANGANESE, SELENIUM, MAGNESIUM, VITAMIN B_6, THIAMIN
  ★   PANTOTHENIC ACID, NIACIN, COPPER

Although grains may look cooked before the specified time, they need to be cooked for the full period to ensure proper breakdown of their nutrients during digestion, so that you can benefit from all of them. To do this without burning the grain, use a heat diffuser and turn heat to its lowest setting, after the pot comes to a boil. In cooking grains, it's best to follow a timer, not your eye.

❧ Pilaf with Brown, Wehani, and Wild Rices ❧

Yield: 6 cups   (4 generous servings plus extra)

For variety of taste, texture, and color, mix grains. Explore your natural food store for unusual kinds. The rices in this recipe are good sources of manganese, selenium, magnesium, molybdenum, niacin, vitamin B_6, thiamin, vitamin B_5 and iron. In contrast, white rice supplies just five of these nutrients and in smaller amounts, and it has no fiber. Don't cheat yourself by eating white rice.

1 cup long-grain brown rice, washed
½ cup short-grain or rose rice, washed
½ cup wehani or black rice, washed
½ cup broken whole wheat udon or spaghetti
1 tablespoon extra-virgin olive oil
1 tablespoon unsalted butter

1 small onion, minced
1½ teaspoons sea salt
¼ teaspoon black pepper
4 cups vegetable or chicken stock (see index) or filtered water
½ cup sunflower seeds, chopped coarsely

1. In a medium, heavy-bottomed pot, begin dry-roasting the wet rices on high heat, stirring occasionally, about 2 to 3 minutes.

2. Lower flame to medium-high, add noodles, oil, and butter, and continue roasting. Stir frequently, especially around the edge of the pot, about 1 to 2 minutes.

3. Add onion, lower flame to medium, and stir continuously to keep pasta from burning until rice is golden and smells fragrant, about another 4 to 5 minutes. Make sure to stir the bottom and edge to prevent burning.

4. Remove pot from the stove, and add salt and pepper. Add stock or water carefully (since pot will be hot and the steam it produces can burn you), return to high heat, and bring to a boil, covered.

5. Reduce flame to low and let pilaf cook undisturbed 50 minutes. (Use a heat diffuser for an electric stove or a thin-bottomed pot.)

6. Fluff with a fork to separate grains, and serve topped with sunflower seeds as a garnish.

VARIATIONS: Add shelled pistachios, walnuts, or pumpkin seeds.

SUGGESTED ACCOMPANIMENTS: Flounder Rolls Stuffed with Salmon and Lemon, and Chinese Napa Cabbage and Celery Salad.

★★★   MANGANESE, SELENIUM, THIAMIN, LINOLEIC ACID, VITAMIN B$_{12}$

There are many rice mixes on the market which contain brown and wild rices, as well as basmati, wehani, rose, and black rice. These are a great convenience or you can make your own mix.

Phytohormones modulate your own body's estrogen level. The grains that contain them are ranked in order of how much is contained in each.

oats   brown rice
barley   whole wheat
rye   cornmeal

❧ Spiced Rice with Pistachios and Flax Seeds ❧

Yield: 5 cups   (4 generous servings plus extra)

Treat yourself to the full range of nutrients available in whole grains. Whole grain basmati has a nutty aromatic flavor and is lighter tasting than regular brown rice, letting the fragrant sweetness from the spices come through.

½ cup brown rice, short or long grain, washed

1 cup brown basmati rice, washed, or additional regular brown rice

3½ cups filtered water

¼ cup pistachio nuts, shelled

2 tablespoons flax seeds or 2 teaspoons flax seed oil

1 teaspoon ground cinnamon or 1 cinnamon stick

2 bay leaves

½ teaspoon sea salt

4 cardamom pods

⅛ teaspoon ground cloves or 4 whole cloves

⅛ teaspoon ground black pepper or 4 whole peppercorns

1 to 2 pinches saffron or ½ teaspoon turmeric (see Note)

1. In a heavy-bottomed, medium saucepan, combine rices and water with remaining ingredients. Bring to a boil over high heat, covered. Reduce flame to low and simmer 55 minutes. (Use a heat diffuser if cooking on an electric stove or using a thin-bottomed pot.)

2. Turn off heat and allow cooked grain to sit covered for 5 minutes.

3. Remove bay leaves (and cinnamon stick if used). With a fork fluff to separate grains.

NOTE: Saffron will give a very slight yellow color and a fragrant taste. The turmeric will give a more intense yellow color and not much taste. Annatto, a Spanish flavoring and coloring agent, can also be used.

SUGGESTED ACCOMPANIMENTS: Grilled shrimp and Composed Salad of Oranges, Avocado, and Endive.

★★★   OMEGA-3 FATTY ACIDS, MANGANESE

★   VITAMIN B$_6$, THIAMIN, MAGNESIUM

❧ Chewy Wheat Berries and Barley ❧ with Rosemary

Yield: 4 generous servings plus extra

Wheat berries are whole grains of wheat. "Cracked wheat," which you'll sometimes see on bread labels, are these grains crushed for faster cooking. Two thirds of the B vitamins and many of the minerals are lost in milling. Wheat berries have 100 percent!

Before you begin, soak ½ cup wheat berries 6 to 8 hours or overnight.

1 **cup soaked wheat berries (from ½ cup)**	2 **teaspoons rosemary**
1 **cup barley, washed (see Note page 161)**	1 **teaspoon sea salt**
3½ **cups filtered water**	2 **tablespoons extra-virgin olive oil**
8 **cloves garlic, 6 cloves coarsely chopped**	1 **tablespoon flax seed oil**

1. Remove wheat berries from soaking water with your hands or a slotted spoon and put in a medium saucepan with a heavy bottom. Add barley, water, 6 cloves coarsely chopped garlic, rosemary, and salt. Bring to a boil, covered, reduce heat to low, and cook for 1 hour. (Use a heat diffuser if cooking on an electric stove or in a thin-bottomed pot.)
2. Mince remaining 2 cloves garlic and in a small bowl mix with olive and flax oils.
3. Fluff surface of the cooked grain to loosen and stir in minced garlic and oils.

Suggested accompaniments: Bluefish Marinated in Plum Vinegar, Greens Four Calcium, and Beverly's Cantaloupe with Freshly Grated Ginger.

★★★   Omega-3 fatty acids, manganese
  ★   Thiamin, magnesium, iron, niacin, potassium

❧ Curried Barley with Caramelized Onions ❧

Yield: 2½ cups   (4 generous servings plus extra)

The barley in this recipe contains potassium, which helps regulate the thyroid. This time-honored grain also contributes B vitamins for energy and boron, an estrogen enhancer.

1 cup barley, washed (see Note)	2 tablespoons extra-virgin olive oil
2½ cups filtered water	2 to 3 onions, sliced
1 teaspoon curry powder	Freshly ground pepper
1 teaspoon sea salt	

1. In a heavy-bottomed, medium saucepan, put barley, water, curry, and ½ teaspoon salt. Bring to a boil over high heat, covered. Reduce flame to low and simmer 55 minutes. (Use a heat diffuser if cooking on an electric stove or using a thin-bottomed pot.)

2. Turn off heat and allow cooked grain to sit covered for 5 minutes.

3. In a medium sauté pan, heat oil and add onions. Cook over a medium-high flame uncovered, stirring frequently until the edges begin to brown. Season with remaining salt and the pepper.

4. With a fork, fluff to separate grains. Pour into a serving bowl and top with caramelized onions.

NOTE: When washing barley, the water will get cloudy from the starch in the barley. Proceed quickly, keeping the barley from staying in the water to preserve as much starch as possible.

SUGGESTED ACCOMPANIMENTS: Butternut Squash and Yam Bisque with Toasted Pumpkin Seeds, Black Bean Loaf, Carrot and Cabbage Slaw with Fresh Fennel, and Banana Refrigerator Cake.

★★★ MANGANESE, THIAMIN, MAGNESIUM
  ★ NIACIN, VITAMIN B₆, COPPER, IRON, ZINC

The bran on barley is hard to separate from the endosperm, so to make it quicker to cook, commercial barley is "pearled," which grinds off the bran until the oval grain becomes round, like a small white pearl. Look for barley that still has an oval shape—a sign the bran is mostly intact. This is preferable to completely rounded barley, the kind that's in the grocery store.

Bulgur, Green Bean, and Walnut Pilaf

Yield: 1 quart   (4 generous servings plus extra)

We start with an easy-to-cook whole grain and add walnuts, the nut of nuts for menopause. Walnuts are the highest in omega-3 fatty acids, which are generally in short supply in our standard diet, and also contain manganese, copper, and magnesium. Walnuts are nourishment for all your vital organs that are busy changing gears.

1 cup bulgur
½ cup walnuts, chopped coarsely
2 cups vegetable or chicken stock (see index) or filtered water

½ teaspoon sea salt
¼ teaspoon black pepper
1 cup green beans, tips removed, cut into ½-inch pieces

1. In a medium pot dry-roast bulgur and walnuts, stirring constantly until aromatic, about 4 or 5 minutes. Be careful not to overheat and burn.

2. Add stock, salt, and pepper. Bring to a boil, covered, then lower flame and cook until water is absorbed, about 15 minutes.

3. Place green beans on top of bulgur mixture and cook, covered, another 5 minutes. Turn off heat and allow pot to stand 5 minutes.

4. With a fork, fluff grain to loosen and stir in green beans. Pour into a serving bowl.

SUGGESTED ACCOMPANIMENTS: Broiled Mackerel in Lime Juice and Classic Candied Yams Revised.

★★★   OMEGA-3 FATTY ACIDS, MANGANESE, LINOLEIC ACID, MAGNESIUM
  ★   VITAMIN K, COPPER, IRON

Bulgur is one of the grains that needs no washing and cooks quickly. The next day, with vinaigrette, this dish becomes salad.

Millet-Rice with Peas and Tomatoes

Yield: 6 cups   *(4 generous servings plus extra)*

Millet is a slow-metabolizing grain that provides a long, steady supply of energy. If you have a lot of work to do, but find with menopause that you can't push your body or mind to work many hours, try this dish for lunch and notice if your energy lasts longer.

1 cup millet, washed
1 cup brown rice, washed
2 tablespoons extra-virgin olive oil
1 tablespoon unsalted butter
1 onion, diced
4 cups filtered water

1 teaspoon sea salt
½ teaspoon black pepper
½ teaspoon basil or oregano
8 sun-dried tomato halves, or 4 plum
   tomatoes, chopped
¼ pound shelled peas

1. Place millet and rice in a medium saucepan and begin heating over high heat until the grains start to dry. Stir occasionally.

2. Add oil, butter, and onion to saucepan and stir to coat grain. Cook over medium heat about 5 to 7 minutes, until golden and fragrant.

3. Add water, salt, pepper, basil, and tomatoes. Bring to a boil, covered, then reduce flame to a simmer and cook 45 minutes.

4. Lift lid and add in peas, cover, and continue cooking for 5 minutes.

5. Turn off flame and allow grain to sit covered for 5 to 10 minutes before removing from pot.

6. Fluff millet-rice with a fork, incorporating cooked peas, place in a bowl, and serve.

SUGGESTED ACCOMPANIMENTS: Greek Lentil and Garlic Soup, baked yams, and Fast Salad of escarole, red cabbage, and scallions.

★★★ MANGANESE, MAGNESIUM
 ★ THIAMIN, FOLIC ACID, VITAMIN B$_6$

Grains can be mixed and cooked together, setting the cooking time for the grain that needs the longest time.

❧ Indian Millet with Currants ❧ and Sunflower Seeds

Yield: 6 cups   (4 generous servings plus extra)

Millet can have a somewhat flat and soapy taste which disappears when you dry roast it or, as we did here, cook it in stock with a little extra salt and fat. Indian cooking from the Asian continent features wonderful grain dishes such as this one for everyday or dressed up for royalty. We enhance ours with menopause-friendly currants and sunflower seeds.

 2 **cups millet, washed**
3½ **cups chicken or vegetable stock**
    (see index)
 ¾ **cup dried currants**
 ½ **cup sunflower seeds**

 2 **tablespoons unsalted butter or flax**
    seed oil
 2 **teaspoons sea salt**
 2 **teaspoons curry powder**

1. Place millet, stock, currants, sunflower seeds, butter, salt, and curry in a medium saucepan with a heavy bottom. Bring to a boil, reduce flame to low, and cook 35 to 40 minutes. (Use a heat diffuser on an electric stove or if using thin-bottomed pot.)

2. Turn off flame and allow cooked grain to sit covered for 5 to 10 minutes.

3. Fluff surface with a fork to loosen and separate grains.

Suggested accompaniments: Indian Chicken with Lemon Slices and Onions, steamed watercress, Poached Pears with Ginger-Kudzu Sauce.

★★★   FOLIC ACID, MANGANESE, MAGNESIUM, COPPER
  ★   RIBOFLAVIN, LINOLEIC ACID, VITAMIN B$_6$

❧ Kasha Loaf with Yam ❧

Yield: 1 loaf   (4 generous servings plus extra)

Magnesium and manganese are needed to build healthy and strong bones and this kasha loaf is a good source of both. Enjoy this satisfying dish after a busy day.

3½ **cups vegetable or chicken stock (see index) or filtered water**
2 **cups whole grain kasha**
1 **large yam, peeled and cubed (about 2 cups)**
1½ **teaspoons sea salt, more as needed**

1 **tablespoon extra-virgin olive oil**
2 **cloves garlic, minced**
1 **onion, minced**
½ **bunch parsley, minced**
¾ **cup whole wheat bread crumbs**
½ **teaspoon white pepper**

1. In a medium pot, put stock, kasha, yam, and salt. Bring to a boil, covered, and simmer 20 minutes.

2. In a small sauté pan, heat olive oil and cook garlic and onion until caramelized, about 10 minutes.

3. Preheat oven to 350°.

4. Fluff kasha with a fork and turn into a large bowl. Add onion mixture, parsley, ½ cup bread crumbs, pepper, and more salt if needed. Mix well, mashing yam and kasha together.

5. Oil a 4-cup loaf pan and sprinkle remaining ¼ cup bread crumbs over bottom of pan. Press kasha mixture into pan. Bake in preheated 350° oven about 45 minutes, until loaf starts to come away from the sides.

6. Use a paring knife to loosen the loaf from the sides of the pan. Place a serving plate on top of the loaf and, holding the plate and pan at the same time, turn upside down. Remove the loaf pan.

7. Slice kasha loaf into ½-inch-thick pieces and serve hot.

SUGGESTED ACCOMPANIMENTS: White bean sauce (see Chick-pea Béchamel) and Your Basic Green Salad with escarole, steamed zucchini, and tangerines.

★★★   MAGNESIUM, MANGANESE
★   FOLIC ACID, VITAMIN B$_6$, COPPER

❧ Quinoa Risotto ❧

Yield: 5 cups   (4 generous servings plus extra)

Quinoa (Keen-wa), a staple of the ancient civilizations of the Andes, is today's gourmet grain. Put this on your shopping list and you support biodiversity. In this recipe we use quinoa as a base for risotto, an Italian cooking technique for making creamy rice. Any grain can be cooked according to this method.

4 tablespoons unsalted butter or extra-virgin olive oil
1 onion, chopped
1½ cups quinoa, washed
4 cups vegetable stock or filtered water (see Note)

2 to 3 pinches saffron threads
1 tablespoon chick-pea miso
Sea salt (optional)
Freshly ground black pepper
Pecorino romano cheese, grated (optional)

1. In a medium saucepan on medium-low heat, melt butter. Add onion and cook until translucent, about 5 to 7 minutes.

2. Add quinoa, and sauté for 4 to 5 minutes.

3. In a small saucepan heat stock over a low flame until warm. Dissolve saffron and miso in the stock and continue heating until the saffron dissolves.

4. Add 1 cup of stock to quinoa, and cook uncovered until the liquid has been absorbed, stirring occasionally. When grain is dry, add more broth as needed, ½ cup at a time, allowing the stock to be absorbed before adding more. Continue this process for at least 30 to 35 minutes until the quinoa is creamy.

5. Season quinoa with salt, if needed, and pepper. The grains will be unevenly cooked, some undercooked and some overcooked.

6. Place cheese in a bowl, and those who would like some can sprinkle their own.

NOTE: A quick way to make a tasty vegetable stock is to add 2 teaspoons of herbal sea salt or 2 tablespoons of miso to 4 cups filtered water and omit salt in the recipe.

SUGGESTED ACCOMPANIMENTS: Escarole and Kidney Bean Soup, Bowl of Antipasto, Soft-Shell Crabs, and Carob Cake with Walnuts.

★★★   MANGANESE, MAGNESIUM, IRON
  ★   PHOSPHORUS, COPPER, OMEGA-3 FATTY ACIDS

> When cooking risotto, the grain may stick to the bottom of the pan, but as stock is added in each stage it will loosen and give a creamy yet chewy consistency to the risotto, which is typical of this dish.

You might be losing iron because of what you eat. Iron depleters include caffeinated and decaffeinated coffee, caffeinated tea, and phosphates in baked goods and soda.

❧ Mexican Rice with Pumpkin Seeds ❧ and Cilantro

Yield: 2 quarts   (4 generous servings plus extra)

Sprinkle seeds into what you're cooking whenever you can to benefit from their ample nutrients. The pumpkin seeds supply magnesium for bone and heart health. Serve this as the main course along with a bean dish for a high-protein meatless meal.

1 tablespoon extra-virgin olive oil
2 onions, minced
8 cloves garlic, minced
8 ripe plum or 3 beefsteak tomatoes, chopped coarsely
1½ cups long-grain brown rice, washed

2 cups filtered water
1½ teaspoons sea salt
½ teaspoon oregano
¼ teaspoon black pepper
¼ cup pumpkin or sunflower seeds
¼ bunch cilantro or parsley, chopped coarsely

1. In a heavy-bottomed medium pot, heat oil and add onions. Cook 2 to 3 minutes, uncovered.

2. Add garlic, tomatoes, and rice to onions. Cook, uncovered, 15 minutes, stirring occasionally, allowing the flavors to be absorbed into the grain.

3. Add water, salt, oregano, pepper, and seeds. Bring to a boil over a high flame, covered. Reduce to low heat (use a heat diffuser if cooking on an electric stove or using a thin-bottomed pot) and cook 45 minutes.

4. When rice is done, fluff with a fork to separate grains. Stir in cilantro. Serve while hot.

SUGGESTED ACCOMPANIMENTS: Twice-Cooked Beans Wrapped in Corn Tortillas, jicama salad with Your Basic Easy Dressing, and chamomile tea.

★★★ MANGANESE, MAGNESIUM
★ VITAMIN C, VITAMIN K, VITAMIN B$_6$, THIAMIN

❧ Roasted Pecans and Wild Rice ❧

Yield: About 4 cups   (4 generous servings)

Wild rice is usually a seed native to America. A lot of wild rice on the market is "tame rice" cultivated in paddies and fertilized with chemicals. But you can also find the original "organic" kind, which has been gathered from shallow waters in Minnesota and dried in the sun.

1 cup wild rice
3 cups filtered water
1 teaspoon sea salt
2 tablespoons extra-virgin olive oil or unsalted butter

2 cloves garlic, minced
1 cup pecans
½ teaspoon thyme
¼ teaspoon black pepper
½ teaspoon herbal sea salt seasoning

1. In a medium saucepan with a heavy bottom, put wild rice, water, and salt. Bring to a boil, covered. Lower flame and simmer for 1 hour.

2. In a medium sauté pan, heat oil and garlic just until mixture starts to bubble. Add pecans, thyme, pepper, and herbal salt. Lower flame to medium and stir constantly until pecans are evenly roasted and smell fragrant. Pour into a small bowl and set aside to cool.

3. Fluff rice with a fork to separate grains. Place in a serving bowl, and just before serving toss pecans on top.

SUGGESTED ACCOMPANIMENTS: Great Northern Ragout Provençal, Butternut Squash Purée, endive and grated carrot salad, and Strawberry Tart with Walnut Crust.

★★★ MANGANESE, OMEGA-6 FATTY ACIDS, OMEGA-3 FATTY ACIDS, MAGNESIUM
  ★ ZINC, COPPER, FOLIC ACID, POTASSIUM

❧ Polenta with Wild Mushroom Sauce ❧

Yield: 1 loaf   (4 generous servings plus extra)

Both cornmeal and shiitake mushrooms contain vitamin B_5, pantothenic acid, necessary for healthy skin. Having enough of this vitamin in your diet can help prevent premature aging and wrinkles. Cook this dish and enjoy it for several meals, including breakfast.

BASIC POLENTA:

6 to 8 cups filtered water
2 cups hi-lysine cornmeal
2 teaspoons herbal sea salt
2 tablespoons unsalted butter or
   extra-virgin olive oil

1 tablespoon salted plum vinegar
   (umeboshi)

1 recipe Wild Mushroom Sauce
   (see recipe)

1. Put 5 cups water in a large, heavy-bottomed pot, and whisk in cornmeal. Add salt. Place pot over high heat.

2. Stir frequently as the water heats. Once the polenta begins to thicken, continuous stirring is required until the polenta boils. Add more water as needed, ½ cup at a time, to keep polenta thick yet a pourable consistency.

3. Once the cornmeal comes to a boil, lower heat. (Be careful to stir enough so that the air bubbles under the surface don't burst and spatter you with hot cornmeal.) Use a heat diffuser if cooking on an electric stove or with a thin-bottomed pot. Cover and continue cooking, stirring every 10 minutes and adding more water as necessary. Let polenta cook for a total of 40 minutes once it has come to a boil.

4. Stir in butter or oil and plum vinegar.

5. Wet the inside of a mold or loaf pan with water. Pour polenta into pan. Set aside to cool and solidify, about 30 to 40 minutes.

6. Unmold polenta, turning onto a serving platter or wooden board. Dip a sharp knife into water and slice polenta. Place on a plate and pour mushroom sauce over.

VARIATIONS: To brown polenta, cut ½-inch-thick slices from cooled loaf. Butter a baking sheet and arrange polenta slices on it. Place several dots of butter on each slice.

Broil 7 to 10 minutes on each side, adding additional dots of butter as needed. Serve with sauce or gravy, or sprinkle with cinnamon and drizzle with maple syrup.

SUGGESTED ACCOMPANIMENTS: French Carrots and Parsnips, and Cannellini and Kidney Beans with Rosemary.

★★★ PANTOTHENIC ACID, VITAMIN A
★ COPPER, RIBOFLAVIN, NIACIN

In scientific studies, Asian mushrooms, including shiitake, have been shown to boost immunity against cancer, as well as lower cholesterol and blood pressure. The common button mushroom has shown no such therapeutic effect, and since these health issues are concerns for women as they age, you have good reason to spend a few extra dollars on the more exotic kinds. You'll also find them much tastier.

❧ Kasha and Red Pepper Timbales ❧

Yield: 12 timbales (½ cup each)   (4 generous servings plus extra)

Kasha, which is toasted buckwheat, is a special food for menopause because it's the grain that contains bioflavonoids. These nutrients ease the anxiety, irritability, and mood swings that many women experience. Here we serve this kasha molded, a decorative option you have whenever you cook a grain.

3½ cups filtered water	1 red pepper, seeded and minced
2 cups kasha	2 teaspoons herbal sea salt
½ cup sunflower seeds	1 teaspoon basil
4 scallions, sliced thin	1 bunch parsley, chopped fine

1. In a medium pot, put water, kasha, sunflower seeds, scallions, red pepper, herbal salt, and basil. Bring to a boil, covered. Lower heat and simmer 10 minutes.

2. Turn off heat and let pot sit 5 minutes. Add parsley, reserving 3 tablespoons, and stir well.

3. Using a ½-cup measure or an ice-cream scoop, dip the measure into a container of water, then fill with kasha mixture, packing it well. Turn cup upside down and tap bottom, unmolding onto plate.

4. Serve, sprinkled with reserved minced parsley.

SUGGESTED ACCOMPANIMENTS: Chicken with Vinegar and Garlic, and onion flowers (from Leg of Lamb with Rosemary and Onion Flowers).

★★★   VITAMIN K, VITAMIN C, MAGNESIUM, LINOLEIC ACID

★   MANGANESE, FOLIC ACID, THIAMIN

❧ Wild Rice Ring ❧

Yield: 1 ring   (4 generous servings plus extra)

Whatever you are cooking, make every dish count nutritionally. Instead of quick-cooking white rice (which has been precooked and dried, further losing nutrients beyond the refining process), prepare this wild rice recipe that's full of magnesium, manganese, and essential fatty acids.

1 cup wild rice, washed	1 onion, minced
5 cups vegetable or chicken stock (see index) or filtered water	¼ teaspoon sage
	¼ teaspoon thyme
1 cup short-grain brown rice, washed	¼ teaspoon marjoram
1 teaspoon sea salt	Pinch ground nutmeg
1 clove garlic, minced	1 cup pine nuts or sunflower seeds
3 tablespoons unsalted butter	

1. In a medium saucepan, put wild rice and 2 cups stock. Bring to a boil, covered, and then lower flame to a simmer. Cook 30 minutes to soften rice.

2. To the wild rice, add the brown rice, remaining 3 cups stock, salt, and garlic. Bring to a boil, covered, lower flame, and cook until all liquid is absorbed, about 50 minutes. Stir every 10 minutes to break up rice.

3. In a small sauté pan, melt butter and add onion, sage, thyme, marjoram, and nutmeg. Cook over medium heat 10 minutes.

4. Preheat oven to 350°.

5. Add pine nuts to onion, turn off flame, and cover. Let sit until rice is ready, then stir into rice mixture.

6. Butter a 10-inch ring mold or loaf pan. Pour in rice mixture and press down with a moistened hand to consolidate. Set mold in a pan of hot water and bake in preheated oven, uncovered, 20 minutes.

7. Remove mold from water and place on a dish towel. To serve, loosen sides with a knife. Place a serving plate on top, slide hand under mold (it may be hot, so wear a gloved pot holder), and flip mold over. Put plate down and lift mold off.

SUGGESTED ACCOMPANIMENTS: After unmolding, fill ring with Wild Mushroom Sauce and serve with French Carrots and Parsnips, and Your Basic Green Salad with Creamy Yogurt Dressing.

★★★   MANGANESE, LINOLEIC ACID, MAGNESIUM, OMEGA-3 FATTY ACIDS, THIAMIN

Short-grain rice is stickier than long-grain rice and, when molded, holds its shape more firmly.

❧ Whole Wheat Linguini with Fresh Tuna ❧

Yield: 3 quarts   (4 generous servings plus extra)

If you are on a diet and have cut back on calories, you won't get so hungry if the foods you're eating are premium and full of nutrients. Choose whole wheat pasta over white-flour pasta and you'll have the advantage of extra vitamins and minerals. This dish is high in selenium—in the pasta, tuna, carrot, and garlic—which keeps your skin supple.

1 tablespoon extra-virgin olive oil
1 pound fresh tuna steak, about 1 inch thick, cut into 1-inch cubes
½ teaspoon sea salt
½ teaspoon black pepper
1 onion, diced
1 carrot, diced
1 stalk celery, diced
4 cloves garlic, minced
8 plum tomatoes, chopped, plus 4 regular tomatoes, cubed (see Note)
1 cup chicken stock (see index), organic preferred
¼ teaspoon thyme or tarragon
Rind of 2 lemons, grated, plus 2 strips zest
2 bay leaves
2 quarts filtered water, boiling
¾ to 1 pound whole wheat linguini or udon
¼ bunch parsley, stems removed, minced

1. In a large skillet heat 2 teaspoons oil over medium-high heat. Add tuna and sauté 2 minutes until browned on outside, turning several times. Inside will still be pink. Remove from pan and set aside in a small bowl. Sprinkle with salt and pepper.

2. Reduce heat to medium and, in the same pan, add remaining 1 teaspoon oil. Sauté onion, carrot, celery, and 3 cloves garlic until vegetables are softened, about 3 to 4 minutes. Add tomatoes, stock, thyme, lemon-zest strips, and bay leaves and bring to a boil. Cook on medium-high heat for about 15 minutes, uncovered, until slightly thickened.

3. Cook linguini in large pot according to package directions. Do not cook al dente. Drain pasta and do not rinse.

4. Return tuna to sauce, reduce to low heat, and simmer uncovered for 5 minutes or longer until the fish flesh is opaque, stirring occasionally.

5. Discard strips of lemon zest and bay leaves. Taste, adding salt and pepper as needed.

6. In a small bowl combine parsley, grated lemon rind, and remaining garlic and set aside.

7. Place pasta in a serving bowl or platter. Spoon the tuna sauce on top. Generously sprinkle with parsley mixture and serve immediately.

NOTE: Pomì brand tomatoes come in an aseptic container which can be found in the canned-tomato section of a store. These have a shorter shelf life but the tomatoes are better tasting since they have not been in cans. We find this type of tomato product fine to use on occasion when fresh tomatoes are not in season.

SUGGESTED ACCOMPANIMENTS: Asparagus Mimosa with Lemon and Flax Seed Oil, and Old-Fashioned Oatmeal Raisin Cookies.

★★★ VITAMIN B$_{12}$, OMEGA-3 FATTY ACIDS
★ SELENIUM, VITAMIN A, MANGANESE, NIACIN, MAGNESIUM

❧ Spicy Almond Udon with Wilted Spinach ❧

Yield: 1 quart   (4 generous servings plus extra)

Udon is Japanese whole wheat pasta. We combine this with spinach, one of the dark leafy greens that are staples of the menopause menu.

1 **quart filtered water for pasta plus ½ cup**
8 **ounces udon**
1 **8- to 10-ounce bag spinach, washed**
¼ **cup almond butter**
2 **cloves garlic, pressed**
½ **teaspoon white pepper**

½ **teaspoon black pepper**
2 **tablespoons salted plum vinegar (umeboshi) or 2 tablespoons lemon juice and ¼ teaspoon sea salt**
2 **tablespoons almonds, toasted and chopped coarsely**

1. In a medium saucepan heat 1 quart water. Cook udon according to package directions until soft, about 10 to 12 minutes.

2. In a separate pot, steam spinach in the water clinging to its leaves after washing; cook until wilted. Remove to a colander and drain. Do not save steaming liquid.

3. In a small bowl, mix together almond butter, garlic, white and black peppers, and plum vinegar.

4. Chop spinach coarsely. To serve, make a ring of spinach on a plate. Fill with cooked udon. Spoon several tablespoons of almond-butter sauce onto udon. Sprinkle with chopped almonds and serve hot.

SUGGESTED ACCOMPANIMENTS: Bowl of Antipasto.

★★★   VITAMIN K, MANGANESE
★   FOLIC ACID, MAGNESIUM, VITAMIN A

We had some of our loyal friends over for dinner to sample sixteen different kinds of whole grain pasta to see which ones they liked. We gave them brown rice pasta, buckwheat noodles (soba), noodles made from wild yam, quinoa shells, kamut spirals, whole wheat linguini, udon, and more. They obediently munched noodles they had never seen before, and everyone found a favorite they wanted to try again. Give whole grain pastas a chance. See our Appendix for brands and sources.

❧ Broccoli Rabe with Tomato and Spirals ❧

Yield: 6 cups   (*4 generous servings plus extra*)

One reason coffee and chocolate may be so popular is for their bitter taste, a flavor popular in other cuisines but not found in many foods we normally eat. Other sources for the bitter taste are dark leafy greens, such as broccoli rabe, that can fulfill your need for this primary flavor.

2   quarts filtered water
2   teaspoons sea salt
8   ounces whole grain spiral pasta
3   tablespoons extra-virgin olive oil
6   cloves garlic, sliced
3   plum tomatoes, seeded and chopped, or ¼ cup sun-dried (see Note)
1   bunch broccoli rabe, washed and chopped into 1-inch pieces (about 1 pound)

2   teaspoons salted plum vinegar (umeboshi) or juice of ½ lemon and several pinches sea salt
1   cup pasta-cooking water
    Red-pepper flakes
    Pecorino romano, grated (optional)

1. In a large stockpot boil water and salt. Add pasta and cook until soft, about 10 to 12 minutes. Drain, reserving 1 cup of liquid, and set aside, covered, in a serving bowl.

2. In a large sauté pan, heat olive oil, adding garlic and tomatoes. Stir 2 or 3 minutes, and add broccoli rabe, cooking several more minutes until vegetable is wilted. Sprinkle with plum vinegar, cover, and cook 10 minutes over medium-low heat.

3. Add pasta water and increase heat, bringing liquid to a boil. Cook 3 minutes. Drain well.

4. Pour broccoli rabe on top of cooked pasta and serve with red-pepper flakes and cheese on the side.

NOTE: In the summer and fall, use fresh tomatoes; in the winter and spring, use sun-dried tomatoes.

VARIATIONS: If you prefer less bitter greens, make this dish with collards, kale, or escarole.

SUGGESTED ACCOMPANIMENTS: Colombian Lima Bean and Corn Stew, steamed carrots, and Carob Cake with Walnuts.

★★★   VITAMIN K, VITAMIN C, VITAMIN A, MANGANESE
  ★   MAGNESIUM, FOLIC ACID, VITAMIN B$_6$, OMEGA-3 FATTY ACIDS, IRON

Sautéing greens will keep their bitter flavor. If you prefer a milder taste, just boil the greens, uncovered, in plenty of water to remove the bitterness and then, if you like, proceed with sautéing (see recipe).

The dark leafy greens that have a bitter flavor are:

broccoli rabe	escarole
chicory	kale
collards	mustard greens
dandelion greens	turnip greens

❧ Vongole and Linguini (Clams and Pasta) ❧

Yield: 1½ quarts   (4 servings)

This classic Italian dish works well for menopause with its vitamin- and mineral-packed shellfish and whole grain noodles. It has a good supply of vitamin B_{12} for healthy nerves and omega-3 fatty acids, which nourish the sex organs and glands.

1 quart filtered water	1 tablespoon extra-virgin olive oil
1 teaspoon sea salt	5 cloves garlic, sliced
8 ounces whole wheat linguini or udon noodles	1 onion, sliced
	1½ cups shrimp or fish stock (see index)
1½ pounds fresh cherrystone clams or vongole in the shell	½ teaspoon herbal sea salt
	½ bunch parsley, chopped coarsely
1 tablespoon unsalted butter	

1. In a large stockpot, bring water and salt to a boil. Add linguini and cook until soft according to package directions.

2. Wash clams in cold water. Remove to a colander.

3. In a large skillet, heat butter and oil. Add garlic and onion and cook over medium-low heat for 5 minutes.

4. Add clams, stock, and herbal salt. Cover and cook 2 minutes. Stir well and continue cooking, covered, another 2 to 3 minutes, until all the clams have opened.

5. Add parsley and stir again. To serve, pour clams and juices over hot pasta.

VARIATIONS: Serve with red-pepper flakes and grated pecorino cheese.

SUGGESTED ACCOMPANIMENTS: Soft-Shell Crabs, Turnips with Tops in Velouté Sauce, and A Quick Cake.

★★★ VITAMIN B_{12}, IRON
★ OMEGA-3 FATTY ACIDS, VITAMIN K, VITAMIN C

❧ Pasta e Fagioli ❧

Yield: 3½ quarts   (4 generous servings plus extra)

Our version of pasta e fagioli, an Italian heritage dish, combines beans and whole grain pasta to create a food for long-term health. It's a source of vegetable protein, good for bone health, and it's low in fat, a plus for the heart. It's also high in fiber, which helps remove excess estrogen, which can cause menopausal symptoms.

Before beginning, sort, wash, and soak ½ cup dried white cannellini beans 6 to 8 hours or overnight.

1 to 1½ cups soaked white cannellini beans (from ½ cup dried)	2 stalks celery, minced
4 cups filtered water, plus 6 cups for pasta	½ bunch Italian parsley, minced
	Pinch red-pepper flakes, to taste
¼ cup extra-virgin olive oil	2 teaspoons sea salt
1 onion, chopped	1 teaspoon basil
4 cloves garlic, minced	½ teaspoon oregano
3 ripe plum tomatoes, seeded and chopped	4 ounces whole grain pasta (see Notes)
	¼ cup grated pecorino romano (optional; see Notes)

1. Lift beans from soaking water with your hands or a slotted spoon and put into a small stockpot. Add 4 cups water and bring to a boil over high heat, covered. Reduce heat and simmer 35 to 40 minutes, until beans just begin to become tender. Discard soaking water.

2. Heat oil in a large stockpot and add onion. Cook for several minutes and then add garlic, tomatoes, celery, and parsley, allowing each to cook for a minute before adding the next.

3. Add red-pepper flakes, 1 teaspoon salt, basil, and oregano. Cook, covered, over a low flame 15 to 20 minutes.

4. In a medium saucepan, heat 6 cups water, to which 1 teaspoon salt has been added, and bring to a boil, covered. Add pasta, leave uncovered, and cook according to package directions. Drain and reserve.

5. Add softened beans and cooking water to the vegetables. Add pasta and stir well. Additional water may be desired, as the pasta absorbs a lot of liquid. The consistency can be soupy or more like stew. Bring to a boil and cook over a medium flame about 10 to 15 minutes. The beans will be completely softened. Serve with grated cheese if desired.

NOTES: **1**. You can choose from a variety of whole grain pastas: broken spaghetti or udon, elbows, quinoa, or kamut shells.

2. For those who do not use cheese, a delicious calcium-rich substitute is toasted sesame seeds with a little added sea salt. Put in a large-holed shaker and use like grated cheese.

VARIATIONS: Cannellini beans are an Italian white kidney bean. They can be substituted with Great Northern, navy, pinto, or kidney beans.

SUGGESTED ACCOMPANIMENTS: Bowl of Antipasto and Italian Almond Cake.

★★★ VITAMIN K, FOLIC ACID, MANGANESE, VITAMIN C, IRON, MAGNESIUM

❧

Pasta e Fagioli can become a soup by adding more water or stock, or kept thick and stewlike by allowing the pasta to absorb most of the liquid. The seasoning may need to be adjusted if more water is added.

❧

❧ Hearty Rigatoni with Sausages, ❧ Garlic, and Broccoli

Yield: 3½ quarts *(4 generous servings plus extra)*

Garlic is a great flavor choice when cooking for menopause. It's good for the heart, immune system, and digestion, and it contains high amounts of vitamin B$_6$, vitamin C, manganese, and selenium, all of which counteract stress. Garlic also contains phytohormones.

Before beginning, sort, wash, and soak 1 cup dried white beans 6 to 8 hours or overnight.

2 to 2½ cups soaked white beans (from 1 cup dried)
10 cups filtered water
1 bay leaf
2 teaspoons sea salt
8 ounces whole wheat rigatoni or other shape pasta
½ pound sausages or meatballs, organic preferred (see Note)

2 teaspoons extra-virgin olive oil
2 teaspoons unsalted butter
2 large onions, chopped coarsely
1 head garlic, peeled (about 15 cloves)
2 teaspoons basil
1 teaspoon oregano
¼ teaspoon thyme
2 stalks broccoli, cut into 4-inch spears
Black or red pepper to taste

1. Remove beans from soaking water with your hands or a slotted spoon and put in a small saucepan. Add 4 cups of water and bay leaf and cook, covered, 40 minutes. Discard soaking water.

2. In a medium stockpot, bring remaining 6 cups water to a boil with 1 teaspoon salt. Add pasta and cook until almost al dente (it will be cooked more later), about 10 minutes. Drain.

3. In a large stockpot, cook sausages over high heat until browned on all sides. Remove to brown paper to drain.

4. Without cleaning pot, add olive oil, butter, onions, whole garlic cloves, basil, oregano, and thyme. Cook 5 minutes, on medium heat, until onions begin to be translucent.

5. With a slotted spoon, remove cooked beans from saucepan and add to onion-garlic mixture. Add ½ cup bean-cooking liquid and sausages. Bring to boil, covered, and cook 10 minutes.

6. Stir pasta and broccoli spears into beans. Cover and let steam 5 minutes, until broccoli is bright green. Season with pepper.

7. Serve immediately on a large platter or in a wide bowl or large pasta platter.

NOTE: If you prefer this dish vegetarian, substitute ½ pound seasoned tempeh and ½ teaspoon fennel seeds for sausage.

VARIATIONS: Leftovers make a great soup.

SUGGESTED ACCOMPANIMENTS: Add a crunchy salad—it's a complete meal.

★★★   VITAMIN K, FOLIC ACID
  ★   VITAMIN C, THIAMIN, MANGANESE, MAGNESIUM, VITAMIN B₁₂

❧ Hungarian Pasta with Cabbage ❧

Yield: 2 quarts   (4 generous servings plus extra)

This recipe is a novel way to include cabbage in your meals. As the cabbage cooks and turns golden brown, it sweetens and becomes quite different from its original self. We think you'll be surprised with how good this tastes.

1 quart filtered water
2 teaspoons sea salt
8 ounces whole grain pasta, such as ribbons
2 tablespoons extra-virgin olive oil
1 red onion, sliced
1 yellow or white onion, sliced

½ head green cabbage, shredded
2 teaspoons herbal sea salt
1 teaspoon oregano
¼ cup walnuts, chopped coarsely
1 cup vegetable stock (see index) or filtered water
½ bunch parsley, chopped coarsely

1. In a medium stockpot, bring water and salt to a boil. Add pasta to water and cook, uncovered, until soft, about 10 minutes.

2. In a large sauté pan, heat olive oil and add onions. Cook, uncovered, over medium-high heat 3 or 4 minutes, until onions start to become translucent.

3. Add cabbage, herbal salt, and oregano. Stir until cabbage is wilted.

4. Add walnuts and stock to cabbage. Cover and continue cooking over medium heat 10 to 12 minutes. Uncover and cook another 5 minutes, until cabbage starts to brown. Add parsley, stir well, and turn off heat.

5. Drain pasta and place on a large platter. Cover with cabbage and serve.

SUGGESTED ACCOMPANIMENTS: Seafood Bisque with Chives, grated pecorino cheese, Pinto Beans and Swiss Chard Patties, Toasted Nuts with Raisins and Apricots.

★★★   VITAMIN C, VITAMIN K, MANGANESE, OMEGA-3 FATTY ACIDS
  ★   MAGNESIUM, LINOLEIC ACID, FOLIC ACID

❧ Asparagus Fusilli ❧

Yield: 3 quarts   (4 generous servings plus extra)

Here's an elegant pasta that delivers vitamin E, a menopause vitamin that revitalizes the entire system. Vitamin E is low in refined and processed foods, but in this dish it's in the asparagus, extra-virgin olive oil, and the whole grain fusilli.

1½ quarts filtered water
2 teaspoons sea salt
8 ounces whole grain fusilli, or other shape pasta
2 tablespoons extra-virgin olive oil
3 cloves garlic, sliced
½ teaspoon basil
¼ teaspoon oregano

¼ teaspoon red-pepper flakes (optional)
Pinch sage
3 tablespoons pine nuts or unhulled sesame seeds
6 sun-dried tomato halves, sliced
1 bunch asparagus, about 1 pound
½ teaspoon herbal sea salt

1. In a medium stockpot, bring water and salt to a boil, covered. Add pasta to water and cook uncovered until soft, about 10 minutes, stirring occasionally.

2. In a large sauté pan, heat olive oil and garlic. Cook 1 minute and add basil, oregano, red-pepper flakes, sage, pine nuts, tomato, and ½ cup water from pasta.

3. Break off woody ends from asparagus and discard. Break off tips and set aside. Cut stems diagonally into three or four pieces. Add stems to sauté pan, stir well, cover, and cook 1 minute. Add asparagus tips, sprinkle with herbal salt, and cook 2 to 3 minutes, uncovered, until the asparagus turns bright green.

4. Drain pasta in a colander (do not rinse). Place in a large serving bowl. Place asparagus sauté on top of pasta and serve while hot.

VARIATIONS: Try other vegetables—zucchini, onions, yams, and green beans.

SUGGESTED ACCOMPANIMENTS: Grated pecorino cheese and Poached Salmon Steaks with Tarragon.

★★★   VITAMIN K, FOLIC ACID
   ★   VITAMIN E, VITAMIN C, MANGANESE, THIAMIN, MAGNESIUM, COPPER

❦

In asparagus season, eat your fill. Asparagus contains glutathione, a compound that once inside your cells snags free radicals before they can do their damage and cause cancer.

❦

❦ Tomatoes Stuffed with Couscous ❦

Yield: 8 tomatoes   (4 generous servings plus extra)

Instead of serving grains in a bowl, serve them inside a vegetable. We stuffed these tomatoes with richly flavored whole grain couscous for a visual and taste treat. Nourishment happens on many levels.

4 cups vegetable stock (see recipe) or
   filtered water
2 teaspoons sea salt
2 cups whole wheat couscous
2 tablespoons unsalted butter or
   extra-virgin olive oil
1 onion, minced
2 cloves garlic, minced

2 teaspoons basil
1 teaspoon mint (see Notes)
   Juice of 1 lemon
½ cup pumpkin seeds
1 bunch parsley, minced
⅛ teaspoon black pepper
8 ripe, firm beefsteak tomatoes
   (see Notes)

1. In a medium saucepan bring stock and salt to a boil, covered. Add couscous, cover, and reduce heat. Simmer 10 minutes.

2. In a small sauté pan, melt butter and cook onion and garlic until onion is translucent, about 5 or 6 minutes.

3. Add basil and mint, and stir well. Cook another 30 seconds. Turn off heat and stir in lemon juice, pumpkin seeds, parsley, and pepper.

4. Cut tops off tomatoes and reserve. Holding tomato firmly in the palm of your hand, scoop out the interior pulp, leaving about ¼ inch of shell. (It should still be firm and hold its shape.) Chop pulp fine and put it in a strainer to allow excess juice to drain. Discard juice and put drained tomato pulp into a large bowl.

5. Preheat oven to 350°.

6. Mix together cooked couscous, onion mixture, and tomato. Stir well. Taste, adding extra salt and pepper, if desired.

7. Spoon couscous mixture into tomato shells. Cover with tomato tops. Place tomatoes in a small enough baking dish so that they are held together tightly and kept upright. Add 1 cup stock to baking dish and carefully place in preheated oven.

8. Bake 30 to 40 minutes, until tomatoes are soft and tops begin to char slightly.

NOTES: **1.** If you don't have fresh mint, remove and use the leaves from a mint tea bag.

2. When choosing tomatoes for this recipe, look for firm tomatoes with very little indenting at the top stem end. For best flavor, be sure they are ripe, but not overripe and soft (these will turn to mush when baked).

VARIATIONS: Add chopped fresh tuna, chicken, or beans to couscous.

SUGGESTED ACCOMPANIMENTS: Collard Greens with White Onions and Three-Bean Salad.

★★★   VITAMIN K, VITAMIN C
  ★   MANGANESE, SELENIUM, MAGNESIUM

❧

Couscous is not so much a grain as a way of treating flour. It's made with fine or coarse semolina, rolled into lumps and then pressed through a sieve to form minute and uniform balls. Couscous is really small-scale pasta.

Couscous made from whole grain semolina flour instead of refined semolina is now available. We love its rich flavor! It is called whole wheat couscous and that's the only one we recommend you use.

❧

❧ Sesame Salad with Buckwheat Noodles ❧ and Fresh Coriander

Yield: 1 quart   (4 generous servings)

Buckwheat noodles, known as soba in Japan, are a traditional Japanese pasta that deserves to be a staple in your kitchen. Buckwheat is the only grain source of bioflavonoids, estrogenic nutrients for female health.

2 **quarts filtered water plus ¼ to ½ cup**
1 **8-ounce package soba noodles**
2 **tablespoons sesame tahini**
3 **tablespoons shoyu soy sauce**
2 **tablespoons brown rice vinegar**
2 **tablespoons unfiltered apple juice**
1 **tablespoon maple syrup**

2 **cloves garlic, peeled and pressed**
1 **teaspoon herbal sea salt**
2 **teaspoons hot sauce**
4 **scallions, minced**
¼ **bunch fresh coriander, leaves only (see Note)**

1. In a large pot bring 2 quarts water to a boil, covered. Add soba and cook uncovered according to package directions, about 12 to 15 minutes. Drain in a colander or remove noodles with a spaghetti fork. Place in a large bowl of cold water to cool for 10 minutes, then drain again in the colander.

2. In a medium bowl, using a whisk, mix tahini with shoyu and rice vinegar until smooth. (It will thicken first before thinning.) Add apple juice and maple syrup and stir again.

3. Add a few tablespoons of water to tahini mixture, stirring well after each addition. (The tahini may separate but that's okay. As more water is added it will emulsify.) Keep adding more water, stirring until mixture is of sauce consistency.

4. Stir in garlic, herbal salt, and hot sauce. (If the sauce sits for more than 30 minutes, then additional water may need to be added to thin it, about 1 tablespoon at a time.)

5. Place noodles in a serving bowl and drizzle with sauce. Toss and then garnish with scallions and coriander leaves. Serve at room temperature or refrigerate 1 hour to serve cold.

NOTE: Depending upon which cultural circles you travel in, you will want to note that fresh coriander is also known as Chinese parsley and cilantro.

SUGGESTED ACCOMPANIMENTS: Chinese Steamed Whitefish with Fresh Coriander, Steamed Spinach, and kiwi and orange slices.

★★★ MAGNESIUM, THIAMIN, LINOLEIC ACID
  ★ VITAMIN K, FOLIC ACID, MANGANESE, SODIUM

❧ 10 ❧
Vegetables

Greens Four Calcium
Easy Onion and Pepper Slices
Steamed Spinach
Classic Candied Yams Revised
Sautéed Mushrooms with Garlic
Roasted Potatoes with Rosemary
Turnips with Tops in Velouté Sauce
Skillet-Roasted Parsnips, Yams, and Squash
Broccoli with Currants
Baked White and Orange French Fries
Puréed Cabbage and Potatoes
Asparagus Mimosa with Lemon and Flax Seed Oil
Plantains Sautéed in Butter
Arame and Cabbage with Mustard Sauce
Gremolata Mashed Potatoes
Butternut Squash Purée
Collard Greens with White Onions
Curried Cauliflower Crown
Kale with Capers and Black Olives
French Carrots and Parsnips
Crusty Baked Tomatoes Topped with Sunflower Seeds
Artichokes Stuffed with Garlic Bread Crumbs

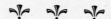

❧

Vegetables are an essential part of a woman's menu because they supply nutrients and fiber that diminish menopause and PMS symptoms and promote long-term health. We cook a wide variety of vegetables and shop for those that are fresh, seasonal, and preferably organic.

Look for produce that is firm, with no signs of bruising, wilting, or decay. There may be minor insect damage or occasional brown spots, but this is normal and doesn't affect the quality of the produce. Look for natural colors—if vegetables have overly bright, cartoonlike colors, chances are the food has been artificially colored.

To wash vegetables: We use a natural fiber brush (also known as a tawashi) and filtered water to clean vegetables. Many vegetables are waxed but peeling removes this. Other vegetables have fungicides sprayed on them to give a longer shelf life. Clean these with a mild soap or peel them. When using organic vegetables, there is no worry about waxes, fungicides, or preservatives.

Root vegetables: Using a brush or a tawashi, wash all vegetables that are going to be peeled; after peeling, rinse again, especially potatoes, carrots, and parsnips.

Dark leafy greens: Fill a large bowl full of water, cut off the bottom ends of the stems, put greens into the bowl of water, and swish around. This allows the sand and dirt to drop to the bottom of the bowl. Lift the leaves out into another bowl or colander. Discard the washing water, rinse the bowl, and repeat this procedure until the water left in the bowl has no sand or dirt particles.

To cut vegetables: Vegetables that are cut in similar sizes cook evenly.

To cook vegetables: Many cooking techniques are used in our vegetable recipes, such as steaming, sautéing, stir-frying, and boiling. A fast way to steam is to put ¼ to ½ inch of water in a saucepan with a tight-fitting lid. Bring the water to a boil and then add the vegetables and steam as usual. A steamer can also be used.

If there's liquid left over after cooking, make sure you drink it or use it as stock for another cooked dish such as grains, beans, or soup. Refrigerated, this liquid stores for 3 to 5 days.

To season: Salt after the vegetables are cooked, otherwise the salt can toughen the vegetables and draw out the nutrients.

❧ Greens Four Calcium ❧

Yield: 1 quart   *(4 generous servings plus extra)*

There's calcium in a wide range of foods beyond dairy—grains, beans, vegetables, fruits, nuts, seeds, and fish all have some. Leafy greens such as chicory, kale, collards, and dandelion are especially high—90 mg in a cup of kale, 218 mg in a cup of collards.

6 cups filtered water
½ bunch of each: chicory, kale,
   collard greens, and dandelion
   (about 2 pounds)
4 tablespoons extra-virgin olive oil
1 onion, sliced

4 cloves garlic, sliced
   Large pinch nutmeg
   Pinch sea salt, to taste
   Juice of 1 lemon
6 black oil-cured or Greek olives,
   pitted (optional)

1. In a large stockpot, bring water to a boil, covered.
2. Wash greens and put in boiling water and cook, uncovered, until tender, between 7 to 12 minutes. (Cooking greens uncovered helps them to retain their green color.)
3. Using a slotted spoon or tongs, remove the greens from the pot to a colander. Let them drain and cool for 5 to 10 minutes. Save the cooking water (see box).
4. In a large skillet, heat 2 tablespoons of the oil over medium heat. Add onion and garlic and cook for 4 to 5 minutes.
5. Chop greens coarsely and add to pan. Add nutmeg and salt. Cook another 5 minutes, uncovered.
6. Place seasoned greens in a bowl, add lemon juice, remaining oil, olives, and salt to taste. Toss well. Serve warm or at room temperature on a platter or in a bowl.

VARIATIONS:
a. Cook only one type of leafy green vegetable.
b. Place cooked greens in warmed whole wheat pita bread for lunch or a snack.
c. Add cooked greens to a grain or bean soup for an all-in-one-bowl meal.
d. Toss greens with pasta for an appetizing and unusual topping. Sprinkle with a little red or black pepper.

SUGGESTED ACCOMPANIMENTS: Colombian Lima Bean and Corn Stew, Kasha and Red Pepper Timbales, and Carob Cake with Walnuts.

★★★   VITAMIN A, VITAMIN K, VITAMIN C
  ★   CALCIUM, FOLIC ACID, MANGANESE, VITAMIN B$_6$, IRON

> While preparing dinner, make a drink of the liquid left after cooking greens, adding some lemon juice or salted plum vinegar. Sipping this helps to calm your hunger, and gives you many easy-to-digest minerals and vitamins. Do not use this liquid for soup stock as it is too bitter.

Overcooked leafy green vegetables that have turned brownish have lost more than their original color. In the process of their color change, they've lost magnesium as well, a mineral you need for the health of your heart and bones. Cook greens in a pot without a lid and the color, along with the magnesium, will be preserved.

❧ Easy Onion and Pepper Slices ❧

Yield: 4 generous servings—plenty!

Here's a tasty way to eat more vegetables—baked with savory bread crumbs. The peppers and parsley in this dish are high in vitamin K, good for bone strength. This recipe goes well in an antipasto, and makes a great addition to a chicken or fish sandwich.

1 large Spanish, Bermuda, or Vidalia
   onion
1 green pepper
1 red pepper
2 tablespoons extra-virgin olive oil
½ cup whole wheat bread crumbs
½ teaspoon basil

¼ teaspoon herbal sea salt
   Fresh black pepper
   Pinch sage
2 pinches paprika or cayenne
   (see Note)
3 tablespoons minced parsley

Preheat oven to 350°.

1. Peel onion, then slice onion crosswise (on the diameter) into ½-inch-thick slices. Cut each pepper in half, remove seeds, and cut in half or quarters lengthwise.

2. Place onion and pepper slices on an oiled or parchment-papered baking sheet or baking dish.

3. Drizzle the slices with oil, then sprinkle with bread crumbs, basil, herbal salt, pepper, sage, and paprika.

4. Bake for 20 minutes, until vegetables are soft when tested with a fork.

5. Lift vegetable slices onto a platter with a spatula, sprinkle with fresh parsley, and serve.

NOTE: Paprika is from a sweet pepper and cayenne from a hot and spicy pepper. Cayenne can substitute for paprika when a spicy flavor is desired.

SUGGESTED ACCOMPANIMENTS: Serve on Bowl of Antipasto, with other tasty morsels such as Sautéed Mushrooms with Garlic, Steamed Summer Squash Salad, Broiled Oysters on the Half Shell with Caviar, and hearty whole grain Italian bread.

★★★   VITAMIN K, VITAMIN C
  ★   FOLIC ACID, MANGANESE, SELENIUM, VITAMIN B$_6$, THIAMIN, IRON

Commercially available bread crumbs can contain dough extenders, conditioners, artificial preservatives, hydrogenated oils, and sugar. Bread crumbs are best when made from whole wheat bread, baked, then sliced and dried, and crumbled. See the Appendix for some suggested brands.

❧ Steamed Spinach ❧

Yield: 2 cups   (4 generous servings plus extra)

As our nutrient list shows, spinach is a multivitamin and mineral supplement in a green leaf. But it's not a source of calcium because oxalic acid in the leaves binds with the calcium before you can absorb it.

1 **pound spinach or Swiss chard, washed well (see Note)**
1 **or 2 cloves garlic, minced**

1 **tablespoon unsalted butter or extra-virgin olive oil**
   Pinch sea salt
   Pinch white pepper

1. After the final washing of the spinach or Swiss chard, put it in a medium saucepan, stuffing the wet vegetable in to allow the lid to fit snugly. Add no additional water—the greens will cook in the water that clings to the leaves.

2. Over medium heat, bring pot to steaming, turn heat to low, and cook until spinach is wilted, about 8 to 10 minutes.

3. Pour spinach and liquid into a colander. The liquid will be a murky green. (Do not save it, since it is high in oxalic acid.) Drain well.

4. Coarsely chop cooked spinach or chard, place in a serving bowl, and add garlic, butter, salt, and pepper. Serve hot or at room temperature.

NOTE: Spinach that is sold in cello-packs is pre-rinsed and takes less time to clean. When spinach comes with the stems intact, cut them off before washing. Make sure that absolutely no sand is left on leaves before cooking.

Swiss chard is available in green and red varieties, both of which are delicious.

VARIATIONS: Grate nutmeg on top for a sweet and fragrant flavor or fresh ginger for a spicy taste, or sauté cooked spinach with garlic. Chopped hard-boiled eggs can add some extra protein and color.

SUGGESTED ACCOMPANIMENTS: Butternut and Yam Bisque with Toasted Pumpkin Seeds, Quinoa Risotto, and Overnight Baked Beans.

★★★ VITAMIN A, VITAMIN E, VITAMIN K, VITAMIN C, FOLIC ACID, MAGNESIUM, IRON,
        MANGANESE, NIACIN, OMEGA-3 FATTY ACIDS
  ★   RIBOFLAVIN, BIOFLAVONOIDS, VITAMIN B_6, IODINE, THIAMIN

⚜ Classic Candied Yams Revised ⚜

Yield: 2 quarts (*4 generous servings plus extra*)

We give you an American favorite, made with mineral-rich blackstrap molasses instead of brown sugar and corn syrup. Yams provide potassium, which is lost in perspiration and which you may be low on if you're having night sweats.

3 **yams, peeled**
1 **cup apple juice**
1 **cup orange juice**
½ **cup dried currants (optional)**
2 **tablespoons unsulphured blackstrap molasses**

2 **tablespoons maple syrup**
2 **tablespoons arrowroot**
½ **teaspoon cinnamon**
¼ **teaspoon ground ginger**
¼ **teaspoon sea salt**

Preheat oven to 375°.

1. Cut yams into ½-inch-thick slices. Place in a roasting pan.

2. Measure and combine apple and orange juices in a 4-cup measuring container. Add currants, molasses, maple syrup, arrowroot, cinnamon, ginger, and salt and stir well. Pour over yams.

3. Place yams in oven and bake 45 minutes, turning with a spatula once or twice, until liquids have become thickened and syrupy.

4. Serve hot.

SUGGESTED ACCOMPANIMENTS: Roast Half Turkey; Chestnut, Pine Nut, and Currant Stuffing; Kale with Capers and Black Olives; and Fresh Blueberry Cobbler.

★★★   VITAMIN C, POTASSIUM, MANGANESE, VITAMIN B$_6$

If you've been listening to the menopause grapevine, you've heard about the wild Mexican yam. It contains a steroid from which the original birth-control pill was made. This same plant is now being used as the source of a natural form of progesterone that in case studies has proven to be remarkably effective in reversing osteoporosis. It grows naturally throughout Central America. The yams you find in the markets are not the same, and unfortunately the tropical version tastes soapy and bitter. It may make good medicine, but it makes terrible eating.

❧ Sautéed Mushrooms with Garlic ❧

Yield: 3 cups   (4 generous servings)

Mushrooms contain pantothenic acid which nourishes the brain, which contains high levels of this B vitamin. Serve leftover mushrooms on whole grain toast for breakfast for a splendid start to the day.

2 **tablespoons filtered water**	½ **pound wild mushrooms (cremini,**
1 **tablespoon extra-virgin**	**shiitake, portobello, oyster, elephant)**
olive oil	**or additional button mushrooms,**
4 **cloves garlic, peeled**	**cut into strips**
½ **pound button**	½ **teaspoon herbal sea salt**
mushrooms,	¼ **bunch parsley, chopped**
cut in half	**Freshly ground pepper**

1. In a small saucepan, place water and oil. Heat and add whole garlic cloves. Stir and let cook, uncovered, 2 or 3 minutes.

2. Add button and wild mushrooms and stir. Add herbal salt and parsley, cover, and let cook 5 to 7 minutes, stirring once or twice. Remove garlic cloves before serving, sprinkled with fresh pepper.

Suggested accompaniments: Roasted Pecans with Wild Rice, Leg of Lamb with Rosemary and Onion Flowers, Collard Greens with White Onions, and Broiled Dates Stuffed with Almonds.

★★★   VITAMIN D, VITAMIN K, PANTOTHENIC ACID

★   COPPER, RIBOFLAVIN, NIACIN, VITAMIN C, FOLIC ACID, SELENIUM, IRON, POTASSIUM

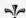

Here's our method for picking and washing mushrooms. Button mushrooms are best when purchased with tightly closed caps. Place several at a time in a bowl of water. Holding the mushroom under water, clasp the mushroom by its stem, and quickly twist it in the palm of your hand. Immediately remove it to a colander. For exotic mushrooms, choose those that have caps that are well opened and quickly rinse their tops under water, trying not to get any on the undersides. Mushrooms absorb water quickly and easily, so if they stay in water for any period of time they will become waterlogged and have less flavor.

❧

❧ Roasted Potatoes with Rosemary ❧

Yield: 1 quart   (4 generous servings plus extra)

Let your oven do the cooking and family and friends will love the results. And when you need fast food, serve any leftover potatoes with a fish fillet or scrambled eggs.

6 to 8 yellow, wax, Peruvian, or
    Eastern potatoes, cut into cubes
8 cloves garlic, peeled
2 teaspoons dried rosemary

½ teaspoon herbal sea salt
2 tablespoons unsalted butter
    Pinch black pepper
    Prepared mustard (optional)

Preheat oven to 475°.

1. In a medium baking pan, put potatoes and garlic. Sprinkle with rosemary and salt. Cut butter into small pieces and dot all over potatoes.

2. Place in preheated oven, uncovered, and lower temperature to 375°. Bake 1 to 1½ hours, turning several times, until golden.

3. Remove from oven and sprinkle with pepper and additional salt if desired. Serve hot with mustard on the side, if you like.

SUGGESTED ACCOMPANIMENTS: Creamless Mushroom Cream Soup, Flounder Rolls Stuffed with Salmon and Lemon, Mesclun Salad, and Apricot-Date-Pecan Bonbons.

★★★   VITAMIN C, VITAMIN B$_6$, POTASSIUM, COPPER
  ★   NIACIN, THIAMIN, MAGNESIUM, CHROMIUM

Look around—you may discover that the common spud is not really so plain anymore. While potatoes are usually marketed as bakers and boilers, there are some interesting varieties available at farmers' markets and in specialty produce departments that will surprise you. Most potatoes have white or yellow flesh, but some varieties are red-streaked or pink, and a few—like the small, sweet-tasting Peruvian—come in exotic blues and purples. Yellow potatoes, like Yellow Finns and Yukon Gold, have a delicious buttery flavor. And any of these can be successfully substituted in this recipe.

❧

Vegetables that contain phytohormones include:

cabbage	green beans	peas
carrots	onions	potatoes
cucumbers	parsley	radishes

❧

❧ Turnips with Tops in Velouté Sauce ❧

Yield: 2 quarts (4 generous servings plus extra)

When you cook these turnips with their tops you gain the folic acid they contain, a tonic to soothe menopause or PMS nerves. This preparation gives you a way to use all parts of a vegetable, reaping the vitamins and minerals that are in each.

**2 bunches turnips with tops
(6 to 8 turnips)**

Filtered water

SAUCE:

**2 tablespoons unsalted butter
2 tablespoons extra-virgin
olive oil
¼ cup whole wheat pastry flour**

**2 to 3 cups vegetable stock (see recipe)
or filtered water
½ teaspoon sea salt
⅛ teaspoon white pepper**

1. Cut off turnip greens and wash turnips and greens separately.
2. Place turnips in a medium saucepan, cover with water, and bring to a boil, covered. Simmer for 25 to 30 minutes, until soft when pierced with a fork.
3. In a large skillet, heat butter, oil, and flour. Stir continuously until golden brown, about 5 minutes. Using a whisk, add ½ cup stock at a time, stirring vigorously until smooth. Continue until mixture has a saucelike consistency. Add salt and pepper. Set aside.
4. Remove turnips with a slotted spoon and place in a bowl to cool. Cut into medium-size cubes or slices.

5. Add more water to saucepan if needed, return to a boil, and put greens in. Simmer, uncovered, 7 to 10 minutes.

6. In a colander, drain greens and let cool a few minutes. Place on a cutting board and, using a sharp knife and fork, cut greens into bite-size pieces.

7. Add turnips and greens to sauce. Warm over low heat 2 or 3 minutes. Add some additional stock if sauce has thickened.

VARIATIONS:
a. Add some pitted Greek or Kalamata olives.
b. Add several pinches of turmeric or saffron to give a yellow hue.
c. Add chopped garlic to sauce.

SUGGESTED ACCOMPANIMENTS: Grilled Fresh Sardines, Portuguese Style; Bulgur, Green Bean, and Walnut Pilaf; and Apricot-Cashew "Mousse."

★★★ FOLIC ACID, VITAMIN C, VITAMIN K
★ VITAMIN A, OMEGA-3 FATTY ACIDS, MANGANESE, COPPER, VITAMIN B$_6$

This velouté sauce is an easy way to get reluctant vegetable-eaters to eat greens. It is also great on cauliflower and carrots, and drizzled over broccoli or used on baked potatoes.

⚜ **Skillet-Roasted Parsnips, Yams, and Squash** ⚜

Yield: 2 quarts   (4 generous servings plus extra)

For a change from white potatoes, try this mix of root vegetables for a fortifying addition to a meal. And if you're staying away from starches because you think you'll gain weight, please don't. These foods are full of vital nutrients they've absorbed from the earth, and they're good for you.

3 medium parsnips, peeled
2 medium yams, peeled
1 medium butternut squash, peeled
3 tablespoons extra-virgin olive oil
1 tablespoon unsalted butter or
 extra-virgin olive oil

1 cup filtered water
1 teaspoon herbal sea salt
2 tablespoons fresh rosemary leaves
 or 2 teaspoons dried

1. Cut parsnips, yams, and squash into bite-size pieces.
2. In a large sauté pan, place the parsnips with oil, butter, water, and herbal salt. Bring to a boil, covered, and cook over high heat for 5 to 7 minutes.
3. Add yams and squash. Return to a boil, then reduce heat to medium-low and continue cooking, covered, for 10 to 15 minutes. As the water evaporates, the vegetables will begin to caramelize and brown.
4. Add the rosemary, stir, and cook several minutes longer.
5. Serve hot or at room temperature.

SUGGESTED ACCOMPANIMENTS: Escarole and Kidney Bean Soup; Delicious Fish Croquettes; Bulgur, Green Bean, and Walnut Pilaf; and slices of fresh fruit.

★★★   VITAMIN A, VITAMIN C
 ★   FOLIC ACID, MANGANESE, POTASSIUM, MAGNESIUM

During the holidays you can usually find sweet potatoes, which can be a nice substitution for the yams. Winter squash, such as buttercup and Hubbard, will go nicely, also. This type of dish gives your palate lots of sweet-tasting vegetables, and often when this is included in a meal, dessert isn't as tempting.

⚜

❧ Broccoli with Currants ❧

Yield: 2 quarts   (4 generous servings plus extra)

Broccoli contains chromium, a mineral essential for keeping your blood sugar stable. When this lowers, your energy and spirits can also drop.

2 red or Spanish onions, peeled
½ cup filtered water or vegetable stock (see recipe)
1 bunch broccoli, preferably with thin stalks
½ cup dried currants
¼ teaspoon oregano

¼ teaspoon marjoram
¼ teaspoon sea salt
½ cup apple juice
2 teaspoons arrowroot or 1 teaspoon kuzu
2 tablespoons extra-virgin olive oil or flax seed oil (optional)

1. Slice onions into ¼-inch rings.
2. In a large sauté pan, heat water over high heat. Add onions. Reduce to medium heat, cover, and cook 5 minutes.
3. Using a paring knife, remove florets from broccoli stalks. Trim or peel stalks of their woody outside and slice into thin diagonal pieces. Add stalks to pan with currants, oregano, marjoram, and salt. Cover and cook 3 to 5 minutes over medium heat.
4. Cut florets into bite-size pieces, and add to pan. Cover and let steam 1 minute.
5. Mix apple juice with arrowroot and drizzle over broccoli. Cover and cook another 4 or 5 minutes, until broccoli is tender and florets are bright green.
6. Remove vegetables to a serving platter and drizzle oil over. Serve while hot.

Suggested accompaniments: Warm Lima Beans with Basil, Tomato, and Chèvre, and Kasha Loaf with Yam.

★★★　VITAMIN K, VITAMIN C, FOLIC ACID
  ★　CHROMIUM, VITAMIN A, OMEGA-3 FATTY ACIDS, VITAMIN B_6, PANTOTHENIC ACID, MAGNESIUM, MANGANESE

Diets high in refined sugar have been shown to increase the excretion of chromium, the very mineral required for sugar metabolism.

❧

❧ Baked White and Orange French Fries ❧

Yield: 4 or 5 cups   (4 generous servings)

We give you a healthy alternative to the deep-fried French fry—the baked French fry. These have crunch and golden color but little fat. Our version is two-toned because we include yams, which are full of vitamin A, as important to your immunity as vitamin C. Take a fresh-made bagful to the movies and enjoy them instead of popcorn.

3 potatoes, peeled
2 yams, peeled
1 egg, organic, free-range preferred
1 tablespoon extra-virgin olive oil

2 tablespoons prepared mustard or brown rice vinegar
Pinch sea salt (optional)

Preheat oven to 450°.

1. Cut potatoes and yams into ½-inch slabs, then cut into sticks.

2. Crack egg into a wide bowl and beat with olive oil. Toss potatoes in egg and oil, coating on all sides. Remove and place potatoes on an oiled baking sheet, spreading them out so that there is room between each stick.

3. Bake for 35 minutes, turning several times after the first 15 minutes. Fries are ready when golden.

4. Serve with mustard or a few drops of vinegar. Sprinkle with salt, if desired.

VARIATIONS: Before baking dust potatoes with chili powder or any other favorite spice.

SUGGESTED ACCOMPANIMENTS: Whole Pompano Baked with Lemon Wedges, Marinated Arame Salad with Horseradish, and Old-Fashioned Oatmeal Raisin Cookies.

★★★   VITAMIN C, POTASSIUM, VITAMIN B$_6$
  ★   COPPER, MANGANESE

The egg helps the un-fries stay moist inside and crispy outside, and lets you use less oil. When oils are heated to high temperatures, trans-fatty acids can form. We also find that the egg helps spices stick to the potatoes.

Especially during menopause, fast foods can be very depleting, so your habits may need to change. In 1994, per person, Americans ate about 30 pounds of French fries (120 4-ounce servings) and 17 pounds of chips and shoestring potatoes. Because these potato products are heated in oil to high temperatures, fried potato consumption is also a measure of the extent of poor-quality oils consumed.

Puréed Cabbage and Potatoes

Yield: 6 cups   (4 generous servings plus extra)

The cabbage-family cruciferous vegetables contain goitrogens that block iodine which your thyroid needs to function, but cooking the vegetables inactivates these compounds. If you are eating lots of cruciferous vegetables raw, also have some seaweed which supplies the iodine you may have lost. Rutabagas and turnips have the highest concentrations of goitrogens.

1 **small or ½ large green cabbage**
   Filtered water
3 **potatoes, peeled and cubed**
2 **cloves garlic**

1 **tablespoon unsalted butter**
½ **teaspoon sea salt**
½ **teaspoon herbal sea salt**
¼ **to ½ bunch parsley, minced**

1. Peel away and discard any damaged leaves from cabbage. Cut into quarters and remove core. Cut into large chunks.

2. In a medium pot, bring ½ inch water to a boil. Add cabbage and potatoes, cover, and steam 15 minutes, until the cabbage is tender and potatoes are soft. (This is our preferred method of steaming rather than using a collapsible steamer insert.)

3. Using a slotted spoon, remove cabbage and potatoes from the pot and purée in a processor or blender. Add garlic, butter, and both salts. Purée until well blended and smooth.

4. Using a rubber spatula, transfer to a serving bowl and sprinkle with parsley. (This can be mixed in, if preferred.)

VARIATIONS: This technique is also great with brussels sprouts and kohlrabi.

SUGGESTED ACCOMPANIMENTS: Persian-Style Peppers Stuffed with Lentils and Bulgur on top of Tomato Sauce, Your Basic Green Salad, and Strawberry Tart with Walnut Crust.

★★★   VITAMIN K, VITAMIN C
 ★   POTASSIUM, FOLIC ACID, VITAMIN B$_6$, COPPER

❧ Asparagus Mimosa with ❧ Lemon and Flax Seed Oil

Yield: 1 quart   (4 generous servings)

Bring out your fine china for this attractive side dish, garnished with a sprinkling of finely chopped egg. Asparagus has boron, the B vitamins, folic acid, riboflavin, thiamin, and vitamin E. Dress with flax seed oil, which has a buttery flavor.

1 **pound asparagus**
  Filtered water
  Juice of 1 lemon
2 **pinches sea salt**

2 **tablespoons flax seed oil**
1 **egg, organic and fertile preferred, hard boiled**

1. Break off woody ends and wash asparagus.
2. Pour ½ inch water in a saucepan, add asparagus, and bring to a boil, covered. Lower heat and cook 5 to 7 minutes, until asparagus is tender.
3. Remove with tongs and place on a plate. Squeeze lemon juice over asparagus, sprinkle with salt, and drizzle with flax seed oil.
4. Peel egg, and just before serving, press through a sieve over the asparagus.

SUGGESTED ACCOMPANIMENTS: Whole grain bread (for dunking into the juices), Black Bean Loaf, Chewy Wheat Berries and Barley with Rosemary, Your Basic Green Salad with Creamy Yogurt Dressing, and Broiled Maple Apples.

★★★   VITAMIN K, FOLIC ACID, OMEGA-3 FATTY ACIDS, VITAMIN C, VITAMIN E
 ★   RIBOFLAVIN, THIAMIN, LINOLEIC ACID, ZINC, BORON

❧ Plantains Sautéed in Butter ❧

Yield: 4 cups   (4 generous servings plus extra)

Discover the sweet pleasures of sautéed plantains, a Latin-American favorite. Plantains contain vitamin B_6, which helps form serotonin, the brain chemical that has a calming effect on your mood.

2 ripe plantains, peeled
½ cup filtered water

1 tablespoon unsalted butter or more
Herbal sea salt

1. In a medium pot, put plantains and water. Bring to a boil and lower flame, simmering plantains about 15 minutes.
2. Remove from water and cut into diagonal slices. Heat a sauté pan with 1 teaspoon butter. Place plantain slices in pan without crowding. Cook until golden on both sides, turning once with a spatula.
3. Remove plantains from pan to a brown bag and add more butter to pan, repeating until all slices are cooked. Keep cooked slices warm in a low oven.
4. Sprinkle with herbal salt and serve.

VARIATIONS: Sprinkle with chili powder, or sprinkle with minced raw garlic, salt, and pepper.

SUGGESTED ACCOMPANIMENTS: Serve with Persimmon Salsa, Twice-Cooked Beans Wrapped in Corn Tortillas, and Old-Fashioned Oatmeal Raisin Cookies.

★★★   VITAMIN C, VITAMIN A, VITAMIN B_6
  ★   POTASSIUM, MAGNESIUM, OMEGA-3 FATTY ACIDS

❧

In the traditional medicine of many cultures, plantains have long been used as a reliable treatment for ulcers. If you sense that the stresses of life are catching up with you, there's no harm in adding plantains to your diet. They stimulate a proliferation of cells and mucus, increasing the natural protective barrier between the acids of your stomach and the lining of your digestive tract.

❧

❧ Arame and Cabbage with Mustard Sauce ❧

Yield: 6 cups   (4 generous servings plus extra)

We combined a sea and a land vegetable to create this sophisticated dish. The seaweed supplies important B vitamins, including niacin. Niacin is not affected by heat, and cooking makes it more absorbable.

½ cup arame	½ teaspoon sea salt
2½ cups filtered water	2 tablespoons prepared grainy
1 tablespoon unrefined sesame oil	mustard
1 onion, sliced	2 tablespoons arrowroot or
½ green cabbage, cored and shredded	1 tablespoon kuzu
1 carrot, sliced diagonally	½ cup sunflower seeds, toasted

1. In a small bowl, soak arame in 2 cups of water for 10 to 15 minutes.
2. In a large sauté pan, heat oil and add onion. Cook over medium heat, uncovered, 4 to 5 minutes. Stir in cabbage, carrot, and salt. Cover and continue cooking for 5 to 10 minutes, until the cabbage has wilted and released water.
3. Lift arame from soaking water with hands and put in pan with vegetables. Discard soaking water. Stir, cover, and continue cooking 5 minutes more.
4. In a measuring cup, mix ½ cup water, mustard, and arrowroot. Add to arame and cabbage mixture, stir, and cook until sauce is clear and shiny, then cook another 30 seconds.
5. Serve with sunflower seeds sprinkled on top.

VARIATIONS: Add herbs of choice such as basil or thyme, or try using spices such as whole caraway or cumin seeds for additional flavor.

SUGGESTED ACCOMPANIMENTS: Tuscan Bread Soup with Basil Infusion, Pinto Bean and Swiss Chard Patties, and Apricot-Date-Pecan Bonbons.

★★★   VITAMIN K, LINOLEIC ACID
  ★   VITAMIN A, VITAMIN C, FOLIC ACID, THIAMIN, MAGNESIUM, CALCIUM, IRON, SELENIUM, MANGANESE, COPPER, POTASSIUM

Arame makes a dramatic garnish on top of salads, mixed with shredded carrot or jicama. It's also nice sprinkled over a bowl of thick soup. Soak it 10 to 15 minutes to soften and bring out its rich, yet mild flavor. It can be eaten as is after soaking or it can be cooked and seasoned.

❧ Gremolata Mashed Potatoes ❧

Yield: 4 cups   (4 generous servings plus extra)

If you're feeling spacy, there's nothing like eating a starchy root vegetable to bring you back to earth. For grounding, try a dish of these garlic mashed potatoes. They really work!

6 medium or large Eastern potatoes, peeled and quartered (see Note)
   Filtered water
2 tablespoons extra-virgin olive oil
1 onion, minced

4 cloves garlic, chopped coarsely
½ teaspoon basil or thyme
1 tablespoon unsalted butter
1 teaspoon herbal sea salt

1. Place potatoes in a medium pot with enough water to cover. Cover, bring to a boil, and let simmer for 15 to 25 minutes, until potatoes are soft when pierced with a fork.

2. Heat oil in a small sauté pan, add onion, garlic, and basil, and cook over medium-low heat until some parts of the onions are translucent and some are golden, about 5 minutes.

3. Remove potatoes from water with a slotted spoon, reserving water, and place in a bowl. Using a potato masher, mash into a paste. Add butter and ½ to ¾ cup potato cooking water as needed to moisten.

4. Add cooked onion-garlic mixture and herbal salt. Mix well. If desired, purée in blender or processor for a smoother texture.

NOTE: Eastern potatoes are thin-skinned, and can be substituted with red Bliss or any other thin-skinned potato. Baking or Idaho potatoes are not recommended.

SUGGESTED ACCOMPANIMENTS: Chicken Paprika with Yogurt Sauce, Bowl of Antipasto, and Fresh Blueberry Cobbler.

★★★ VITAMIN C, VITAMIN B$_6$
  ★ POTASSIUM, NIACIN, MANGANESE, MAGNESIUM, CHROMIUM

Vegetables that contain vitamin C, in descending order of concentration:

green and red peppers	mustard greens	parsley
broccoli	cabbage	oyster plant
brussels sprouts	kale	rose hips
snowpeas	potatoes	

❧ Butternut Squash Purée ❧

Yield: 1 quart   (4 generous servings plus extra)

Winter squash are effortless to cook when you bake them, and they tend to slightly caramelize on the edges, making them extra sweet. This is one of those comforting dishes you'll be glad to have when you're frazzled.

1 butternut squash (about 1½ pounds)   ¼ teaspoon sea salt
2 tablespoons unsalted butter   ½ cup unfiltered apple juice (optional)

Preheat over to 450°.
1. Cut squash in half lengthwise. Place cut side down, unseeded, on an unoiled baking sheet. Cook 45 to 60 minutes, until soft when pierced with a fork.
2. With a spoon, remove seeds and discard or save them to toast and munch on later. Scrape pulp out of skin and place in bowl of a processor or in a blender. Discard skin.
3. Add butter and salt to squash and purée until smooth. If using a blender, add up to ½ cup of apple juice, a few tablespoons at a time.

VARIATIONS: Baked yams can be used instead of, or with, squash. Steamed rutabaga or carrots can be added, up to half of volume. The purée can be made into soup:

Heat 1 teaspoon unsalted butter with 1 teaspoon curry powder and cook until foamy, about 30 seconds. Add purée and water or stock and heat, seasoning to taste.

SUGGESTED ACCOMPANIMENTS: Oven-fried Chicken with Herbs, Kasha and Red Pepper Timbales, Three-Bean Salad, and Peach Crumble.

★★★ VITAMIN A, VITAMIN C
★ FOLIC ACID, MAGNESIUM, OMEGA-3 FATTY ACIDS, THIAMIN

Winter Squash Varieties

Here's a list of winter squash that can substitute for each other. Butternut squash has always been easy to find, and now these others are becoming more common. Try them out for their sweet taste, unusual shapes, and variety of textures.

acorn	delicata	longneck
buttercup	Golden Delicious	turban
butternut	Hubbard	

When you eat foods in a range of colors, you supply yourself with a variety of nutrients. Buy fruits and vegetables that are red, orange, yellow, green, brown, and white.

❧ Collard Greens with White Onions ❧

Yield: 1 quart   (4 generous servings plus extra)

In Chinese diet therapy, leafy greens such as collards are thought to benefit the lungs because the structure of the leaf resembles the system of vessels and arteries that channel through this organ. From our western point of view, these vegetables contain potassium and folic acid, which increase our oxygen-carrying capacity. Either way, collards bring oxygen to the brain and can help clear up a menopausal muddle.

½ cup filtered water
2 tablespoons extra-virgin olive oil
1 white or Vidalia onion, sliced

1 bunch collards (about 1 to 1½ pounds)
½ teaspoon sea salt
Juice of 1 lemon

1. In a large sauté pan, add water and oil and heat over medium heat. Add onion and cook 4 to 5 minutes.
2. Wash collards, slice stems thin, and cut leaves into 1-inch pieces.
3. Add stems and salt to sauté pan, stirring well. Cover and let steam 5 to 7 minutes. Add leaves and cook uncovered, turning frequently until wilted and soft.
4. Place collards and onions in a serving bowl and add lemon juice. Toss and serve.

SUGGESTED ACCOMPANIMENTS: Shrimp and Crabmeat with Pasta, Fast Salad, and Banana Refrigerator Cake.

★★★   VITAMIN A, VITAMIN C
  ★   MANGANESE, FOLIC ACID, VITAMIN E, VITAMIN B$_6$, POTASSIUM, LINOLEIC ACID

❧ Curried Cauliflower Crown ❧

Yield: 3 cups   (4 generous servings plus extra)

Like other cruciferous vegetables, cauliflower helps block cancer. Vitamin C is the active ingredient; when it is present, it prevents nitrates from converting into nitrites, which are the chemicals present in bacon and processed meats that you're warned can cause cancer.

1 head cauliflower, leaves trimmed
1½ cups filtered water
1 tablespoon unsalted butter
2 teaspoons curry powder
¼ cup dried currants

1 tablespoon arrowroot or 2 teaspoons kuzu
¼ teaspoon herbal sea salt
¼ teaspoon black pepper

1. In a medium saucepan that will comfortably hold the cauliflower, put the vegetable with ½ cup of water. Cover and bring to a boil over high heat. Lower flame and steam until soft when pierced with a fork, about 8 to 10 minutes. Do not overcook.

2. In a small saucepan, heat butter and curry powder over medium heat until bubbly, about 1 minute. Reduce heat to low and add currants and ½ cup water.

3. Mix remaining ½ cup water with arrowroot and herbal salt. Add to pot with curry and currants. Bring to a boil over high heat, stirring constantly until thickened and clear. Cook another 30 seconds. Turn off flame and add black pepper.

4. Using a slotted spoon and tongs, carefully remove cooked cauliflower from pot and place on a serving platter or in a wide bowl. Spoon sauce over top, allowing it to drip down the sides. Serve while hot.

SUGGESTED ACCOMPANIMENTS: Indian Chicken with Lemon Slices and Onions, Red Lentil Dhal, Tomatoes Stuffed with Couscous, and Frothy Mango Lassi.

★★★   VITAMIN C, FOLIC ACID
★   VITAMIN B$_6$, PANTOTHENIC ACID, OMEGA-3 FATTY ACIDS, VITAMIN K

❧ Kale with Capers and Black Olives ❧

Yield: 1 quart   (4 generous servings plus extra)

If you now need glasses for driving at night, foods with beta-carotene are for you. In your body beta-carotene converts to vitamin A, which becomes part of your photoreceptor cells that allow you to see light and dark.

3 tablespoons extra-virgin olive oil	2 tablespoons capers
1 onion, sliced	½ cup black or Greek olives, pitted
1 teaspoon oregano	Juice of 1 lemon
1 teaspoon thyme	Sea salt
1 bunch kale	

1. Heat a heavy-bottomed sauté pan with 2 tablespoons olive oil. Add onion, oregano, and thyme, stir, and cook 3 or 4 minutes. Add washed kale, cover, and bring to steaming over medium-high heat. Lower flame and, after the kale has wilted, remove cover. Stir several times, cooking about 10 to 15 minutes.

2. Add capers and cook uncovered for another minute.

3. Remove to a serving bowl and toss with remaining 1 tablespoon of olive oil, olives, lemon juice, and salt. Serve hot or at room temperature.

VARIATIONS: For a spicy taste, serve with a shaker of red-pepper flakes or hot sauce on the side.

SUGGESTED ACCOMPANIMENTS: Venison Shish Kebab, Carrot and Cabbage Slaw with Fresh Fennel, and Peach Crumble.

★★★   VITAMIN A, VITAMIN C, VITAMIN K
★   VITAMIN E, OMEGA-3 FATTY ACIDS, FOLIC ACID, VITAMIN B_6, MANGANESE, CALCIUM, MAGNESIUM, POTASSIUM, THIAMIN

> The best way to buy olives is at a store that has an assortment, where you can ask to taste them. If they have been cured too long and taste of too much salt or vinegar, when you get home, store them in water, which will leach these out. If they are still salty after one or two days, change the water again. Store in refrigerator.

Beta-carotene is actually a pigment, the color orange, as in carrots, but green vegetables also contain beta-carotene. It's just that you can't see it, because the color is covered up by the green chlorophyll.

The green vegetables with beta-carotene, ranked in order of concentration:

parsley	bok choy
broccoli	asparagus
scallion	

Leafy greens:

lamb's quarters	collards
spinach	beet greens
dandelion	mustard
turnip	chicory
kale	carrot greens

❧ French Carrots and Parsnips ❧

Yield: 5 cups   (4 generous servings plus extra)

Keep those carrot tops—they're on the menu for women—and by chopping both top and root, with little effort you'll create a vegetable dish with two brightly contrasting colors. Carrots are part of the parsley family and their greens are pleasantly mild tasting. The tops become your leafy green vegetable for the meal.

½ cup filtered water
4 carrots with tops, sliced diagonally, tops removed and reserved (see Note)

2 parsnips or parsley roots, sliced diagonally
2 tablespoons unsalted butter
¼ teaspoon sea salt

1. In a medium saucepan, bring water to a boil. Add carrots and parsnips. Cover and steam until tender, about 10 minutes.
2. Chop carrot greens fine. Put in a bowl and set aside.
3. Pour off carrot and parsnip cooking water, keeping the vegetables in the pot.

4. Place saucepan over low heat and add butter and salt, stirring to coat carrots and parsnips. Add minced carrot tops, stir again, and cook 1 minute. Place in a serving bowl and eat while hot.

NOTE: You can substitute parsley or cilantro for the carrot tops.

SUGGESTED ACCOMPANIMENTS: Poached Salmon Steaks with Tarragon, Wild Rice Ring, and Apricot-Date-Pecan Bonbons.

★★★   VITAMIN A, VITAMIN K, VITAMIN C
★   MAGNESIUM, FOLIC ACID, POTASSIUM, IRON, MANGANESE

Raw food gives you crunch and fiber, and living enzymes, but some foods are better eaten cooked. The carotenoids in carrots that convert to vitamin A in your body are more available once the carrot has been heated and softened.

❧ Crusty Baked Tomatoes Topped ❧ with Sunflower Seeds

Yield: 6 halves   (4 servings plus extra)

Eating vegetables when they are in season gives you the most nutrients and the best flavor. Tomatoes are at their peak in summer and early fall, and their mealy off-season counterparts are no substitute.

3 ripe beefsteak tomatoes
¼ cup filtered water
2 tablespoons extra-virgin olive oil or unsalted butter

½ cup whole wheat bread crumbs, plain or seasoned
½ teaspoon herbal sea salt
2 tablespoons sunflower seeds

1. Cut tomatoes in half crosswise (around the diameter). In a wide skillet over medium-low heat, heat water and olive oil. Place tomato halves in skillet, cut side down. Cover pan and cook over medium heat for 5 minutes.

2. Using a metal spatula and a fork to keep tomato from slipping, flip each tomato. Sprinkle cut sides with bread crumbs, herbal salt, and seeds (don't worry if some of these fall into the pan). Tilt skillet, and with a large spoon lift several spoonfuls of the liquid from bottom of pan onto each tomato half. Cover and cook 4 to 5 minutes, until sunflower seeds are moist and tomatoes are soft and the skins begin to split or slip down.

3. Remove tomatoes to a serving plate, seed side up.

VARIATIONS: Instead of sunflower seeds, try chopped pecans or walnuts.

SUGGESTED ACCOMPANIMENTS: Smelts Sautéed in Butter; Composed Salad of Oranges, Avocado, and Endive; and Poached Pears in Ginger-Kuzu Sauce.

★★★   VITAMIN C, LINOLEIC ACID
  ★   THIAMIN, SELENIUM, MANGANESE, VITAMIN K, VITAMIN E

❧ Artichokes Stuffed with Garlic Bread Crumbs ❧

Yield: 5 artichokes   (4 generous servings plus extra)

Globe artichokes are a wonderful menopause vegetable because of the range of vitamins and minerals they contain. Already-cooked artichokes are a great snack break, munched leaf by leaf.

5 globe artichokes
1 cup whole wheat bread crumbs
½ bunch parsley, minced
3 cloves garlic, minced

½ teaspoon sea salt
¼ cup extra-virgin olive oil
1 cup filtered water, more as needed

1. To prepare artichokes: Cut off stem and ¼ to ½ inch of the bottom of the globe and set aside. Cut off top and discard. Discard the tough bottom row of outer leaves. Open up core by pulling leaves apart from one another to expose center spiny area. With a grapefruit knife or a spoon, remove the light-colored core and discard. Peel stem, removing woody exterior and leaves. Repeat with remaining artichokes. Place artichokes and stems in a medium pot.

2. In a small bowl mix together bread crumbs, parsley, garlic, and salt. Spoon several tablespoons of bread crumbs into the center of each artichoke. Drizzle olive oil on each.

3. Pour water into pot alongside the artichokes and bring to a boil, covered. Lower heat and cook about 30 minutes. Check once or twice to see if the water has evaporated, and add more if necessary.

4. Using a spatula and a fork, carefully turn each artichoke over onto the bread-crumb side. Cover pot and continue cooking for 15 minutes, until crumbs have soaked up liquid and are slightly golden. Artichokes should be tender when a fork is inserted.

5. Remove artichokes to a serving platter and serve hot or at room temperature.

EATING INSTRUCTIONS: Artichokes are meant to be eaten with your fingers. Pull off a leaf and scrape it with your teeth to extract the soft area at the bottom inside part of the leaf. When you reach the core, there will be a fuzzy part that will detach easily from the heart. Remove this and discard. Now that you've reached the heart, eat it slowly and savor its unique taste. The stems taste very much like the hearts, without all of the effort!

SUGGESTED ACCOMPANIMENTS: Polenta with Wild Mushroom Sauce, Cannellini and Kidney Beans with Rosemary, and Frozen Banana Maple-Walnut Whip.

★★★ VITAMIN K, FOLIC ACID, VITAMIN C, MAGNESIUM, IRON, MANGANESE, COPPER, VITAMIN E

★ POTASSIUM, OMEGA-3 FATTY ACIDS

❦ 11 ❦
Fish and Shellfish

Grilled Fresh Sardines, Portuguese Style
Swordfish Steaks Marinated in Curry Powder Rub
Broiled Mackerel in Lime Juice
Whole Pompano Baked with Lemon Wedges
Delicious Fish Croquettes
Chinese Steamed Whitefish with Fresh Coriander
Smelts Sautéed in Butter
Poached Salmon Steaks with Tarragon
Flounder Rolls Stuffed with Salmon and Lemon
Bluefish Marinated in Plum Vinegar
Russian Whiting
Shrimp and Crabmeat with Pasta
Soft-Shell Crabs
Steamed Scallops Seviche Style
Oyster-Pot Stew
Bouillabaisse Brimming with Greens
Broiled Oysters on the Half Shell with Caviar

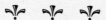

❧

In the Far East, fish contributes almost 30 percent of the protein in the average diet, while fish makes up only about 7 percent of protein intake for Americans. Fish is a wonderful source of minerals, including potassium, iodine, zinc, and copper, plus omega-3 fatty acids, all in low amounts in the standard American diet.

There are three categories of fish—freshwater, saltwater, and shellfish. They each differ slightly in nutritional value, freshwater fish supplying magnesium, phosphorus, iron, and copper and saltwater fish and shellfish providing high amounts of iodine, fluorine, and cobalt. While the unsaturated fat content of fish and shellfish changes depending on the season and species, fatty fish such as mackerel, halibut, and salmon are good sources of vitamins A and D year round.

Shellfish are high in cholesterol, but many types—particularly crab, scallops, clams, mussels, and lobster—are actually slightly lower in cholesterol than chicken. And although shrimp and crayfish have about twice as much cholesterol as meat, they contain much less fat and most of it is unsaturated.

Fish and shellfish are available fresh, frozen, salted, dried, canned, and smoked. Although we prefer fresh fish and shellfish to any other kind, you do need to handle it with special care so the possibility of bacterial infection remains low. Purchase fish and shellfish as a last errand on your way home, making sure that the items do not stay unrefrigerated for more than a half hour. In the warm weather, have the fish packed in ice. Once home, place the fish and shellfish in the back of the refrigerator and use the same day or within 24 hours.

Buying Fresh Fish: What to Look For

1. Whole fish:
   skin glistens, scales intact;
   gills are red or pink (not gray,
   brown, or green); eyes are firm
   and convex (not sunken);
   flesh is somewhat resistant
   when gently pressed

2. Fillets:
   luminous and translucent;
   firm and elastic to the touch

3. The fish store should not smell
   very fishy.

Concerns about the effect of polluted water on fish and shellfish are very legitimate in these times. For safety's sake, eat a variety of species of fish and shellfish and have these just two or three times a week.

❧ Grilled Fresh Sardines, Portuguese Style ❧

Yield: 10 sardines   (4 generous servings plus extra)

The beauty of sardines, even fresh ones, is that you can eat them whole, calcium- and magnesium-rich bones and all, giving you minerals which your own bones need for repairing and rebuilding.

10 whole sardines, cleaned, with head
     and tail intact
3 lemons

1 teaspoon sea salt
10 metal or wooden skewers
     (see Note)

1. Using two skewers side by side, an inch or two apart, skewer two sardines, one at a time, leaving at least ½ inch between sardines. Repeat with the remaining sardines.

2. Place in a stainless-steel or enamel baking pan. Squeeze the juice of 2 lemons over, and sprinkle with salt.

3. Broil until browned on one side. Then, holding both skewers, carefully turn over and broil on the other side, about 5 to 7 minutes total, depending on the size of the sardines. The sardines will start to fall apart and will be flaky when cooked.

4. Serve each person their own set of skewered sardines with remaining lemon cut into wedges.

NOTE: If using wooden skewers, soak in water for at least 30 minutes before skewering fish, to keep skewers from burning under the broiler.

SUGGESTED ACCOMPANIMENTS: French Carrots and Parsnips, Your Basic Green Salad, and Frozen Banana Maple-Walnut Whip.

★★★   VITAMIN B_{12}, OMEGA-3 FATTY ACIDS
★   VITAMIN C, MANGANESE, PHOSPHORUS, ZINC, PANTOTHENIC ACID, MAGNESIUM, CALCIUM, POTASSIUM, IRON, COPPER, VITAMIN B_6

❧

There is really no substitute for the taste of fresh sardines, which is why we recommend them over canned. When canned sardines are the only choice, we prefer sardines canned in water over those in oil. Choose the variety with the bones and skin.

❧

❧ Swordfish Steaks Marinated in ❧ Curry Powder Rub

Yield: 4 generous servings

The essential fatty acids found in fish can help maintain beautiful skin. The wonderful fish oils originate in the algae and plankton of the sea, which is eaten by fish and, finally, you.

1 pound swordfish steaks

CURRY POWDER RUB (also see chart opposite)**:**

2 tablespoons turmeric
1 teaspoon ground ginger
1 teaspoon ground coriander

¼ teaspoon ground cloves
Pinch asafetida or hing (see box)

1. Wash fish in cold water and put into an enamel or stainless-steel baking pan. Mix together all ingredients of curry rub and sprinkle on both sides of fish, using all of the rub.

2. Place in refrigerator for 25 to 45 minutes, depending upon the thickness of the fish steak. Preheat oven to 350°.

3. Using a butter knife, scrape off excess rub. Bake or broil until fish begins to flake when tested with a fork—about 20 to 30 minutes if baked, or 10 to 20 minutes if broiled, depending upon the thickness. Turn once during cooking.

VARIATIONS: Substitute flounder, halibut, or salmon—either steaks or fillet.

SUGGESTED ACCOMPANIMENTS: Spring Greens Potage with Asparagus, Curried Cauliflower Crown, Raisin-Ginger Chutney, tomato slices with sea salt and pepper, and Crispy Walnut and Seed Bars.

★★★   VITAMIN B$_{12}$, NIACIN, OMEGA-3 FATTY ACIDS
  ★   PHOSPHORUS, VITAMIN B$_6$, IRON, MAGNESIUM, ZINC, POTASSIUM, RIBOFLAVIN, COPPER, MANGANESE

Asafetida, which is also known as hing, bonds the flavors in curry and is considered to have a truffle-like taste when cooked. It comes as a powder and one small container will last many years. Don't be frightened off by the smell!

This handy guide will help you build a variety of curry powders—plain, sweet, or spicy and hot. Add anywhere from a couple of pinches to several teaspoons of the additional spices to the curry base. For expediency, create your own mix and store it in a covered jar for easy use.

For marinating times see page 259.

Curry Powder Base

2 tablespoons turmeric
1 tablespoon cumin
1 tablespoon ground ginger
2 teaspoons ground coriander
1 teaspoon fenugreek
pinch asafetida (hing)

Sweet Spice Additions

cinnamon
cardamom
cloves
allspice
nutmeg

Hot and Spicy Additions

cayenne
freshly ground black pepper
freshly ground white pepper
fresh ginger
chili powder
dry mustard
red-pepper flakes

❧ Broiled Mackerel in Lime Juice ❧

Yield: 4 generous servings

Animal foods, especially fish, are high in phosphorus—important for healthy nerves, mental agility, and the metabolizing of food. With the high meat, dairy, and soda intake of the standard American diet, phosphorus deficiency is rare and not a concern in menopause. (In fact, too much phosphorus is more of a problem for us.) Really fresh mackerel is a treat, but it's important to buy it and eat it within 24 hours—the rule we follow for all fish dinners.

1　**1-pound mackerel, cleaned and split down center (butterflied), with head**
½　**cup lime or lemon juice plus 1 lime or lemon cut into wedges**

1　**teaspoon salted plum vinegar (umeboshi)**
¼　**teaspoon sea salt**

1. Wash fish in cold water. Place mackerel skin side up in a stainless-steel or enamel pan.

2. Mix lime juice, plum vinegar, and salt. Pour over mackerel. Lift fish up slightly to allow marinade to run under it. Cover and marinate for 1 hour, refrigerated, spooning marinade over fish after 30 minutes.

3. Broil about 7 to 10 minutes, spooning marinade over top every 2 minutes. Be careful that the skin does not burn. Do not turn over.

4. Serve immediately with lime wedges.

Suggested accompaniments: Puréed Cabbage and Potatoes, French Carrots and Parsnips, and Carob Cake with Walnuts.

★★★　VITAMIN B$_{12}$, OMEGA-3 FATTY ACIDS, VITAMIN C, VITAMIN B$_6$, PHOSPHORUS
　★　PANTOTHENIC ACID, NIACIN, RIBOFLAVIN, THIAMIN, POTASSIUM, MAGNESIUM

❧ Whole Pompano Baked with Lemon Wedges ❧

Yield: 4 generous servings

You may have heard that fish is a brain food and indeed it is. The brain is about 60 percent fat and the most abundant are the polyunsaturated omega-3 fatty acids. The oilier the fish, the more fat there is; it's concentrated around the gills, fins, and belly, so eat all the parts. And when you use lemons, you add bioflavonoids, which help balance your estrogen.

3 teaspoons extra-virgin olive oil
1½ to 2 pounds whole pompano, cleaned with head intact

1 teaspoon herbal sea salt
1 teaspoon oregano
1 or 2 lemons, organic preferred

Preheat oven to 350°.

1. Drizzle 1 teaspoon of oil into a stainless-steel or enamel baking pan large enough to comfortably fit fish. Wash fish in cold water and place in pan.

2. Using a sharp knife, make four or five slits, about 2 inches long, evenly spaced across the body of the fish. Sprinkle salt and oregano in the slits and on the inside cavity of the fish. Drizzle remaining 2 teaspoons of oil on fish.

3. Cut lemon in half, lengthwise. Squeeze one half over top and inside, and leave inside the fish. Cut the other half into four or five pieces and press these into the slits, rind side up.

4. Bake for 20 to 30 minutes, until a fork can slide in easily when inserted.

5. Place on a serving platter and serve immediately. Extra lemon wedges may be offered.

VARIATIONS: Red snapper, talapia, porgy, and flounder are among the more common ones we choose.

SUGGESTED ACCOMPANIMENTS: Gremolata Mashed Potatoes, Mesclun Salad, and Banana Refrigerator Cake.

★★★ VITAMIN B_{12}, OMEGA-3 FATTY ACIDS, PHOSPHORUS, NIACIN, POTASSIUM, PANTOTHENIC ACID

★ VITAMIN B_6, MAGNESIUM, THIAMIN, RIBOFLAVIN

❧ **Delicious Fish Croquettes** ❧

Yield: 8 croquettes   (4 generous servings)

Both the fish and the whole wheat bread crumbs contain selenium, a mineral linked to a lower rate of heart disease because it helps keep arteries free of plaque. This is a good recipe to have when you tire of eating fish fillets.

1 **pound fish fillets, salmon, cod or scrod, turbot, catfish, or flounder**
2 **stalks celery, quartered**
2 **scallions**
1 **egg, organic, free-range preferred**
1 **tablespoon prepared mustard**
2¾ **cups whole wheat bread crumbs**

½ **teaspoon sea salt**
½ **teaspoon brown rice vinegar or cider vinegar**
¼ **teaspoon oregano**
⅛ **teaspoon thyme**
Pinch cayenne or white pepper
1 **lemon, cut into wedges**

1. Check fillets for small bones by running fingers over them. Wash and place in the bowl of a processor or chop fine. Add celery, scallions, egg, mustard, ¾ cup bread crumbs, salt, vinegar, oregano, thyme, and cayenne. Blend until smooth.

2. Pour remaining 2 cups bread crumbs into a small, shallow bowl. Using a small bowl of water to keep hands wet, mold fish mixture into patties or balls. Put patty in bowl with bread crumbs and turn to coat all over. Arrange on a buttered baking pan. Repeat until all the fish mixture is used.

3. Broil 4 to 5 minutes on each side, until golden. (Or bake 20 minutes at 350°, turning once.)

4. Serve with lemon wedges.

Suggested accompaniments: Classic Potato Salad Revisited, Asparagus Mimosa with Lemon and Flax Seed Oil, Fresh Summer Fruit Compote.

★★★ SELENIUM, VITAMIN B_{12}, OMEGA-3 FATTY ACIDS, MANGANESE, VITAMIN K, PHOSPHORUS, MAGNESIUM, NIACIN

★ FOLIC ACID, THIAMIN, IRON, VITAMIN D, RIBOFLAVIN, PANTOTHENIC ACID, VITAMIN B_6

The essential fatty acids in fish oils deteriorate easily. To insure you're eating the freshest, choose fish in this order: fresh-caught fish first, fresh farm-raised fish second, and quick-frozen fish third.

Chinese Steamed Whitefish with Fresh Coriander

Yield: 4 servings

We emphasize eating whole foods because you have a better chance of getting all the nutrients nature provides. By cooking fish whole you protect the somewhat fragile essential fatty acids from light and oxygen and at the same time create a showy presentation dish as we do here—a whole fish on a platter adorned with stems of lacy green coriander.

1½ pounds whole fish or 1 pound fish
    fillets (see Note)
    Sea salt
 4 scallions or spring onions, sliced
    thin
 1 1-inch piece fresh ginger, cut into
    fine matchsticks or minced

 2 cloves garlic, slivered
 2 tablespoons shoyu soy sauce
 1 tablespoon unrefined sesame oil
 2 tablespoons dark sesame oil
10 to 15 fresh coriander leaves
    (cilantro)

1. Wash fish or fillets in cold water, sprinkle with salt, place on a dish, and let sit in refrigerator, covered, 30 minutes.

2. Wash salt off fish. Heat a wok (or frying pan) with 2 cups water. Place fish on a plate and, using wok stand or two chopsticks, put plate in wok, over water. Spread scallions, ginger, and garlic over the fish. Sprinkle with soy sauce and unrefined sesame oil.

3. Cover and steam until flesh flakes, about 10 to 15 minutes, depending upon thickness of fish.

4. Carefully remove fish to a serving platter and season with dark sesame oil; top with coriander leaves.

NOTE: For the whole fish you may choose flounder, blackfish, sea bass, sole, fluke, pompano, red snapper.

SUGGESTED ACCOMPANIMENTS: Sesame Salad with Buckwheat Noodles and Fresh Coriander, and steamed broccoli with Teriyaki Marinade.

★★★ VITAMIN B$_{12}$, OMEGA-3 FATTY ACIDS
★ VITAMIN K, VITAMIN B$_6$, LINOLEIC ACID, RIBOFLAVIN, PHOSPHORUS, MAGNESIUM, POTASSIUM, MANGANESE

Since dark sesame oil can deteriorate with heat (it's already been toasted), we first cook the fish and then add the oil, which lends a regal flavor.

⚜ Smelts Sautéed in Butter ⚜

Yield: 4 generous servings

Smelts are convenient quick foods because it is not necessary to fillet or debone them—even the backbone is soft enough to eat. The bones give you calcium, which helps lower high blood pressure and elevated fats in the blood, both indicators of potential heart disease. The oil in smelts is also very high in heart-healthy monounsaturates. Think of it as olive oil from the sea.

16 smelts, cleaned, with head and tail intact (about 1 pound)
½ cup whole wheat flour or hi-lysine cornmeal

½ teaspoon sea salt
4 to 5 tablespoons unsalted butter
1 lemon, cut into wedges

1. Wash smelts in cold water. Place flour or cornmeal and salt in a wide bowl and mix well. Dust a few fish at a time in the flour. Set aside on a dish. Repeat with remaining fish.

2. Melt 2 tablespoons butter in a large skillet over medium heat. Place several fish in pan (do not crowd pan) and cook until golden on both sides, 4 to 5 minutes, turn-

ing once. Remove fish to brown paper, melt 2 more tablespoons butter, and continue until all fish are cooked.

3. Remove smelts from paper to a serving platter. Serve immediately with lemon.

SUGGESTED ACCOMPANIMENTS: Roasted Potatoes with Rosemary, Fast Salad of escarole and grated carrots, and Light Lemon Pudding Parfait with Kiwi Slices.

★★★ VITAMIN B_{12}, OMEGA-3 FATTY ACIDS, MANGANESE, PHOSPHOROUS, CALCIUM, MAGNESIUM

★ PANTOTHENIC ACID, ZINC, SELENIUM, NIACIN, IRON

✤ Poached Salmon Steaks with Tarragon ✤

Yield: 4 generous servings

Salmon is high in vitamin D, which helps to limit phosphorus and increase the absorption of calcium, minerals that must be in balance for bone health.

4 salmon steaks, ½ inch thick	**1 teaspoon tarragon**
(about 4 to 5 ounces each)	**½ teaspoon herbal sea salt**
½ cup filtered water	**1 lemon, cut into wedges**

1. Wash salmon in cold water and place in a large skillet with filtered water. Sprinkle with tarragon and herbal salt.

2. Heat on high, covered, and when steaming, lower to medium heat. Cook about 5 to 8 minutes, until fish flakes when a fork is inserted. Do not overcook.

3. Using a metal spatula, remove the steaks to individual plates. Serve immediately with lemon wedges.

SUGGESTED ACCOMPANIMENTS: Wild Rice Ring with Wild Mushroom Sauce, Artichokes Stuffed with Garlic Bread Crumbs, Carrot and Cabbage Slaw with Fresh Fennel, and Apricot-Cashew "Mousse."

★★★ VITAMIN D, VITAMIN B_{12}, NIACIN, SELENIUM, OMEGA-3 FATTY ACIDS

★ VITAMIN E, VITAMIN B_6, PANTOTHENIC ACID, VITAMIN C, THIAMIN, POTASSIUM, MAGNESIUM, IRON

Fish with high amounts of essential fatty acids, ranked in order of concentration from highest:

fish roe	sardines
mackerel	salmon
anchovies	tuna
herring	

Fish with moderate amounts:

turbot	oysters
shark	swordfish
bluefish	pompano
striped bass	

❧ Flounder Rolls Stuffed with ❧ Salmon and Lemon

Yield: 8 rolls   (4 generous servings)

If you're making an effort to eat fish, but fillets have become boring, wrap this flounder around some colorful salmon and you'll have a new dish. This presentation turns a family meal into dinner-party food.

3 tablespoons extra-virgin olive oil
8 Dover sole or flounder fillets
1 4-inch salmon fillet, cut into 8 strips
   Herbal sea salt

2 lemons, organic preferred, each cut into 8 wedges
4 teaspoons unsalted butter, cut into 8 pieces

Preheat oven to 350°.

1. Drizzle 1 tablespoon olive oil on the bottom of a baking dish. Wash sole and salmon and pat dry with a paper towel.

2. Lay one fillet down on a plate and cover with one strip of salmon, a sprinkle of herbal salt, one lemon wedge, and ½ teaspoon butter. Roll wide end toward narrow end and place rolled end down in a baking dish. If you like, the rolls can be fastened with a toothpick. Repeat with remaining fillets.

3. Drizzle remaining 2 tablespoons olive oil over top of rolled fillets. Place in oven and bake 15 to 20 minutes, until fish flakes.

4. Serve immediately with extra lemon wedges on the side.

SUGGESTED ACCOMPANIMENTS: Millet-Rice with Green Beans and Tomatoes, Marinated Arame Salad with Horseradish, and fresh apple slices.

★★★ OMEGA-3 FATTY ACIDS, VITAMIN B_{12}, VITAMIN E
★ VITAMIN D, VITAMIN C, SELENIUM, LINOLEIC ACID, VITAMIN K

❧ Bluefish Marinated in Plum Vinegar ❧

Yield: 4 generous servings

Fish dishes such as this broiled bluefish have enough fat to be satisfying but are still a low-calorie source of protein—a good choice if you've put on more pounds than you want at menopause.

1 **pound bluefish fillets**	2 **cloves garlic, sliced**
½ **cup filtered water**	2 **slices fresh ginger**
¼ **cup salted plum vinegar (umeboshi)**	1 **bay leaf**

1. Wash fillets in cold water and place in a medium stainless-steel or enamel pan.

2. In a measuring cup, put water, plum vinegar, garlic, ginger, and bay leaf. Mix well and pour over fish. Using a fork, raise fish on both sides so that the marinade runs under. Place in refrigerator and marinate at least 30 minutes.

3. Broil on medium heat until fish flakes, about 12 to 15 minutes.

SUGGESTED ACCOMPANIMENTS: Hungarian Pasta with Cabbage; Fast Salad of endive, scallions, and red radishes; and Beverly's Cantaloupe with Freshly Grated Ginger.

★★★ VITAMIN B_{12}, OMEGA-3 FATTY ACIDS, NIACIN, VITAMIN B_6, PHOSPHORUS
★ VITAMIN A, MAGNESIUM, VITAMIN K, ZINC, PANTOTHENIC ACID, RIBOFLAVIN

⚜ Russian Whiting ⚜

Yield: 4 generous servings plus extra

Both vitamin A and the oils in fish are required for vision, and whiting is a great source of both. Leftovers are terrific served cold the next day; try them with a few tablespoons of yogurt on the side.

1 tablespoon extra-virgin olive oil
2 onions, chopped
2 cloves garlic, minced
2 carrots, chopped
2 stalks celery, chopped
4 ripe beefsteak or 8 plum tomatoes, seeded
½ bunch dill, stems removed

½ teaspoon sea salt
A few grinds freshly ground black pepper
½ cup whole wheat bread crumbs
½ teaspoon herbal sea salt
1 pound whiting fillets
2 tablespoons unsalted butter

1. In a large sauté pan, heat olive oil and add onions, garlic, carrots, celery, tomatoes, dill, salt, and pepper. Simmer covered for 30 to 40 minutes, stirring occasionally.

2. Mix bread crumbs and herbal salt in a wide bowl. Wash fillets in cold water, and then coat with crumbs. Set on a plate.

3. Heat a heavy-bottomed frying pan (preferably cast iron) and melt 1 tablespoon butter. In several batches, gently cook fillets in pan on medium-low heat, turning once, until golden on both sides. Add more butter as needed. Remove to a brown paper bag to drain.

4. To serve, place fillets on a serving platter. Spoon tomato and vegetable sauce on top and serve hot.

SUGGESTED ACCOMPANIMENTS: Broiled Oysters on the Half Shell with Caviar, Easy Onion and Pepper Slices, and fresh raspberries, strawberries, and blueberries.

★★★ VITAMIN A, VITAMIN B$_{12}$, OMEGA-3 FATTY ACIDS, VITAMIN C, PHOSPHORUS
★ FOLIC ACID, MANGANESE, VITAMIN B$_6$, VITAMIN K, POTASSIUM

❧ Shrimp and Crabmeat with Pasta ❧

Yield: 6 cups   (4 generous servings)

Cooking shellfish the way we do in this recipe allows you to keep all of the nutrients and flavors because their juices become the sauce. Serve in individual broad-rimmed earthenware bowls and sprinkle some chopped parsley around the edges, making a showy presentation for company.

½ to ¾ pound shrimp
2 quarts filtered water
1 teaspoon sea salt
8 ounces quinoa or spelt pasta
1 cup shrimp stock (see Notes)
½ teaspoon marjoram or other herb of choice

½ teaspoon herbal sea salt
½ pound fresh crabmeat (or 1 container frozen)
Fresh black pepper
2 tablespoons extra-virgin olive oil or flax seed oil
¼ bunch parsley, chopped coarsely

1. Shell and clean shrimp. Set aside, saving shells for stock, if desired.

2. In a large stockpot bring water and salt to a boil.

3. Add pasta and cook, uncovered, according to package directions.

4. In a medium sauté pan, heat stock to a boil. Add marjoram and herbal salt. Cook over high heat about 10 minutes, reducing stock to about half.

5. Stir in shrimp and crabmeat. Cook, uncovered, 3 to 4 minutes, until shrimp turns pink. Add several grinds of fresh pepper.

6. Drain pasta in a colander. Place in a large serving bowl or platter.

7. Pour shrimp, crab, and stock over pasta. Drizzle with oil and sprinkle parsley on top. Serve immediately.

NOTES: 1. To clean shrimp: Pull off outer shell and set aside for stock (see below). Using a paring knife, cut through back of shrimp, exposing the vein. Remove vein, wash area, and proceed with recipe.

2. A fast fish stock can easily be made from shrimp shells. Place shells in a small pot with 2 cups water. Cover and bring to a boil. Uncover and cook 5 minutes, strain, and use. An alternative vegetarian stock can be made by dissolving 1 tablespoon white miso or 1 teaspoon herbal sea salt in 1 cup filtered water.

VARIATIONS: Leftover Shrimp and Crabmeat with Pasta is great used as an appetizer or side dish for your next meal. Or add water, sea salt, and an herb and have a quick bowl of nutritious soup.

SUGGESTED ACCOMPANIMENTS: Leafy Greens Vietnamese Style and steamed carrots.

★★★ VITAMIN B$_{12}$, OMEGA-3 FATTY ACIDS, SELENIUM, MANGANESE, PHOSPHORUS
★ MAGNESIUM, NIACIN, COPPER, FOLIC ACID, THIAMIN, VITAMIN D, VITAMIN K, ZINC

❧ Soft-Shell Crabs ❧

Yield: 4 delicious servings

These special crabs are a delicacy. Because you eat them in their entirety, including the shell and legs, these crabs are a good source of calcium, which is in these parts. A deficiency in calcium can cause irritability and insomnia. The fresh crabs are available May through September, primarily in areas near the sea.

1 cup hi-lysine corn flour or meal
1 teaspoon herbal sea salt
1 teaspoon basil
4 soft-shell crabs (see opposite)

2 tablespoons unsalted butter
2 tablespoons extra-virgin olive oil
Juice of 2 lemons, plus 1 lemon cut into wedges

1. Mix the corn flour, herbal salt, and basil in a wide bowl. Wash the crabs in cold water and toss to coat with corn mixture. Set aside on a plate until all crabs are coated.

2. In a large sauté pan (large enough to fit all the crabs at once), heat the butter and olive oil. Add crabs and cook over medium heat until crabs start to turn pink and white. (Use a spatter shield or stand far back, as the pan will sometimes spit hot oil as the crabs cook.) Carefully turn over and cook on the other side, about a total of 7 to 10 minutes.

3. Pour lemon juice all over crabs and immediately cover and steam for 2 minutes. Serve immediately with lemon wedges.

VARIATIONS: If there are any left over, they make a great sandwich with mustard and a pickle on the side.

SUGGESTED ACCOMPANIMENTS: Vongole and Linguini, romaine and red-onion salad, steamed fresh corn, and Apricot-Cashew "Mousse."

★★★ VITAMIN B$_{12}$
★ CALCIUM, VITAMIN C, IRON

Purchase soft-shell crabs as your last errand, let the fishmonger clean them for you (the eyes and gills are removed), and immediately go home and refrigerate them. They should be used the same day they are purchased, preferably within hours, because they spoil quickly. One large crab will feed one person. If they are small or medium-sized, 1½ or 2 crabs per person may be required, depending upon the diners' appetites.

❧ Steamed Scallops Seviche Style ❧

Yield: 1 quart   (4 generous servings plus extra)

Here's a traditional hot-weather dish from far south of the border, good for summer or a day of hot flashes. Seviche is traditionally "cooked" by letting the raw fish sit in lime juice for 6 to 12 hours. To be safe, we've lightly steamed the scallops and then let them marinate in the juices and flavorings.

Juice of 2 limes
Juice of 2 lemons
½ cup filtered water
1 pound bay scallops
2 cloves garlic, minced
½ bunch parsley, chopped

3 tablespoons extra-virgin olive oil
½ teaspoon sea salt
Several grinds fresh pepper
½ red or green pepper, seeded and minced
2 scallions, minced

1. Place lime and lemon juices in a medium bowl.
2. In a covered sauté pan, heat water to a boil. Add scallops and cover for 20 seconds. Immediately remove with a slotted spoon and submerge in lime and lemon juices, stirring well. Refrigerate until cool, at least 30 minutes—longer is even better.
3. Add garlic, parsley, olive oil, salt, fresh pepper, red pepper, and scallions to scallops. Stir and return to refrigerator to marinate for at least 30 minutes.

VARIATIONS: Use shrimp, squid, blue snapper, cod, or mussels.

SUGGESTED ACCOMPANIMENTS: Garlic bruschetta (see Garlic Soup with Bruschetta), Collard Greens with White Onions, and Beverly's Cantaloupe with Freshly Grated Ginger.

★★★   VITAMIN K, VITAMIN C, OMEGA-3 FATTY ACIDS
  ★   VITAMIN B$_6$, PHOSPHORUS, MAGNESIUM, PANTOTHENIC ACID, VITAMIN A, VITAMIN B$_{12}$, FOLIC ACID, NIACIN, THIAMIN, VITAMIN E

⚜ Oyster-Pot Stew ⚜

Yield: 4 quarts   (4 generous servings plus extra)

The RDA for zinc is 15 mg per day and there are 76.4 mg of zinc in just six medium-size oysters. High levels of zinc are closely associated with high levels of blood histamines. When histamine levels are high, women have orgasms more easily. (And if that doesn't convince you to eat oysters, nothing will!)

4 tablespoons whole wheat pastry flour	2 carrots, diced
3 tablespoons unsalted butter or extra-virgin olive oil	5 black peppercorns or ½ teaspoon ground
1 yellow onion, diced	5 allspice berries or ½ teaspoon ground
4 cloves garlic	6 scallions
6 cups filtered water, boiling	1 tablespoon herbal sea salt
1 red onion, diced	½ bunch fresh parsley, leaves only
2 potatoes, peeled and diced	1 quart shucked oysters, in their liquor

1. In a heavy-bottomed stockpot, heat flour, stirring constantly until it turns a light golden brown. Add butter and continue roasting until flour paste smells nutty, about 2 to 3 minutes. Be careful not to burn and, if it seems as if it might, remove pot from heat for a moment but keep stirring. (Once the fat becomes hot, it continues cooking even though it is not on the flame.)

2. Add the yellow onion and garlic, lower heat to medium and continue to stir frequently until onions are translucent, about 5 minutes.

3. Add boiling water, onion, potatoes, and carrots, bringing the entire contents back to a boil. Reduce to a simmer and cook about 20 minutes partially covered.

4. Place the black peppercorns and allspice berries in a tea ball (or tie in cheese-cloth) and add to pot. If using ground spices, stir in now.

5. Dice scallions into ½-inch pieces, separating the white from the green parts. Add the white parts to the stew; set the green aside. Add herbal salt and stir.

6. Simmer stew until vegetables are soft, about 45 minutes, stirring occasionally.

7. Add scallion greens, parsley leaves, and oysters and their liquor. Turn off heat.

8. Remove tea ball with spices and taste stew, adjusting seasoning if needed. Serve steaming hot with hot sauce or hot peppers for those who dare.

SUGGESTED ACCOMPANIMENTS: Crostini with Almond Romesco Sauce, Your Basic Green Salad, and Yogurt Cheesecake with Loganberry Glaze.

★★★ VITAMIN D, VITAMIN B$_{12}$, COPPER, IRON, SELENIUM, ZINC, OMEGA-3 FATTY ACIDS
  ★ VITAMIN C, MAGNESIUM, MANGANESE, PHOSPHORUS, FOLIC ACID, NIACIN, THIAMIN, POTASSIUM, VITAMIN B$_6$, VITAMIN E

When choosing oysters, make sure their shells are firmly closed and that they have been stored at 45°, on ice or in the refrigerator. (If you buy them without the shells, make sure the liquid is clear. If it is milky, discard.)

To shuck an oyster: Place a large strainer over a bowl. Over the strainer, hold oyster with the hinge part firmly in the palm of your hand. Push the blade of an oyster knife between the two halves of the shell near the hinge and twist the knife to force the hinge open, cutting the muscle that holds the shell halves together. Carefully pull the top of the shell off, leaving the oyster in the bottom half and holding it upright to retain the natural juices. The juices can be used for cooking, or they can be poured back into the half shell. (The opened oysters are placed in a bed of coarse salt to keep them level so that they don't spill their juices.)

❧ Bouillabaisse Brimming with Greens ❧

Yield: 3 quarts   (4 generous servings plus extra)

We created this version of bouillabaisse to include leafy greens. Inside every molecule of green chlorophyll is some heart-friendly magnesium, which keeps arteries from narrowing, lowers cholesterol, and prevents blood clots.

Have on hand: cotton cheesecloth and string.

2 tablespoons extra-virgin olive oil or unsalted butter
4 cloves garlic, minced
1 onion, chopped
1 stalk celery, sliced
1 leek, cleaned and chopped
1 fish head and bones
12 shrimp, shelled and deveined, shells reserved
1 bay leaf
½ teaspoon fennel seeds
1 sprig thyme
5 black peppercorns
5 cups filtered water
2 potatoes, peeled and sliced ½ inch thick

2 teaspoons lemon juice
1 pound mixed greens, such as spinach, escarole, collards, scallions, and watercress, chopped into 1-inch pieces
1 to 1½ pounds cod fillet, cut into large chunks
1 pound flounder fillet, cut into large chunks
1½ teaspoons sea salt
1 tablespoon salted plum vinegar (umeboshi)
White pepper to taste
20 Italian flat-leaf parsley leaves

1. In a large stockpot, heat oil over medium heat and sauté garlic, onion, celery, and leek until wilted and soft, about 10 minutes.

2. Tie fish head and bones in cheesecloth with shrimp shells, bay leaf, fennel seeds, thyme, and peppercorns. Add to stockpot with water (or replace this step with seasoned and strained fish stock). Bring to a boil, covered.

3. Add potatoes and lemon juice, return to a boil, then lower heat and simmer 30 minutes, uncovered.

4. Using a pair of tongs, remove cheesecloth bag, let cool, and then discard, squeezing any liquid back into the pot.

5. Add chopped greens. Cook, uncovered, 5 to 7 minutes.

6. Add cod, flounder, and shrimp and cook another 4 to 5 minutes, until fish becomes flaky and shrimp curl and turn pink.

7. Add salt, plum vinegar, and white pepper to taste. Serve in broad bowls topped with 4 or 5 parsley leaves.

SUGGESTED ACCOMPANIMENTS: A basket of crostini with Almond Romesco Sauce or garlic bruschetta (see Garlic Soup with Bruschetta), and Peach Crumble.

★★★   VITAMIN K, OMEGA-3 FATTY ACIDS, SELENIUM, VITAMIN B$_{12}$
★   VITAMIN C, FOLIC ACID, VITAMIN B$_6$, VITAMIN A, MAGNESIUM, VITAMIN D

We have used fish that's easy to find and handle. Other seafood that's good in this bouillabaisse is lobster, clams, mussels, halibut or grouper steak, monkfish, catfish, eel, and almost any other kind except oily and strong-tasting fish that will overpower the delicate flavors. (This dish is also known as zuppa di pesce, chowder, and San Francisco's cioppino.)

❧ Broiled Oysters on the Half Shell with Caviar ❧

Yield: 4 servings

Oysters belong on a woman's menu because of the remarkable variety of nutrients they contain, a luxurious way to fulfill your daily requirements.

2 cups kosher salt
12 fresh oysters in the shell
1 lemon

1 ounce fresh black caviar, such as
oestra or sevruga (about ¼ cup)

1. Spread salt evenly in a metal or enamel baking pan with sides.
2. Open or shuck oysters (see page 234) and place each in the salt bed, keeping the natural juices from spilling out.
3. Squeeze a few drops of lemon on each oyster and place under the broiler, cooking only until the edges curl. Do not overcook.
4. Remove oysters from broiler and place 1 teaspoon of caviar on each oyster. Serve immediately.

SUGGESTED ACCOMPANIMENTS: Whole Wheat Linguini with Fresh Tuna, Your Basic Green Salad, and Poached Pears with Ginger-Kuzu Sauce.

★★★   VITAMIN D, VITAMIN B_{12}, COPPER, IRON, SELENIUM, ZINC, OMEGA-3 FATTY ACIDS

★   MAGNESIUM, PANTOTHENIC ACID, SODIUM, PHOSPHORUS, VITAMIN A, RIBOFLAVIN, THIAMIN, CALCIUM, FOLIC ACID, MANGANESE, VITAMIN B_6, VITAMIN E, NIACIN

✿ 12 ✿
Poultry

Fresh Chicken Dinner and Soup, Too
Chicken with Garlic and Vinegar
Roasted Chicken with Barley-Mushroom Stuffing and Pears, Turnips, and Garlic
Moroccan Chicken with Cashews and Chick-peas Served with Couscous
Chicken Paprika with Yogurt Sauce
Stir-Fried Chicken with Bok Choy and Black-Bean Sauce
Oven-Fried Chicken with Herbs
Braised Chicken with Kale
Indian Chicken with Lemon Slices and Onions
Roast Half Turkey
Organic Chicken Liver Pâté
Teriyaki Chicken and Vegetables
Chicken Marinated in Chili Powder Rub
Chicken Salad

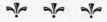

᪲

Poultry is a good source of protein that is versatile, flavorful, and comparatively low in animal fats. It also contains the B-complex vitamins, especially niacin, iron, and phosphorous. White meat is easier to digest because it contains less fat and connective tissue, and is particularly high in niacin, while dark meat is especially high in thiamin and riboflavin. Eating some of each is preferred to eating only white or only dark meat.

Raw poultry must remain chilled in the coldest part of the refrigerator and will keep one or two days. If frozen, thaw poultry in the refrigerator on a plate. It will take from two to four days for it to thaw, depending upon the size. Make sure that it is completely thawed before cooking, to ensure thorough cooking. Once cooked, it is best to consume the bird within 5 days. If it has been stuffed, remove the stuffing and store in a separate container.

Organic and free-range poultry are raised without the use of added hormones or antibiotics. These birds have been allowed to grow naturally, with sunlight and exercise, and they are much lower in fat. They are becoming more widely available (see our Appendix for sources). This is why we always recommend the use of organic, free-range poultry in our recipes. The free-range chicken may be the "haute poulet" of the moment, but in reality, they are the same delicious barnyard bird our forefathers (and mothers) ate for Sunday suppers long before the age of technology and chemicals.

❧ Fresh Chicken Dinner and Soup, Too ❧

Yield: 1 chicken dinner and lots of soup   (*4 generous serving plus extra*)

This idea of making two meals in one came from a neighbor. Cook the whole chicken in a pot to produce a rich-tasting soup and afterwards brown the chicken in the oven to provide a delicous dinner. Add some barley or pasta to the broth and have a bowl of this old-fashioned remedy, which traditional Chinese medicine also considers a curative. According to this ancient system, energies that flourished during a woman's years of fertility in menopause become unbalanced or blocked, and eating chicken is thought to help restore harmony.

3 **quarts filtered water**
1 **tablespoon cider vinegar or brown rice vinegar**
1 **2- to 3-pound chicken, organic preferred**
2 **carrots**
2 **onions, peeled**
3 **stalks celery**

2 **potatoes, peeled**
2 **bay leaves**
5 **peppercorns**
2 **teaspoons herbal sea salt**
2 **teaspoons sage powder**
2 **lemons**
2 **teaspoons sea salt**

1. In a large stockpot begin heating water and vinegar.
2. While the water and vinegar heat, wash chicken, removing innards. Unwrap, setting liver aside, and wash neck, gizzard, and heart. Pull off any excess fat from chicken and neck and discard. Place chicken and innards—except liver—in pot with water. Refrigerate liver for future use.
3. Add uncut, washed carrots, onions, celery, and potatoes.
4. Put bay leaves and peppercorns into a tea ball. Add to pot. Bring to a boil, uncovered, skimming off any foam as it comes to the top. Lower flame to a simmer and cook, covered, 35 minutes. After 20 minutes cooking time, preheat oven to 350°.
5. Using a large fork and tongs, carefully remove chicken from pot and place in a roasting pan. Sprinkle with herbal salt and sage. Cut one lemon in half, squeeze juice all over chicken, and place rinds of lemon inside of chicken. Bake 15 to 20 minutes until golden brown.
6. Remove tea ball from soup and discard contents. Using tongs, remove vegetables to a bowl. Season soup with salt and juice of the other lemon to taste.
7. Cut carrots, onions, celery, and potatoes into pieces. Place in a serving bowl.

(Or return vegetables to pot and serve with broth.) Pour broth into a soup tureen and serve with the bowl of vegetables.

8. Remove roasted chicken to a cutting board. Cut into pieces, place on a platter and serve.

NOTE: If not using organic chicken, discard neck and liver.

SUGGESTIONS FOR USE: Utilize broth in any recipes that call for stock, except those that specify fish stock. Use remaining chicken for salad or sandwiches.

SUGGESTED ACCOMPANIMENTS: Curried Barley with Caramelized Onions, Your Basic Green Salad, and Old-Fashioned Oatmeal Raisin Cookies.

★★★ SELENIUM, NIACIN, VITAMIN A
★ OMEGA-3 FATTY ACIDS, LINOLEIC ACID, VITAMIN B_6

❧ Chicken with Garlic and Vinegar ❧

Yield: 4 generous servings plus extra

This family favorite became our soul food as we wrote the book. Serve a platter of this mouthwatering combination of savory chicken and crispy garlic and every last morsel will be eaten. Our dish contains niacin, a B vitamin that benefits your love life and sexual functioning. Chew on the bones for their flavor and nutrients, including calcium in the marrow.

1 **2- to 2½-pound chicken, organic preferred, cut into 8 pieces**	**Herbal sea salt**
2 **tablespoons extra-virgin olive oil**	**Freshly ground black pepper**
15 **cloves garlic, unpeeled**	⅓ **cup cider vinegar**
	¼ **cup filtered water**

1. Wash chicken pieces in cold water. Pat dry.
2. In a heavy-bottomed nonreactive skillet, such as enamel, heat olive oil and add chicken in a single layer. Cook on medium-high heat until browned on all sides.
3. Add garlic cloves and sprinkle with salt and pepper. Cook on medium heat, uncovered, turning pieces as they brown. (Use a splatter guard.) Cook chicken until it no longer releases any pink juices when pricked with a fork, about 30 minutes.
4. Mix together vinegar and water. Turn skillet flame to high and let pan heat for

1 to 2 minutes. Pour vinegar solution all over chicken and quickly cover with lid. Steam for 3 to 4 minutes, until all the water has evaporated.

5. Place on a serving dish and serve while hot.

Suggested accompaniments: Quick Salad of shredded romaine lettuce and red radishes, Puréed Cabbage and Potatoes, and Steamed Summer Squash Salad.

★★★   Niacin, Selenium
★   Vitamin B₆, Omega-3 fatty acids, Linoleic acid

Think of garlic as a staple food, not just a seasoning. Because of the phytohormones it contains, garlic has estrogenic properties and it is especially important in postmenopause because it reduces blood pressure and blood-cholesterol levels.

❧ Roasted Chicken with Barley-Mushroom ❧ Stuffing and Pears, Turnips, and Garlic

Yield: 4 generous servings plus extra

When eating chicken, always have some of the breast or a drumstick, since these two parts of the bird are a good source of selenium. This is a whole meal in one recipe.

Before you begin, prepare cooked barley and millet (see Notes) or use already cooked grain.

½ pound button mushrooms
3 apples, cored and quartered
1 onion
2 cloves garlic
2 teaspoons herbal sea salt
½ teaspoon paprika
¼ teaspoon sage
1 to 1½ cups cooked barley and millet (see Notes)

1 3-pound chicken, organic preferred
1 lemon
1 or 2 teaspoons rosemary
½ teaspoon sea salt
¼ teaspoon black pepper
8 cloves garlic, peeled
2 white turnips, quartered
1 Bosc pear, cored and quartered

Preheat oven to 350°.

1. In a processor (or by hand), pulse-chop mushrooms, apples, onion, and garlic. Remove to a medium mixing bowl.

2. Add herbal salt, paprika, sage, and cooked barley and millet. Mix well.

3. Wash chicken in cold water. Stuff cavity with mushroom stuffing (see Notes), and truss the chicken. Place in a roomy baking pan. Squeeze lemon juice all over outside of chicken. Sprinkle with rosemary, salt, and pepper. Place garlic, turnips, and pear pieces around chicken.

4. Put chicken in oven. Place another baking pan filled with water on the bottom shelf of the oven. Bake for 50 to 60 minutes, until juices run clear when thigh is pierced with a fork.

5. Using a slotted spoon, remove pears, turnips, and garlic; place in a processor and purée (or put in a bowl and mash with a potato masher).

6. Remove stuffing to a covered serving bowl, cut chicken with a poultry shears or knife, and place on a heated platter. Serve with vegetable purée.

NOTES: **1.** Cook ¼ cup barley and ¼ cup millet in a small pot with 1½ cups filtered water or stock and a pinch of sea salt. Bring to a boil, covered, and simmer for 50 minutes. Any previously cooked grain will work well also.

2. The stuffing can be baked in a separate covered container instead of in the chicken. Before serving drizzle some chicken drippings over it.

SUGGESTED ACCOMPANIMENTS: Your Basic Green Salad and Strawberry Tart with Walnut Crust.

★★★   SELENIUM, NIACIN
  ★   OMEGA-3 FATTY ACIDS, LINOLEIC ACID, VITAMIN B$_6$

❧ Moroccan Chicken with Cashews and ❧ Chick-peas Served with Couscous

Yield: 4 generous servings plus extra

This traditional dish of Morocco is infused with sweet and savory spices—ginger, cinnamon, cumin—and we've adapted it to include whole wheat couscous. The robust nutty flavor of this grain is superior to its refined-flour version and gives you a wider range of vitamins and minerals.

Before you begin, soak 1 cup dried chick-peas 6 to 8 hours or overnight in filtered water, and drain.

2 to 2½ cups soaked chick-peas (from 1 cup dried)
5 cups filtered water
2 bay leaves
1 tablespoon extra-virgin olive oil
1½ teaspoons turmeric
1 2½- to 3-pound chicken, organic preferred, washed and cut into quarters
3 onions, chopped
4 cloves garlic, minced
2 teaspoons ground ginger

1 teaspoon cinnamon
1 teaspoon cumin
¼ cup black currants
½ cup cashew pieces, toasted
5 cups chicken stock (see index), organic preferred
2 tablespoons lemon juice
1½ teaspoons sea salt
¼ teaspoon black pepper
1 teaspoon herbal sea salt
2 cups whole wheat couscous

1. Remove beans from soaking water with your hands or a slotted spoon and put into a medium saucepan with water and bay leaves. Bring to a boil, covered, and simmer for 60 minutes. (Pressure cook for 40 minutes.)

2. In an ovenproof casserole, heat olive oil and 1 teaspoon turmeric on medium-high and add chicken pieces, bone side up. Cook about 10 minutes, until browned, turning once. Remove chicken to a brown paper bag. Keep oil in casserole.

3. Preheat oven to 350°.

4. Cook onions in the same pot as chicken (without adding any more fat) until translucent. Add ½ teaspoon turmeric, garlic, ginger, cinnamon, cumin, and currants. Cook 2 to 3 minutes on low heat.

5. Drain chick-peas (reserve liquid for soup stock) and discard bay leaves. Add chick-peas, cashews, and 3 cups stock to spices in casserole and stir. Add chicken pieces, lemon juice, salt, and pepper. Bring to a boil, cover, and place in preheated oven to cook until juices run clear when thigh is pricked with a paring knife, about 45 minutes.

6. About 10 minutes before the chicken is cooked, in a small pot bring remaining 2 cups chicken stock and herbal salt to a boil. Slowly add couscous to pot. Do not stir. Return to a boil, covered, and turn off heat. Let sit covered 10 minutes.

7. Spoon couscous onto a serving platter and arrange the chicken, chick-peas, onions, and cashews on top and around. Pour the juices into a gravy boat and serve on the side.

SUGGESTED ACCOMPANIMENTS: Fast Salad of steamed asparagus and red pepper strips, yogurt infused with mashed garlic, and Fresh Blueberry Cobbler.

★★★   NIACIN, SELENIUM
★   LINOLEIC ACID, OMEGA-3 FATTY ACIDS, VITAMIN B$_6$

⚜ Chicken Paprika with Yogurt Sauce ⚜

Yield: 4 generous servings plus extra

The quick-cooked yogurt sauce for this chicken casserole is fresher tasting and tangier than the traditional sour cream version and lower in fat, and the bacteria in the yogurt even aids digestion—an improvement in every way.

1 tablespoon extra-virgin olive oil	1 cup chicken stock (see index) or
1 3-pound chicken, organic preferred,	filtered water
cut into 4 to 8 pieces	2 tablespoons paprika
2 onions, chopped	½ teaspoon sea salt
2 carrots, chopped	2 cups plain bacteria-active yogurt
2 stalks celery, chopped	2 scallions, minced

1. In a large, heavy-bottomed casserole or skillet, heat oil over medium-high heat. Add as many chicken pieces as will fit without crowding. Saute until browned on both sides, about 8 minutes. Remove to a brown paper bag to drain and repeat with remaining pieces.

2. Reduce heat to low and add onions, carrots, and celery. Cook, stirring occasionally, until the onions turn translucent, about 10 minutes.

3. Add stock and chicken pieces. Sprinkle with paprika and salt. Bring liquid to a boil, reduce heat, and cover. Simmer until juices run clear when thigh is pierced with a fork, about 30 minutes.

4. Line a strainer or colander with a paper towel or coffee filter. Place in a container so liquid can drip through. Pour yogurt into strainer and let drain.

5. With tongs, remove chicken from casserole to a heated platter.

6. Skim any fat from the liquid in casserole. Reduce stock to about ½ cup, boiling for about 3 or 4 minutes.

7. In a small bowl place drained yogurt, discarding paper towel. Add several tablespoons cooking liquid and whisk. Reduce heat under casserole to low and whisk yogurt into pan. Cook for 1 minute, then pour sauce over the chicken, sprinkle with scallions, and serve immediately.

SUGGESTED ACCOMPANIMENTS: Hungarian Pasta with Cabbage, Your Basic Green Salad with arugula and chicory, and Light Lemon Pudding Parfait with Kiwi Slices.

★★★ NIACIN, SELENIUM, VITAMIN A
★ OMEGA-3 FATTY ACIDS, LINOLEIC ACID, VITAMIN B$_6$

❧ Stir-Fried Chicken with Bok Choy ❧ and Black-Bean Sauce

Yield: 2 quarts (*4 generous servings plus extra*)

Stir-frying is an ancient quick-cooking technique and still a great way to save time and energy in the kitchen. If you've run out of steam, toss these ingredients together and take advantage of their vitamin C, good for fatigue.

1 medium bunch bok choy
3 tablespoons fermented black beans, soaked in ¼ cup boiling filtered water
1 to 2 tablespoons shoyu soy sauce
1 tablespoon arrowroot or kuzu
½ cup vegetable stock (see recipe) or filtered water
2 tablespoons filtered water

2 tablespoons unrefined sesame oil
1 onion, sliced
3 cloves garlic, sliced
8 to 12 ounces chicken, cut into strips (see Note)
2 teaspoons dark sesame oil
4 sprigs fresh coriander (cilantro)

1. Slice bok choy stems into ¼-inch pieces, and greens into ½-inch pieces. Set them aside in separate bowls.

2. Drain black beans, discarding liquid. Place in a small bowl with soy sauce, arrowroot, and stock and mash with a fork or back of a spoon. Mix well. Set aside.

3. Heat 2 tablespoons water and sesame oil in wok or sauté pan, add onion, and sauté for 1 minute. Add garlic and cook for another 30 seconds.

4. Add chicken to wok and cook for 3 to 4 minutes.

5. Add bok choy stems to chicken and stir constantly, turning with the chicken until all of the stems have been coated with the oil and flavorings. Cover and cook for 3 minutes.

6. Add bok choy leaves to wok, stirring well. Add black bean mixture to wok, stir well on high heat until liquid has thickened and is clear, then cook 30 seconds more.

7. Add dark sesame oil and toss once more.

8. Serve on a platter topped with coriander sprigs.

NOTE: Bone half of a chicken and cut meat into strips or chunks, or use chicken breast.

SUGGESTED ACCOMPANIMENTS: Millet-Rice with Peas and Tomatoes, and Crispy Walnut and Seed Bars.

★★★ VITAMIN C, LINOLEIC ACID, VITAMIN A, FOLIC ACID
★ NIACIN, VITAMIN B$_6$

When stir-frying, put water in the pan first, then the oil. This will keep the temperature at 212° and reduce the risk of the oil breaking down at higher temperatures, producing toxic substances.

❧ Oven-Fried Chicken with Herbs ❧

Yield: 4 servings plus extra

Many people love the taste and crunch of crispy fried foods. So here's a baked version of fried chicken that uses a minimum of fat yet has the same appeal.

¾ cup hi-lysine cornmeal or whole wheat flour
1½ teaspoons sea salt
1 teaspoon black pepper
2 eggs, organic, fertile preferred
2 tablespoons filtered water
2 teaspoons oregano

2 teaspoons basil
1 cup whole wheat bread crumbs
¼ cup unhulled sesame seeds
1 teaspoon herbal sea salt
1 3-pound chicken, organic preferred, cut into quarters
2 tablespoons unsalted butter or extra-virgin olive oil

Preheat oven to 325°.

1. In a wide bowl, mix cornmeal, salt, and pepper.
2. In a medium bowl, whisk eggs and water, add oregano and basil.
3. In a third bowl, put bread crumbs, sesame seeds, and herbal salt.
4. Trim any large pieces of fat from chicken and, if preferred, remove skin. Wash chicken pieces in cold water. Dredge in cornmeal mixture, dip in the egg mixture, and lastly coat with bread crumbs.
5. Heat a heavy-bottomed, ovenproof skillet, large enough to hold chicken pieces in a single layer. Add butter, coating bottom and sides of skillet. Place chicken in skillet bone side up and brown, about 2 minutes. Turn pieces over and place skillet in preheated oven. Bake for 60 minutes.
6. Remove skillet and increase oven temperature to 450°. Wait about 5 minutes, then place skillet in oven to allow the coating to crisp for 4 or 5 minutes.

SUGGESTED ACCOMPANIMENTS: French Carrots and Parsnips; Roasted Potatoes with Rosemary; Carrot and Cabbage Slaw with Fresh Fennel; and Banana Refrigerator Cake.

★★★ SELENIUM, NIACIN
★ LINOLEIC ACID, OMEGA-3 FATTY ACIDS, VITAMIN B₆

❧ Braised Chicken with Kale ❧

Yield: 4 generous servings plus extra

Vitamin K is found in leafy green vegetables, including the kale in this dish. We hear little about this vitamin, but it does important work—assisting in liver function and the storage of glucose for energy. Vitamin K lessens the symptoms of perimenopause.

1 tablespoon extra-virgin olive oil or cold-pressed safflower oil
1 red onion, sliced
1 yellow or Spanish onion, sliced
2 cloves garlic, crushed
1 bunch kale (about ¼ to ⅓ pound), chopped coarsely

1 3-pound chicken, organic preferred
1 teaspoon sea salt
  Fresh pepper
4 cups vegetable or chicken stock (see index) or filtered water
1 teaspoon thyme
3 potatoes, peeled and quartered

1. In a large, heavy-bottomed casserole, heat oil over medium-high heat. Add onions, garlic, and kale, and sauté until kale begins to wilt, about 5 minutes.

2. Wash chicken in cold water. Sprinkle inside and out with ½ teaspoon salt and a few grinds pepper. Set aside.

3. Add stock, ½ teaspoon salt, a few grinds of pepper, and thyme, and stir. Place chicken in casserole. Bring stock to a boil, covered, reduce heat to a simmer, and cook about 50 to 60 minutes.

4. Using a large fork and tongs, lift chicken from casserole to a serving platter. Cover with parchment paper and foil to keep warm.

5. Skim off any visible fat in casserole. Add potatoes and simmer until tender, about 10 minutes.

6. Arrange vegetables around chicken. Pour braising liquid into a gravy boat and serve on the side.

SUGGESTED ACCOMPANIMENTS: Millet-Rice with Peas and Tomatoes, and Fast Salad of scallions and plum tomatoes.

★★★   VITAMIN K, NIACIN, SELENIUM
  ★   VITAMIN C, VITAMIN B$_6$, OMEGA-3 FATTY ACIDS, LINOLEIC ACID

❧ Indian Chicken with ❧ Lemon Slices and Onions

Yield: 2 quarts   (4 generous servings plus extra)

Here's an elegant dish to serve to company, that combines a luxurious rich yogurt sauce with subtle spices. Present the chicken from a silver platter, and decorate with the menopause fruit, lemon slices, high in bioflavonoids. Then don't forget to eat the garnish!

1 **3- to 3½-pound chicken, organic preferred, skinned and cut into 8 pieces**	1 **teaspoon cumin**
3 **onions**	½ **teaspoon turmeric**
6 **tablespoons filtered water plus 1½ cups**	2 **tablespoons plain bacteria-active yogurt**
1**-inch piece fresh ginger, minced**	1½ **teaspoons sea salt**
4 **cloves garlic**	¼ **teaspoon cinnamon**
2 **plum tomatoes, seeded**	¼ **teaspoon cloves**
5 **tablespoons unrefined safflower oil**	⅛ **teaspoon cayenne**
1 **tablespoon ground coriander**	1 **whole lemon, organic preferred, sliced and seeded**
	⅛ **teaspoon freshly ground pepper**

1. Wash chicken and then, with paper toweling, pat dry.

2. Chop 2 onions coarsely and put into a blender with 6 tablespoons water, ginger, garlic, and tomato, blending until a smooth paste.

3. Slice remaining onion. Heat 1 tablespoon oil in a medium stockpot. Add sliced onions and cook until caramelized and golden brown, about 15 minutes. Remove onions to a bowl and set aside.

4. In the same pot, add 2 tablespoons oil, if needed, and put in half the chicken pieces. Brown on all sides until golden, then remove to a brown paper bag to drain. Add remaining 2 tablespoons oil to pot. Brown remaining chicken and drain.

5. Pour in onion paste from blender. (This can splatter, so keep face averted.) Stir and cook on medium-high heat for about 10 minutes, until golden brown.

6. Add coriander, cumin, and turmeric and cook another 2 minutes, stirring continuously. Add yogurt 1 tablespoon at a time, stirring well. Add salt, cinnamon, cloves, cayenne, and 1½ cups water. Bring to a boil, covered, lower heat to a simmer, and cook 10 minutes.

7. Add lemon slices, chicken, caramelized onion, and fresh pepper to pot, stirring to incorporate all of the flavors. Bring to a boil, covered, lower heat to a simmer, and cook 20 to 25 minutes, adding more water as necessary. You will end up with a very thick sauce.

8. Serve in a shallow platter or bowl, arranging lemon slices on top.

SUGGESTED ACCOMPANIMENTS: Red-Lentil Dhal, Tomatoes Stuffed with Couscous, Your Basic Green Salad, and a bowl of yogurt.

★★★   NIACIN, SELENIUM
★   LINOLEIC ACID, OMEGA-3 FATTY ACIDS, VITAMIN E, VITAMIN B$_6$, BIOFLAVONOIDS

❧ Roast Half Turkey ❧

Yield: 4 generous servings plus extra

It's not just for Thanksgiving! This low-fat meat is high in zinc, a mineral your body chemistry depends on. After you've enjoyed the turkey for dinner, there's plenty left to make soup, sandwiches, and salad.

½ turkey (7 to 9 pounds), organic preferred (see Note)
1 lemon, organic preferred

1 tablespoon sage or rosemary
2 teaspoons sea salt
1 teaspoon black pepper

Preheat oven to 325°.

1. Place turkey in a Dutch oven or baking pan, and sprinkle inside and out with lemon juice, sage, salt, and pepper. Put lemon halves inside turkey. Place bone side up and cover or wrap with parchment paper and foil.

2. Put into oven and cook covered for 1 hour. Turn turkey over, with bone side down. Cover and cook another hour.

3. Uncover turkey, baste with juices that are in the pan. (If there are very little juices, add some water or stock.) Return to oven, uncovered, and cook until skin side is browned, about 30 minutes. If further cooking is needed, turn turkey over so that breast side is sitting in the juices and cover with parchment and foil until done (see cooking times opposite).

4. Remove turkey from oven, let cool for 5 minutes. Remove from pan to a cutting surface. Using a carving knife and fork, slice enough turkey for the meal. Allow the remaining turkey to cool for easier cutting.

NOTE: Have turkey cut in half by your butcher or meat manager. If buying at a farm, let them know in advance that you want it split in half. Freeze the other half.

COOKING TIMES: 20 minutes per pound. For a half turkey of 9 pounds, a total of 3 hours of cooking will be needed.

SUGGESTED ACCOMPANIMENTS: Classic Candied Yams Revised; Chestnut, Pine Nut, and Currant Stuffing; Asparagus Mimosa with Lemon and Flax Seed Oil; Your Basic Green Salad; and Peach Crumble.

★★★ SELENIUM, NIACIN, ZINC, VITAMIN B$_6$
★ OMEGA-3 FATTY ACIDS, PANTOTHENIC ACID, IRON

Sage has estrogenic properties that makes it useful for menopause. It has been used medicinally to stop sweating and reduce hot flashes. Sage can also fortify a debilitated nervous system. Pour some boiling water over the leaves, steep, and you have sage tea.

❧ Organic Chicken Liver Pâté ❧

Yield: 1 quart　(*4 generous servings plus extra*)

Pâté is really easy to make, lasts a long time in the refrigerator, and freezes well. It can be used as an hors d'oeuvre on a cracker, as a sandwich spread, or mixed into a cooked grain. One of the benefits of chicken liver is the folic acid it provides, a vitamin that elevates blood histamine levels. Higher levels of histamines are associated with an increase in sexual responsiveness.

Before beginning, hard-boil 2 eggs.

2　tablespoons extra-virgin olive oil
2　onions, diced (or pulse-chopped in processor)
2　stalks celery, chopped (or pulse-chopped in processor)
¼　cup chicken or vegetable stock (see index) or filtered water
1　pound chicken or turkey livers, organic only (see Note page 257)

2　teaspoons herbal sea salt
1　teaspoon ground allspice or nutmeg
½　teaspoon black pepper
2　eggs, organic, free-range preferred, hard-boiled and shelled
½　cup walnuts, chopped

1. In a large sauté pan, heat olive oil and onions. Cook several minutes, add celery, and cook, uncovered, over moderate heat until onion and celery begin to caramelize and turn golden, about 10 minutes. Remove to a bowl.

2. In the same sauté pan, add stock, chicken livers, herbal salt, and allspice, cooking until no pink juice is released when liver is pricked with a fork. Turn off flame.

3. In a processor or meat grinder, put caramelized onions, celery, and cooked livers with pepper and eggs. Blend well.

4. Using a cake spatula, shape the liver mixture into an oval mound on a serving plate. Press nuts into pâté, cover with plastic, and chill at least 1 hour or overnight.

Suggested uses: Stuff into celery or hollowed cherry tomatoes or cucumbers. Spread on crackers or use as a filling for sandwiches. Extra can be frozen for future use.

Suggested accompaniments: Whole Grain Crackers with Four Seeds, and Creamless Mushroom Cream Soup.

★★★　VITAMIN A, VITAMIN B$_{12}$, FOLIC ACID, RIBOFLAVIN, OMEGA-3 FATTY ACIDS
★　PANTOTHENIC ACID, IRON, LINOLEIC ACID

A rich relative of meat-loaf lineage, pâtés are really no harder to make than a meat loaf. Their distinguishing characteristics are their luxurious ingredients, which classically can include ground meats, diced pork fat, sliced tongue, chicken or game, cream, eggs, spices, brandy, nuts, truffles, and endless other combinations. Our recipe is, of course, a delicious yet healthful version of the more richly made classic French pâté.

❧ Teriyaki Chicken and Vegetables ❧

Yield: 2 quarts   *(4 generous servings plus extra)*

In menopause, quick solutions to dinner are a blessing at the end of a tiring day. Here's a recipe that takes advantage of a mouthwatering sauce that you can keep on hand. Enjoy this with brown rice rather than the usual white.

1 **2½- to 3-pound chicken, preferably organic, cut into 8 pieces**
2 **onions, sliced**
2 **carrots, sliced diagonally**
1 **green pepper, seeded and cut into large pieces**
1 **double recipe Teriyaki Marinade, without thickener (see recipe)**

1. In a wide pot or deep sauté pan, brown chicken on all sides. Remove to a brown paper bag to drain.

2. Remove excess chicken fat (more than 1 tablespoon). Sauté onions, carrots, and green pepper in the pot for several minutes.

3. Return chicken to pot with vegetables. Pour teriyaki marinade all over. Cover and let cook until chicken no longer releases any pink juices when pricked with a fork.

To serve: Place chicken and vegetables on a wide platter. Serve remaining teriyaki marinade on the side.

SUGGESTED ACCOMPANIMENTS: Basic Brown Rice, Your Basic Green Salad, and orange wedges.

★★★   VITAMIN C, LINOLEIC ACID, VITAMIN A
  ★   FOLIC ACID, NIACIN, VITAMIN B₆

❧ Chicken Marinated in Chili Powder Rub ❧

Yield: 4 generous servings

Rubs are spice and seasoning mixtures that you sprinkle over meats to flavor them before cooking. After marinating a short time, they give food intense flavors. And as the meat cooks, the rub seals in the juices of the meat and the nutrients it contains.

1 **2½-to 3-pound chicken,**   **½ cup chili powder rub**
   preferably organic, quartered   **(see chart opposite)**

1. Wash chicken quarters in cold water. Put into an enamel or stainless-steel baking pan. Sprinkle rub on both sides of chicken, using all of the rub.
2. Place in refrigerator for 25 to 45 minutes (see chart page 259).
3. Using a butter knife, scrape off excess rub.
4. Bake or broil until chicken is tender when a fork is inserted and no pink juices come out. Cook about 30 minutes, baked, or 20 minutes, broiled. Turn at least once during cooking.

SUGGESTED ACCOMPANIMENTS: Puréed Cabbage and Potatoes, tomato slices with sea salt and pepper, and Banana Refrigerator Cake.

★★★   NIACIN, SELENIUM
  ★   OMEGA-3 FATTY ACIDS, LINOLEIC ACID, VITAMIN B₆

Chili Powder Rub

You can use this chart to make ½ cup of rub. Start with the chili powder base and add your own special spices in varied amounts. For marinating times, see recipe.

Chili Powder Base

¼ cup chili powder	2 teaspoons oregano
1 tablespoon cumin	2 teaspoons ground ginger
1 tablespoon garlic powder	1 teaspoon sea salt

Mild Spicy | *Hot and Spicy*

Mild Spicy	*Hot and Spicy*
white pepper	cayenne
black pepper	ancho chilies
mulato chilies	pasilla chilies
dry mustard	negro chilies
jalapeño peppers*	chipotle chilies

---

*Seed jalapeños, chop, and use. For a spicier flavor chop with seeds intact.

❦ Chicken Salad ❦

Yield: about 3 cups   (4 sandwiches)

We give you a version of this favorite made without commercial mayonnaise so that you can avoid the hydrogenated or refined oils these may contain.

3 cups cooked chicken, shredded or cut into small pieces
2 tablespoons extra-virgin olive oil
2 stalks celery, minced (about ½ cup)
4 scallions or ½ red onion, minced

Juice of 1 lemon
¼ teaspoon herbal sea salt
1 teaspoon prepared mustard
⅛ teaspoon white pepper
1 bunch watercress

1. Place chicken in a medium bowl. Add olive oil, celery, onion, lemon juice, herbal salt, mustard, and pepper. Toss well.

2. Serve on a bed of watercress.

VARIATIONS: This recipe can also be used for turkey salad, shrimp or fish salad, or tempeh salad.

SERVING SUGGESTIONS: Serve on bread, with crackers, or in Boston lettuce-leaf cups.

★★★   VITAMIN K, NIACIN, SELENIUM
★   LINOLEIC ACID, OMEGA-3 FATTY ACIDS, VITAMIN B_6

13

Meat and Game

Beef Liver with Onions and Portobello Mushrooms
Beef Ribs with Black and White Pepper Rub
Great Meat Loaf
Full-of-Vegetables Beef Stew
Lamb with Apricot, Figs, and Almonds
Leg of Lamb with Rosemary and Onion Flowers
Rabbit in Fresh Red Sauce
Venison Shish Kebab
Beef Sukiyaki with Ginger and Garlic

We've included fewer recipes for meat than other foods since meat recipes fill so many other cookbooks and because, in the interest of health, we de-emphasize this kind of protein in favor of plant foods. But there are times when, if you are not a vegetarian, only a piece of meat will satisfy. Meat provides B vitamins and a variety of minerals for menopause—it's the best source of iron—and gives energy that lasts for hours.

When you have meat, a piece the size of your palm is close to the 3.5-ounce serving of meat generally recommended for health—not large by American standards. High amounts of animal protein in the diet have been associated with heart disease because of the saturated fat and cholesterol that meat contains. And the type of protein in meat may be a contributing factor in osteoporosis.

The quality of the meat you eat is also important. We prefer to cook with organic beef, pork, and lamb to limit our exposure to hormones and antibiotics. Organic meats are more expensive, but we think they're worth it.

Game: We recommend special meats since they're much lower in fat than standard meats, and a source of omega-3 fatty acids, which are especially good for female health. Eating game varies the diet and increases your chance of getting a range of nutrients. Since most of today's game is farm-raised, not hunted in the wild, the meat is not as tough or "gamey" as it used to be. Try our venison and rabbit recipes.

✣ Beef Liver with Onions and ✣ Portobello Mushrooms

Yield: 4 cups   (4 generous servings)

Liver is low in fat and, while it tends to be high in cholesterol, that's no reason to avoid it altogether. (Cholesterol is an essential part of every cell wall, and it is the source molecule from which all of your hormones are made—including estrogen.) We're not saying you should eat liver every day, but if your cholesterol level is normal, once or twice a month have some of this exceptionally nutritious food.

2 tablespoons unsalted butter or extra-virgin olive oil
1 Spanish onion, sliced
2 portobello mushrooms, stems removed, caps sliced
¼ teaspoon sea salt

1 pound beef liver, organic only (see Note)
¼ teaspoon thyme
½ teaspoon herbal sea salt
Freshly ground black pepper (optional)

1. In a large skillet, melt 1 tablespoon butter and add onion and mushrooms. Cook 4 or 5 minutes over medium heat, uncovered.

2. Sprinkle with sea salt, cover, and cook on low flame another 5 minutes.

3. Remove onion and mushrooms to a bowl and cover to keep warm. Heat remaining tablespoon butter, add liver, and sprinkle with thyme and herbal salt. Cook about 4 minutes, turning once.

4. Put onion and mushrooms on top of liver in skillet, cover, and cook another 1 or 2 minutes. If desired, sprinkle with pepper and serve immediately.

NOTE: Liver is the only meat that we insist be organic, since liver is the processing organ for the chemicals and toxins that pass through the animal. We'd rather you never eat liver if it is going to be non-organic.

SUGGESTED ACCOMPANIMENTS: Butternut Squash and Yam Bisque with Toasted Pumpkin Seeds, Basic Brown Rice, Your Basic Green Salad, and fresh apple and pear slices.

★★★   VITAMIN A, VITAMIN K, VITAMIN B_{12}, FOLIC ACID, NIACIN, PANTOTHENIC ACID, RIBOFLAVIN, COPPER, SELENIUM

★   VITAMIN B_6, VITAMIN C, IRON, ZINC, THIAMIN

❧ Beef Ribs with Black and White Pepper Rub ❧

Yield: 4 generous servings

Here's a quick and easy technique to flavor meats. Use a dry mixture of spices that can be made in minutes, is quickly applied, and yields a complex and rich flavor. With a jar of premixed spices on hand this technique requires little brain power when you're feeling fuzzy-headed from menopause.

3 to 4 pounds beef ribs or country-style pork ribs	1 tablespoon dry mustard
2 tablespoons ground black pepper	1 tablespoon paprika
2 tablespoons ground white pepper	1 teaspoon ground coriander
	1 cup filtered water

1. Wash ribs in cold water and put into a baking dish. In a small bowl combine black and white peppers, mustard, paprika, and coriander. Coat ribs with rub and then press onto both sides, using all of the mixture.

2. Place in refrigerator for 25 to 45 minutes (see chart opposite).

3. Preheat oven to 375° (see Note).

4. Scrape some of the rub off the ribs with a butter knife before cooking. Add water to pan, and place in oven. Bake until ribs are tender and meat begins to fall off the bone, about 35 to 45 minutes. If you are cooking a rack of ribs, after the first 20 minutes they can be cut apart to speed cooking, using tongs and a sharp knife. (Waiting until they are partially cooked keeps the ribs from drying out.) Turn ribs over several times during cooking.

NOTE: To avoid carcinogens that can be generated when grilling fatty foods, we chose to bake this American favorite.

VARIATIONS: The rub can be used on different cuts of meat, such as steaks, London broil, and even chicken, tempeh, and fish.

SUGGESTED ACCOMPANIMENTS: Tomatoes Stuffed with Couscous; Steamed Spinach; Carrot and Cabbage Slaw with Fresh Fennel; and Light Lemon Pudding Parfait with Kiwi Slices.

★★★ VITAMIN B$_{12}$
★ IRON, ZINC, NIACIN, VITAMIN B$_6$

Basic marinating time for rubs:	
Type of Meat	*Marinating Times*
Fillets and other thin cuts	10 to 15 minutes
Medium cuts	15 to 25 minutes
Thick cuts	25 to 45 minutes
Refrigerate, covered. Broil, bake, or sauté.	

❧ Great Meat Loaf ❧

Yield: 1 loaf   (4 generous servings plus extra)

Meat loaf is fast and easy to make and ours is extra nutritious because we've added oatmeal, a phytohormone grain. Meat loaf is a versatile food and a slice can be used for any meal. For dinner serve sliced meat loaf with tomato sauce and mashed potatoes: for lunch put a slice in a whole grain bun with lettuce, mustard, and sprouts, and serve with soup on the side. And for breakfast try a little meat loaf with twice-cooked beans and tortillas. You'll finish this meat loaf in no time at all!

1 **pound ground sirloin beef or turkey, organic preferred**
½ **cup oatmeal**
½ **cup whole wheat bread crumbs**
1 **egg, organic preferred (optional)**
3 **cloves garlic, minced**
1 **onion, minced**

¼ **bunch parsley, minced**
1 **teaspoon sea salt**
1 **teaspoon basil**
1 **teaspoon oregano**
¼ **teaspoon black pepper**
Pinch cinnamon

Preheat oven to 350°.

1. In a medium bowl combine ground meat, oatmeal, bread crumbs, egg, garlic, onion, parsley, salt, basil, oregano, pepper, and cinnamon. Mix well.

2. Shape mixture into an oval, or press into a lightly oiled 4-cup loaf pan. Bake until firm, about 45 minutes.

3. Cool 10 minutes. Slice and serve.

VARIATION: Turn this into meatballs by forming into walnut-sized balls; place on a baking sheet, and broil under medium heat. Using tongs, turn several times until all sides are golden.

SUGGESTED ACCOMPANIMENTS: Tomato Sauce, Artichokes Stuffed with Garlic and Bread Crumbs, Beet and Potato Salad, and Frozen Banana Maple-Walnut Whip.

★★★   VITAMIN B$_{12}$, VITAMIN K, SELENIUM
★   ZINC, NIACIN, IRON

❧ Full-of-Vegetables Beef Stew ❧

Yield: 3 quarts   (4 generous servings plus extra)

We're tipping the balance of this standard dish in favor of vegetables to give you a start on your daily quota. Leftover stew is easily made into a hearty soup with the addition of stock or water, plus seasonings.

½ cup whole wheat flour
1 pound beef-stew cubes, organic preferred
3 tablespoons extra-virgin olive oil
4 stalks celery, diced large
3 carrots, chopped into pieces
3 potatoes, peeled and cubed
2 onions, chopped into pieces
1 to 2 parsnips, chopped into pieces
½ butternut squash or yam, peeled and cubed

3 cups vegetable stock (see recipe) or filtered water
2 bay leaves
½ teaspoon sea salt
½ teaspoon herbal sea salt
½ teaspoon black pepper
½ bunch parsley, minced
½ cup plain bacteria-active yogurt (optional)

1. Put flour into a small bowl and thoroughly coat beef cubes. Heat oil in a large Dutch oven and add beef. Brown over medium heat for 2 to 3 minutes.

2. To stewpot add any remaining flour that has not coated the meat and all the vegetables. Stir in stock, bay leaves, salt, and pepper. Cover and cook 1 hour, stirring once or twice.

3. Garnish with parsley and serve yogurt on the side.

VARIATIONS: Tempeh, chicken pieces, and other meats can be used instead of, or with, beef chunks.

SUGGESTED ACCOMPANIMENTS: Mesclun Salad with Mustard Vinaigrette, Garlic Bruschetta, and Apricot-Cashew "Mousse."

★★★   VITAMIN A, VITAMIN B_{12}
  ★   VITAMIN C, VITAMIN K, VITAMIN B_6

There's an easy way to remember that animal foods contain cholesterol and that there's none in foods from plants. Only a liver can make cholesterol, and a plant doesn't have one! If you see a label on vegetable oil made from nuts and seeds that states it contains "no cholesterol," you'll know they are just stating the obvious. The beef in this stew contains cholesterol; the vegetables do not.

❧ **Lamb with Apricots, Figs, and Almonds** ❧

Yield: 4 quarts *(4 generous servings plus extra)*

Many traditional cuisines in other countries routinely include nuts and fruit in their cooking. Here is a lamb dish from the Middle East that incorporates these luxurious ingredients.

1 tablespoon extra-virgin olive oil
2 pounds lamb shank, cubes, or shoulder steaks, organic preferred
2 onions, diced
2 carrots, diced
1 turnip, diced
½ rutabaga, peeled and diced
10 unsulphured apricots, quartered

10 unsulphured black or white figs, quartered
½ cup almonds
1 cinnamon stick
1 tablespoon rosemary or 3 fresh sprigs
2 teaspoons herbal sea salt
1 cup filtered water

1. In a medium stockpot, heat oil. Add lamb and braise until golden on all sides. Remove to a plate.

2. Add onions, carrots, turnip, and rutabaga, stirring after each addition. Return lamb to pot, and add apricots, figs, almonds, cinnamon stick, rosemary, herbal salt, and water. (Be sure that the cinnamon stick is covered by the liquid.)

3. Bring to a boil, covered. Lower heat and simmer until lamb begins to fall off the bones, about 45 to 60 minutes.

SUGGESTED ACCOMPANIMENTS: Couscous, Leafy Greens Vietnamese Style, a bowl of yogurt, and Sunflower-Nori Snack.

★★★   VITAMIN B$_{12}$
★   VITAMIN A, NIACIN, RIBOFLAVIN, ZINC, IRON

To thicken cooking liquids, in a small sauté pan roast ¼ cup whole wheat pastry flour until it turns golden and smells nutty, stirring continuously, about 5 to 7 minutes. Gradually add cooking liquids from the lamb to flour, continuing to cook and stirring with a whisk until this becomes a thick sauce. Then make a well in the lamb pot, pushing the vegetables and meat aside, and add sauce to the liquids in the stockpot. Stir flour mixture and meat liquids together. Then mix through the lamb stew to make a slightly thickened sauce, cooking another 2 or 3 minutes.

Leg of Lamb with Rosemary and Onion Flowers

Yield: 4 generous servings plus extra

Cooking large cuts of meat is a convenient way to make food for several meals—a good solution when you're busy and have many mouths to feed. Lamb supplies niacin that your body needs to generate energy and you'll get the maximum if you serve the lamb au jus. As meat cooks, it releases moisture and niacin along with it, which ends up in the juice.

LAMB:

5-pound leg of lamb	Sea salt
6 cloves garlic	Black pepper
4 teaspoons rosemary, more as needed	

ONION FLOWERS:

4 medium onions, peeled	Herbal sea salt

Preheat oven to 450°.

LAMB:

1. Wash lamb in cold water. Remove the fell membrane (papery white outside). Using a sharp, pointed paring knife, cut six 1-inch crosscuts in the fatty side of the lamb. Into each crosscut, put 1 clove of garlic and some rosemary, salt, and pepper, pressing each item deep into the cut.

2. Sprinkle salt and pepper over the outside of lamb. Place on a rack in a roasting pan, fat side up.

3. Place in oven and reduce heat to 325°. Roast 30 minutes per pound, about 2½ hours. Do not cover or baste.

4. Slice and serve while hot.

ONION FLOWERS: (Prepare 1 hour before lamb is finished cooking.)

1. Place onion root side down on a cutting board. Using a paring knife, cut in quarters from the top and then again to make eighths, without going through the root (so that the root of the onion holds the pieces together). Sprinkle each onion with a little herbal salt.

2. Wrap onions individually in parchment paper, twisting or pinching the ends to keep the wrapping closed.

3. Place in a baking dish and put into oven with lamb. Bake for 40 to 45 minutes.

4. Unwrap onions and arrange around lamb on serving platter.

SUGGESTIONS FOR USE: Lamb sandwiches with tomato slices and mustard.

SUGGESTED ACCOMPANIMENTS: Wild-Rice Ring; Steamed Spinach; Fast Salad of carrot, radishes, and cucumber; and Crispy Walnut and Seed Bars.

★★★   VITAMIN B_{12}
★   NIACIN, ZINC, RIBOFLAVIN, IRON

We've seasoned this roast with rosemary because it is one of the herbs well-suited to menopause. It's used medicinally to stimulate the circulation and nerves, to ease tension, and is recommended as an antidepressive, combined with other herbs and taken as a tea.

❧ Rabbit in Fresh Red Sauce ❧

Yield: 3 quarts   (4 generous servings plus extra)

Rabbit is a long-standing and common staple in Europe, but it is becoming available here fresh in specialty stores or frozen in the supermarket. For a varied diet, whenever game is on the menu, go ahead and order it.

5 pounds ripe tomatoes, plum preferred, or 2 26-ounce boxes tomatoes (see Note page 173)
Sea salt
3 tablespoons extra-virgin olive oil
1 3- to 5-pound rabbit, cut into pieces (see Note)

1 onion, chopped
4 cloves garlic, sliced
3 sprigs fresh parsley
2 teaspoons basil
1 teaspoon oregano
1 bay leaf
Fresh black pepper

1. Cut tomatoes in half crosswise (along the diameter). Sprinkle cut sides generously with salt. Place cut side down on a cutting board and let sit at least 15 minutes. Juices will begin running out of the tomato.

2. Heat 2 tablespoons olive oil in a narrow, medium stockpot, and braise rabbit until golden on all sides. Remove to a plate.

3. Squeeze each tomato half, just enough to eject the seeds and any further juice. Using a spoon, scrape the seeds off the tomato as they are pushed out. (Leave the inner pulp intact.) Chop tomatoes.

4. In the same pot, add 1 tablespoon remaining olive oil and onion, and cook 2 minutes. Add garlic, parsley sprigs, basil, oregano, bay leaf, and tomato. Stir, cover, and cook over moderate heat, covered, 15 minutes, stirring every 5 minutes or so. This will give you a light tomato sauce.

5. Return rabbit to pot and spoon tomato sauce over to cover; add several grinds of pepper. Cook, covered, over moderate heat for 1½ to 2 hours, until the meat is tender and starts to fall off the bones.

6. Season to taste with salt, pepper, and extra-virgin olive oil. If you prefer a smoother sauce, press tomato sauce through a food mill. Serve on a platter on top of fresh polenta.

NOTE: You will need 2 to 3 pounds of rabbit if it has been boned, and 4 to 5 pounds with the bone in.

VARIATIONS: Chicken can be substituted for rabbit.

SUGGESTED ACCOMPANIMENTS: Polenta, grated pecorino romano cheese, Broccoli with Black Currants, and fresh blackberries and blueberries.

★★★   VITAMIN B$_{12}$
   ★   VITAMIN B$_6$, VITAMIN C, NIACIN, OMEGA-3 FATTY ACIDS, IRON

⚜ Venison Shish Kebab ⚜

Yield: 4 generous servings—maybe leftovers!

If you are low in iron and you need to add iron-rich food to your diet, the iron in meats such as venison is more easily absorbed than the kind in vegetables. Even at that, your body only absorbs about 10% of the iron you eat. To boost absorption, combine iron with vitamin C—have fresh oranges for dessert.

Have on hand: metal or wooden skewers. (Soak wood or bamboo skewers several hours before using.)

1½ **pounds venison, cut into 1½-inch cubes (see Variations)**
 2 **cups Teriyaki or Lemon-Lime-Orange Marinade (see recipes)**
 4 **tomatoes, quartered**
 2 **onions, quartered and separated**
 1 **green pepper, seeded and cut into 16 cubes**
 ½ **pound button mushrooms**

1. Wash the meat in cold water. Dry with paper towels and place in a shallow, flat container with marinade, tomatoes, onions, pepper, and whole mushrooms. Cover and refrigerate at least 1 hour—3 hours would be even better.
2. Thread meat and vegetables onto skewers, alternating the two. Wider spacing will allow more thorough cooking for well-done meat; tight spacing will result in meat which is less done.
3. Grill or broil 3 inches from heat source and brush frequently with leftover marinade. Turn to brown evenly and cook until done, about 8 to 10 minutes. (To bake, put the skewers and marinade in a shallow baking pan and place in a preheated 375° oven. Bake about 30 minutes, or until meat is done to your likeness.)
4. Pull meat and vegetables off skewers and onto a platter. Or give each person their own skewer of meat and vegetables. Serve immediately.

VARIATIONS: Shish kebab can also be made with lamb, beef, pork, chicken, or seafood such as shrimp, scallops, or monkfish. Marinated tofu and tempeh chunks will also skewer just fine.

SUGGESTED ACCOMPANIMENTS: Millet-Rice with Peas and Tomatoes, Fig Sauce with Basil, Your Basic Green Salad, and sliced blood oranges.

★★★ RIBOFLAVIN, IRON, NIACIN
 ★ VITAMIN C, COPPER, ZINC, THIAMIN

❧ Beef Sukiyaki with Ginger and Garlic ❧

Yield: 3 quarts   (4 generous servings plus extra)

A high-protein diet has been associated with an increase in osteoporosis, and it's protein from animal foods that particularly draws the calcium from bones. This dish lets you enjoy the wonderful flavor of beef but uses only modest amounts.

It is best to cook this dish in two batches.

2 tablespoons unrefined sesame oil
2-inch piece fresh ginger, minced
4 cloves garlic, minced
1 pound beef—sirloin tip, eye of round, or fillet, organic preferred, sliced ⅛ inch thick (see Note)
6 scallions, sliced thin
1 onion, sliced thin

½ pound button mushrooms, sliced
1 bunch watercress
½ cup filtered water
¼ cup shoyu soy sauce
1 teaspoon unsulphured blackstrap molasses
¼ pound snow peas or shelled peas

1. Heat 1 tablespoon of the oil in wok or a large sauté pan. Add half the ginger and garlic, cooking briefly, then add half the beef and cook about 2 minutes, turning frequently.

2. Push the beef up on the side of the wok, and sauté half of each vegetable in sequence—first scallions, then onion, mushrooms, and watercress—adding one and letting it cook a little before adding the next one. In total, sautéing time will take about 7 to 10 minutes.

3. In a small bowl mix together water, soy sauce, and molasses, stirring well.

4. Push the meat and vegetables back into the center of the wok, add half the soy sauce mixture, and snow peas. Stir and cook about 4 more minutes. The vegetables should retain their color and crispness.

5. Remove sukiyaki to a bowl, cover, and make a second batch, or else serve the first batch while preparing next one.

NOTE: Place the meat in the freezer for 20 minutes to make slicing easier. Cut against the grain. The meat and all the other ingredients should be at room temperature for cooking.

VARIATIONS: Instead of beef, use chicken, tempeh, or shrimp.

SUGGESTED ACCOMPANIMENTS: Vegetable-Trimmings Stock with miso, Basic Brown Rice, steamed green beans and carrots with garlic, and fresh persimmons with strawberries.

★★★   VITAMIN K, VITAMIN B$_{12}$, SELENIUM
  ★   ZINC, NIACIN, IRON, RIBOFLAVIN

❧ 14 ❧

Breakfast Foods and Whole Grain Muffins

BREAKFAST FOODS

Old-Fashioned Oatmeal
Brown Rice Congee (Chinese Rice Porridge)
Homemade Granola
Millet with Currants and Sunflower Seeds
Polenta French Toast with Blackberry Syrup
Salmon and Brown-Rice Patties
Fresh Herb Frittata
Open-Faced Nut-Butter Sandwiches
Homemade Fresh Yogurt

WHOLE GRAIN MUFFINS

Hearty Oatmeal-Apple Muffins
Breakfast Corn Muffins
Savory Corn Muffins with Onion and Poppy Seeds
Whole Grain Muffins with Sunflower and Flax Seeds

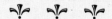

❧

Breakfast is an important meal to eat because it gives you fuel to run on for the day. If you're not accustomed to eating breakfast, begin to form the habit; when you reach menopause, breakfast is more important than ever. Include complex carbohydrates, protein, and fat in this meal because these break down at different rates. When you've run out of carbohydrates to burn, the protein kicks in and finally the fat, to give you a three- to four-hour supply of energy.

For complex carbohydrates, eat cooked whole grain cereals and breads. For protein, have an egg or some of last night's beans, fish, chicken, or meat. And for fat (and some protein), use nuts, seeds, or butters made from these or put some butter or flax seed oil on your hot cereal or toast.

Whole Grain Muffins

Our muffins are full of good ingredients, a nutritious addition to eat at lunch or dinner or as snacks and mini-meals. In our recipes, we use nuts, seeds, dried fruit, and healthy fats and oils for long-lasting energy. Enjoy sweet versions flavored with spices and maple syrup and savory muffins with the chewiness of seeds. Homemade muffins freeze, defrost, and reheat well.

Buying Breakfast Foods

Read the ingredients! When you buy cereal, look for whole grains and avoid all sugars (refined white sugar, cane sugar, honey, corn syrup, fructose, dextrose) and hydrogenated oil. Even scrutinize the products that sound healthy. Stores sell "granola," a term sometimes used as loosely as the word "natural." Muffins also sound homey and good for you, but store-bought ones are usually made with lots of sugar and poor-quality fats. We include four muffin recipes that are truly healthy.

And see the following for suggestions beyond the standard breakfast foods.

AT BREAKFAST, FOR A CHANGE, CONSIDER HAVING

Cold cereal: Try varieties made with whole grains and without refined sugar and preservatives—and instead of milk, eat with yogurt, juice, or nut and seed milks.

Hot cereal: Use a variety—cream of kasha, brown rice, millet, and oatmeal.

Fruit: Fresh and unsulphured dried fruits, compote with nuts and seeds.

Meats: Cooked or naturally smoked fish, organic liver, hamburger or steak pieces, natural and sugar-free sausages.

Soup: Vegetable, bean, or grain.

Dinner foods: Reheat leftovers such as grain pilafs, casseroles, stews, or twice-cooked beans with tortillas.

❧ Old-Fashioned Oatmeal ❧

Yield: 2½ cups   (4 generous servings)

One whole grain many of us have eaten since childhood is oatmeal. For flavor and texture we prefer it in its most unadulterated form—old-fashioned rolled oats.

2 cups filtered water	**¼ cup flax seeds**
¾ cup old-fashioned rolled oats	**¼ teaspoon sea salt**

1. In a small saucepan, heat water, oatmeal, flax seeds, and salt. Bring to a boil, lower heat, and simmer, uncovered, 15 minutes.

2. Pour into four bowls and top each with any of the suggested toppings below. Serve hot.

SUGGESTED TOPPINGS: Chopped nuts, maple syrup, or pumpkin or sunflower seeds.

VARIATIONS:

For Sweet Oatmeal: To this recipe, add 1 teaspoon cinnamon and ¼ cup black currants or raisins. Toasted nuts and maple syrup will also go well.

For Savory Oatmeal: To this recipe, add 1 tablespoon miso, 2 tablespoons tahini or almond butter, and raw or toasted seeds.

SUGGESTED ACCOMPANIMENTS: Almonds and herbal tea.

★★★   VITAMIN B$_6$, THIAMIN, OMEGA-3 FATTY ACIDS
  ★   MANGANESE, MAGNESIUM, RIBOFLAVIN, PANTOTHENIC ACID, COPPER, IRON

Oatmeal can be made to have a creamy or more chewy texture. The technique in this recipe—starting the oatmeal in cold water and bringing it to a boil—produces creamy oatmeal. To make a chewier oatmeal, first bring the water and salt to a boil, then add the oatmeal and cook for 15 minutes. Try both ways and you'll see quite a difference!

❦ Brown Rice Congee (Chinese Rice Porridge) ❦

Yield: 7 cups   (4 generous servings plus extra)

This dish is a long-cooked soupy grain that is easy to digest and particularly fortifying. It's a staple of Chinese cooking and often served with added protein—a raw egg dropped into the hot congee (which cooks the egg) or fish, pork, beef, or tofu. Try this porridge when you need reviving.

½ cup short-grain brown rice, washed
6 to 8 cups filtered water
⅛ teaspoon sea salt
2 scallions, sliced

Shoyu soy sauce
Hot sauce
Assorted additions (see Note)

1. In a medium saucepan, put rice, water, and salt. Bring to a boil, covered. Lower heat and simmer 4 to 6 hours or overnight.

2. Serve in bowls and top with scallions. Serve with soy sauce, hot sauce, and breakfast meats on the side.

NOTE: Serve congee with organic liver, meat, or fish slices, crumbled hard-boiled eggs, seasoned tempeh, cooked vegetables, cooked chestnuts, seaweed, hot sauce, sunflower or pumpkin seeds.

VARIATIONS: Any raw or precooked whole grain can be used instead of rice to make this dish, which is distinguished by the procedure used to cook the grain. Also, long-grain or sweet brown rice make a good variation.

★★★   MANGANESE, VITAMIN K
★   MAGNESIUM, SELENIUM, PHOSPHORUS, THIAMIN, PANTOTHENIC ACID, NIACIN, VITAMIN B_6

❦

In natural-food and Japanese grocery stores look for condiment shakers filled with a mix of sesame seeds, seaweed, and even bonito (fish) flakes—all high in calcium and other important minerals. These seasonings are great on congee and many other dishes. Keep a shaker on the table and use these flavorings instead of salt.

❦

❧ Homemade Granola ❧

Yield: about 10 cups   (20 ½-cup servings)

We've packed loads of good ingredients into this granola, a highly nutritious cereal that makes every calorie count. This substantial breakfast can help you reach your natural weight as it cuts your hunger for sugary morning snacks.

7   cups old-fashioned rolled oats
½ to 1 cup walnuts, almonds, or
    pecans, chopped coarsely
½   cup sesame seeds
½   cup sunflower or pumpkin seeds
½   cup unsweetened coconut (optional)
1   teaspoon sea salt
1½ teaspoons cinnamon
½   teaspoon ground ginger
½   cup flax seed oil

½ to 1 cup filtered water, as needed
1   teaspoon pure vanilla extract
1   cup apple butter (optional)
½   cup maple syrup or barley malt
¼   cup unsulphured blackstrap
    molasses
1   cup currants or raisins
½   cup unsulphured dates or apricots,
    chopped

Preheat oven to 350°.

1. In a large bowl, mix oats, nuts, sesame and sunflower seeds, coconut, salt, cinnamon, and ginger.

2. In a medium bowl, whisk together flax seed oil, ½ cup water, vanilla, apple butter, maple syrup, and molasses. Pour wet ingredients into dry mixture and stir well. Add more water as needed to moisten oatmeal.

3. Spread oatmeal mixture in non-oiled baking pans or, for easy cleanup, first cover pans with parchment paper. Bake until golden, turning several times while baking, about 30 minutes.

4. Remove to a large bowl to cool and add raisins and dates.

5. Store in an airtight container.

VARIATIONS: Add other dried fruits such as apricots, pears, peaches, or prunes.

SUGGESTED ACCOMPANIMENTS: Ripe banana, Almond Milk, and mint tea.

★★★   OMEGA-3 FATTY ACIDS
★   MANGANESE, LINOLEIC ACID, THIAMIN, MAGNESIUM

Molasses is the byproduct of the final extraction of sugar refining. Blackstrap molasses is high in minerals. Purchase the unsulphured kind, as the preservative sulphur dioxide can cause adverse reactions. Think of it as a liquid mineral supplement you can cook with.

❧ Millet with Currants and Sunflower Seeds ❧

Yield: 1 quart   (4 generous servings)

This cereal-seed mix gives you premium fuel to run on until lunch. It stabilizes blood sugar and provides thiamin, riboflavin, and niacin to ward off low energy and depression.

2 **cups millet, washed**	2 **tablespoons unsalted butter or flax**
3½ **cups filtered water or nut milk**	**seed oil**
½ **cup sunflower seeds**	1 **tablespoon sea salt**
¼ **cup dried currants**	

1. In a medium, heavy-bottomed pot, put millet, water, sunflower seeds, currants, butter, and salt. Bring to a boil, reduce heat to low, and cook, covered, 30 minutes. (Use a heat diffuser with an electric stove or thin-bottomed pot.)
2. Fluff with a fork to loosen and separate grains.

VARIATIONS: Add spices such as ground cloves, cinnamon, or even saffron. Substitute walnuts or almonds for the sunflower seeds.

SUGGESTED ACCOMPANIMENT: Herbal tea.

★★★   LINOLEIC ACID, FOLIC ACID
★   THIAMIN, MANGANESE, MAGNESIUM, COPPER, IRON, VITAMIN B$_6$

❧ Polenta French Toast with Blackberry Syrup ❧

Yield: 8 slices   (4 generous servings)

If you are unfamiliar with the delights of cornmeal for breakfast, try a slice of browned polenta topped with fruit syrup, a recipe inspired by French toast. The berry syrup provides estrogenic bioflavonoids and no refined sugar.

Have on hand: 1 recipe polenta, cooled in a loaf pan (see recipe)

POLENTA:

2 tablespoons unsalted butter or flax seed oil

8 slices polenta, ½ inch thick
1 teaspoon cinnamon

SYRUP:

1 cup unfiltered apple juice
4 ounces all-fruit blackberry preserves
2 tablespoons maple syrup (optional)

¼ cup filtered water
2 tablespoons arrowroot powder

POLENTA:

1. Melt 1 tablespoon butter or oil in a large, heavy-bottomed skillet or pancake griddle. Arrange polenta slices in pan with a little room between each slice. Sprinkle with cinnamon.

2. Cook 5 to 10 minutes on each side, turning only once when the first side has turned golden. Add remaining butter as needed.

SYRUP:

1. In a small pot heat apple juice, preserves, and maple syrup. In a small container mix together water and arrowroot until dissolved. Pour into apple-juice mixture, stirring constantly, until juice clears and thickens, then cook for another 30 seconds.

2. Serve polenta slices with syrup on the side.

VARIATIONS: You can add fresh berries to the syrup for a texture and taste change. Or mix maple syrup and water (two to one), pour over slices while still in the pan, and cook down for a few minutes before serving. Or even add a little molasses, if you like the flavor, for some vital nutrients.

SUGGESTED ACCOMPANIMENTS: Caffix grain beverage.

★★★ THIAMIN, IRON, MANGANESE, PHOSPHORUS

❧ Salmon and Brown-Rice Patties ❧

Yield: 4 generous servings plus extra

Fondly known as "hot-flash hash" in our kitchens, this dish has nutrients that keep you cool. These patties supply you with vitamin E, selenium, and magnesium, all known to reduce hot flashes.

4 cups spinach, washed
1 pound salmon fillet, skin removed
4 teaspoons sesame seeds
4 teaspoons sunflower seeds
1 egg, organic, free-range preferred
1 teaspoon herbal sea salt

2 cups cooked brown rice
½ cup whole wheat bread crumbs
1 tablespoon flax seed oil
1 tablespoon unsalted butter
1 lemon, cut into wedges

1. Place wet spinach in a medium saucepan. Cover, bring to a boil, and simmer until spinach is wilted, about 5 to 7 minutes. Drain in a colander and cool.

2. Cut salmon into chunks, removing any bones. Place in processor with cooked spinach, sesame and sunflower seeds, egg, and herbal salt. Pulse a few times until seeds are chopped and everything is mixed.

3. Put salmon mixture in a bowl and add rice. Mix well. Add ¼ cup bread crumbs, stir, and add more if needed to hold in patty shape.

4. Heat one-half of oil and butter in a medium sauté pan. With wet hands form small patties and place in heated oil. Cook for 5 to 7 minutes, turning once. (If you prefer, you can cook this as hash, sautéing loose mixture until done, about 5 minutes. The patties can also be baked for 20 minutes at 350°.

SUGGESTED ACCOMPANIMENTS: Herbal tea, such as rose hip.

★★★ VITAMIN D, VITAMIN K, VITAMIN B$_{12}$, SELENIUM, OMEGA-3 FATTY ACIDS
★ VITAMIN E, FOLIC ACID, NIACIN, VITAMIN A, MAGNESIUM, PHOSPHORUS

❧ Fresh Herb Frittata ❧

Yield: 4 servings

A frittata is an omelette with flair, quickly whisked together and cooked with pieces of vegetables. This technique is handy to know when you want an easy meal.

1 teaspoon unsalted butter or extra-virgin olive oil
1 onion, minced
5 eggs, organic, free-range preferred
1 bunch watercress, chopped coarsely

½ bunch parsley, chopped coarsely
½ bunch scallions, sliced
¼ teaspoon sea salt
⅛ teaspoon pepper

1. In a medium, oven-safe frying pan, melt ½ teaspoon of the butter over medium heat. Add onion and cook until translucent. Remove onion to a small plate or bowl.

2. Into a medium bowl, break eggs and beat with a whisk until fluffy. Add onion, watercress, parsley, scallions, salt, and pepper.

3. Heat remaining ½ teaspoon butter in frying pan, making sure it coats the sides and bottom of the pan. Pour in eggs, and allow to cook 2 or 3 minutes, until the edges begin to dry a little.

4. Turn on broiler. Place frying pan under broiler for 1 or 2 minutes, until eggs puff and the top turns golden.

5. Slide a knife around the edge to loosen frittata. Slip out onto a large serving platter and cut into quarters. Eat while hot.

SUGGESTED ACCOMPANIMENTS: Whole grain toast or waffles, and herbal tea.

★★★ VITAMIN K, VITAMIN C
★ SELENIUM, FOLIC ACID, VITAMIN B$_{12}$, RIBOFLAVIN

Organic Eggs

Good things do come in small packages. Case in point: the egg. In spite of its bad rap because of a high cholesterol content, the egg is a wonderful source of high-quality protein, plus iron, zinc, and vitamins A, B$_2$, D, E, and K. In moderation, it's a great whole food.

We recommend buying organic eggs, which are free of antibiotics and added hormones that can burden your system, and we prefer eggs from free-range chickens who eat a more natural diet. Eggs from naturally raised chickens tend to have thick shells, bright yellow-orange yolks, and a richer flavor.

❧ Open-Faced Nut-Butter Sandwiches ❧

Yield: 2 sandwiches

Here is an unpretentious, gourmet whole food—a grown-up PB&J!

2 slices whole wheat bread or 1 bagel, English muffin, or pita	2 to 3 teaspoons almond, cashew, or hazelnut butter (see Appendix) 2 teaspoons all-fruit jam

Toast bread. Spread nut butter thinly on top of each slice and then spread jam.

SUGGESTED ACCOMPANIMENTS: A cup of herbal tea or grain coffee substitute.

★★★   MANGANESE, SELENIUM, MAGNESIUM, FOLIC ACID, LINOLENIC ACID
  ★   IRON, NIACIN, RIBOFLAVIN, THIAMIN, COPPER

We recommend eating a variety of nuts—our two nutritional favorites, almonds and walnuts, plus cashews, hazelnuts, pecans and pistachios. Peanuts are fine if eaten raw, but so often the peanuts being served are processed and have added ingredients. "Roasted" peanuts are actually fried, usually in coconut oil, and then salted. "Dry-roasted" peanuts are salted and may contain sugar, honey, and preservatives.

High-quality nut "butters"—really just nuts ground to a paste—are a nutritious convenience food. The most widely eaten nut butter is peanut butter, but unfortunately manufacturers of peanut butter usually add sugar, salt, and hydrogenated oils to their product. If you are craving peanut butter, look for a natural-foods store that grinds its own and enjoy some fresh made.

❧ Homemade Fresh Yogurt ❧

Yield: 2 quarts

The active bacteria lactobacillus acidophilus in the yogurt we recommend helps metabolize estrogen in the colon, lowering body estrogen levels and possibly the risk of breast cancer.

2 quarts whole milk, preferably organic

¼ cup prepared plain bacteria-active or homemade yogurt (see Note)

1. In a medium saucepan, over medium heat, scald milk.
2. Thin yogurt in a cup with several tablespoons of the warm milk. Pour into the saucepan and stir well.
3. Pour yogurt with added culture into a large bowl (preferably ceramic) or individual glass containers. Cover with plastic and set in a warm place (such as an oven with a pilot light or a warm attic or garage) until yogurt is set, about 6 to 8 hours or overnight. (Moisture may accumulate on the top of the yogurt; if desired, this can be removed with paper toweling.) Chill yogurt.

NOTE: Before using up yogurt, save ¼ cup to start a new batch.

★★★   IODINE, VITAMIN B$_{12}$
  ★   CALCIUM, SELENIUM, PHOSPHORUS, RIBOFLAVIN

❧

To make a thicker or cheese-style yogurt, line a colander with cotton cheese-cloth, unbleached paper towels, or coffee filters. (Bleached paper towels have dioxin, a toxic substance.) Place the colander in a bowl and pour in the yogurt. Allow to sit for several hours or overnight in the refrigerator. Yogurt cheese can be seasoned with an infinite variety of fresh or dried herbs and spices to make a terrific dip for vegetables or a spread for crackers.

❧

❧ Hearty Oatmeal-Apple Muffins ❧

Yield: 16 muffins

One way you can take good care of yourself during menopause is by carrying good food with you. These muffins are perfect minimeals for your car and office.

Have on hand: oiled or paper-lined muffin cups.

2 **eggs, organic, fertile preferred (see Note)**
¼ **cup sweet butter, at room temperature, or flax seed oil**
⅓ **cup maple syrup**
1 **tablespoon pure vanilla extract**
½ **teaspoon sea salt**
1 **apple, grated (about 1 cup)**
    Rind of 1 orange or lemon, organic preferred
½ **cup almond, cashew, rice, or soy milk**

2 **cups oatmeal**
1 **cup whole wheat pastry flour**
½ **cup walnuts or pecans, chopped coarsely**
½ **cup sunflower seeds**
½ **cup dried currants or raisins**
2 **tablespoons flax seeds**
1 **teaspoon cinnamon**
½ **teaspoon aluminum-free baking powder (optional)**

Preheat oven to 375°.

1. In a medium bowl, using a whisk (or blender or electric beater), whip eggs and butter together.

2. Add maple syrup, vanilla, salt, grated apple, and orange rind and mix well. Stir in nut milk and mix well.

3. In a large bowl mix oatmeal, flour, walnuts, sunflower seeds, currants, flax seeds, cinnamon, and baking powder.

4. Stir butter-maple mixture into flour mixture, stirring just enough to moisten.

5. Spoon batter into prepared muffin tins, filling cups three-fourths full, or use an ice-cream scoop dipped in water to give muffins a rounded top.

6. Place in preheated oven and bake 20 minutes until golden on top.

7. Remove muffins to a cooling rack or turn upside down in muffin pan to cool bottoms and keep tops moist.

NOTE: If you prefer to omit eggs, add 1½ tablespoons (instead of ½ teaspoon) aluminum-free baking powder and 3 tablespoons filtered water. To eliminate the baking powder completely, the eggs must be used.

VARIATIONS: Add chopped dates, apricots, or prunes.

SUGGESTED ACCOMPANIMENTS: All-fruit jam and almond butter.

★★★   OMEGA-3 FATTY ACIDS, MANGANESE, THIAMIN, LINOLEIC ACID
  ★   SELENIUM, MAGNESIUM, PHOSPHOROUS, IRON

❧ Breakfast Corn Muffins ❧

Yield: 8 muffins

These morning muffins are full of manganese, nourishment for the nerves and brain—good wake-up food.

Have on hand: oiled or paper-lined muffin cups.

2 eggs, organic, fertile preferred (see Note)
¼ cup sweet butter, at room temperature
½ cup maple syrup
½ cup almond, cashew, rice, or soy milk

2 tablespoons pure vanilla extract
1 cup hi-lysine cornmeal
1 cup whole wheat pastry flour
2 tablespoons flax seeds, ground or whole
½ teaspoon sea salt

Preheat oven to 350°.
1. In a medium bowl, using a whisk or blender, whip eggs and butter together.
2. Add maple syrup, milk, and vanilla and mix well.
3. In a small bowl, mix together cornmeal, flour, flax seeds, and salt.
4. Add egg mixture to cornmeal combination, stirring until dry ingredients are just moistened. Do not overmix.
5. Pour into prepared muffin tins, filling cups three-fourths full, or use an ice-cream scoop dipped in water to give muffins rounded tops.
6. Place in preheated oven and bake until tops are golden, about 30 minutes.
7. Remove muffins to a cooling rack or turn upside down in muffin pan to cool bottoms and keep tops moist.

NOTE: If you prefer to omit eggs, use 1 tablespoon arrowroot powder and 1 tablespoon baking powder, plus an additional ¼ cup water or milk.

SUGGESTED ACCOMPANIMENTS: Herbal tea and Almond and Apple Butter Spread.

★★★ OMEGA-3 FATTY ACIDS, MANGANESE
★ SELENIUM, THIAMIN, VITAMIN B$_6$, RIBOFLAVIN

❧ Savory Corn Muffins with Onion ❧ and Poppy Seeds

Yield: 12 muffins

Restaurant corn muffins are usually made with sugar and are as sweet as cake. Ours feature the flavor of the corn itself and are sweetened with just a bit of mineral-rich molasses. We added poppy seeds as a bonus. A batch of these muffins made in the morning will fill the air with a wonderful aroma and they reheat well all week.

Have on hand: oiled or paper-lined muffin cups.

2 teaspoons plus ¼ cup unsalted butter
1 onion, diced
1 cup hi-lysine stone-ground cornmeal
½ cup whole wheat pastry flour
3 tablespoons poppy seeds
2 teaspoons aluminum-free baking powder

½ teaspoon sea salt
1 tablespoon unsulphured blackstrap molasses
1 egg, organic, free-range preferred
¾ cup nut or rice milk, or filtered water
3 ears corn, kernels removed, about 1 cup (see Note)

Preheat oven to 375°.

1. In a small frying pan, heat 2 teaspoons butter and onion, cooking over medium-high heat until golden, about 10 minutes.

2. In a medium-size bowl, mix together cornmeal, pastry flour, poppy seeds, baking powder, and salt.

3. Place ¼ cup butter in a small metal bowl and put into the oven to melt. Once butter is melted, whisk in molasses, egg, and milk. Stir in caramelized onion and corn. Pour into cornmeal mixture and stir until moistened.

4. Spoon batter into muffin cups, filling each three-quarters full. Bake until golden on top, about 25 to 30 minutes.

5. Remove muffins to a cooling rack or turn upside down in muffin pan to cool bottoms and keep tops moist.

NOTE: To remove corn kernels from the cob, break corn in half and rest the broken end on a cutting board, so that the cob end points up. Carefully hold the corn and with a knife cut down the side, turning corn after each cut until all kernels have been removed. (The cobs are great for soup stock.)

SUGGESTED ACCOMPANIMENTS: Full-Of-Vegetables Beef Stew and leafy green salad.

★★★ MANGANESE, OMEGA-3 FATTY ACIDS
  ★   THIAMIN, IRON, SELENIUM, LINOLEIC ACID, BORON

Hi-lysine cornmeal has higher amounts of lysine as well as other amino acids, which extend its shelf life by keeping it from going rancid. This type of cornmeal retains the sweet, nutty flavor of corn. As with all whole grain flours, purchase this cornmeal in small quantities, store in the refrigerator or freezer, and use up quickly.

❧ Whole Grain Muffins with ❧
Sunflower and Flax Seeds

Yield: 12 muffins

Here's breakfast in a muffin, a handful of good things to eat as you run out the door, with whole grains and a variety of seeds.

Have on hand: oiled or paper-lined muffin cups.

2 cups oatmeal
1 cup whole wheat pastry flour
½ cup sunflower seeds
¼ cup flax seeds
1 teaspoon caraway or cumin seeds
   (optional)

2 teaspoons aluminum-free baking
   powder
½ teaspoon sea salt
1 egg, organic, free-range preferred
¼ cup unsalted butter, melted
1 cup nut or rice milk

Preheat oven to 350°.

1. In a medium bowl, mix together oatmeal, flour, sunflower, flax, and caraway seeds, baking powder, and salt.

2. In a small bowl, whisk together egg, butter, and milk. Pour the liquid ingredients into the oatmeal mixture and stir until blended.

3. Spoon into prepared muffin cups, filling each three-fourths full. Bake in preheated oven until tops are golden, about 30 minutes.

4. Remove muffins to a cooling rack or turn upside down in muffin pan to cool bottoms and keep tops moist.

SUGGESTED ACCOMPANIMENTS: Split Pea and Barley Soup with Spices, and Butternut Squash Purée.

★★★ OMEGA-3 FATTY ACIDS, LINOLEIC ACID, MAGNESIUM, VITAMIN E
★ VITAMIN B$_6$, MANGANESE, THIAMIN, SELENIUM

If a muffin is going to be your portable breakfast, then also pack some fruit. Keep some on hand, already washed.

❧ 15 ❧
Appetizers, Sauces, and Marinades

APPETIZERS

White Bean Spread with Vegetables
Taramasalata (Greek Caviar Spread)
Butternut Babaganoush
Greek Cucumber and Yogurt Dip

SAUCES

Chick-pea Béchamel
Basil-Parsley Pesto
Wild Mushroom Sauce
Latin Cilantro-Garlic Sauce
Quick Barbecue Sauce
Almond Romesco Sauce
Cilantro Salsa
Persimmon Salsa
Fig Sauce with Basil
Tomato Sauce
Tofu Alfredo Sauce

MARINADES

Lemon-Lime-Orange Marinade
Teriyaki Marinade

❧

Made with nutritious ingredients chosen for women, these appetizers are simple enough for everyday, but elegant enough for entertaining. Try the Taramasalata, made with salt-cured cod roe. It's full of vitamin E, which tempers hot flashes and moistens skin. Or sample the White Bean Spread, high in fiber for a healthy heart.

The sauces and marinades are also based on foods we recommend—nuts with essential fatty acids, citrus with bioflavonoids, figs with all their vitamins and minerals, estrogenic tofu, and wild mushrooms recognized by traditional Chinese medicine as a food that stimulates fundamental energies postmenopause.

Just as important is the ingredient that's absent—sugar, the usual sweetener in recipes such as Teriyaki Marinade. We use maple syrup and nutrient-rich blackstrap molasses instead.

❧ White Bean Spread with Vegetables ❧

Yield: 2 cups spread   (4 generous servings plus extra)

A healthy menopause diet leans toward the vegetarian, and beans are a staple of this way of eating. If you're not in the habit of making them a major part of your meal, have beans as a starter course or snack instead, and begin with this delicious White Bean Spread.

BEANS:

2 cups cooked navy or Great Northern beans (see page 120)
2 teaspoons salted plum vinegar (umeboshi)
2 teaspoons brown rice vinegar

2 cloves garlic
3 tablespoons extra-virgin olive oil
½ onion
½ teaspoon sea salt

VEGETABLES:

2 stalks celery, cut into sticks
8 cherry tomatoes
1 red pepper, seeded and cut into strips

2 carrots, cut into sticks
4 mushrooms, cut in half
4 scallions

1. In a blender or processor, place beans, vinegars, garlic, olive oil, onion, and salt. Purée until smooth. Place in a serving bowl, and add a serving spoon.

2. Arrange vegetables on a platter, making room for dip bowl.

VARIATIONS: Any kind of leftover beans will whiz right up and make this delicious dish.

SUGGESTED ACCOMPANIMENTS: Serve with whole grain crackers or warmed whole grain pita bread.

★★★   VITAMIN A, VITAMIN K, VITAMIN C, FOLIC ACID

❧ **Taramasalata (Greek Caviar Spread)** ❧

Yield: 2 cups

Tarama is primarily a Greek and Turkish product, made from the roe of mullet. Carp, mackerel, or codfish roe can be substituted. This egg-paste is a pale orange and is sold in jars, refrigerated, at Greek, other ethnic, and imported-food stores. Serve taramasalata with bread sticks, celery and carrot sticks, or hearty whole grain bread. Or place a dollop inside a baked potato, or thin with water and use as a sauce over steamed vegetables.

1 **potato, peeled and quartered (see Note)**	1 **cup extra-virgin olive oil**
2 **cups filtered water**	**Juice of 3 lemons, plus 1 lemon cut into wedges**
⅓ **cup tarama**	10 **kalamata or Greek olives**
2 **tablespoons grated red onion**	

1. Place potato and water into a small saucepan, bring to a boil, and simmer until potato is soft when pierced with a fork, about 15 minutes. Drain and place in cold water to cool completely.

2. Place tarama and potato in a processor. Pulse until completely blended. (Or pound tarama with potato in a mortar, remove to a medium bowl and then proceed.) Add onion and several tablespoons of olive oil, beating with a whisk or pulsing.

3. Keep adding small amounts of oil and lemon juice, beating or pulsing in between additions, until all the oil and juice have been used. The mixture will be cream-colored and the consistency of mayonnaise.

4. Pour into a small serving bowl and garnish with olives and lemon wedges.

NOTE: Soft whole wheat bread crumbs can be used instead of potato. Moisten them in lemon juice first.

★★★   VITAMIN E, VITAMIN K, VITAMIN C
  ★   OMEGA-3 FATTY ACIDS, LINOLEIC ACID

Taramasalata from Fresh Roe

Unlike tarama, fresh roe hasn't been cured with salt, but it is equally delicious. Steam ¼ pound fresh mullet roe in ¼ cup filtered water, covered, about 2 minutes. Remove roe to a plate, detach and discard the membrane, and let roe cool. Follow instructions, adding sea salt and freshly ground pepper to taste.

❧ Butternut Babaganoush ❧

Yield: 2½ to 3 cups   (4 generous servings plus extra)

Babaganoush, a classic Middle Eastern appetizer, is usually made with eggplant but we've used squash instead for its vitamin A, which maintains your skin as you age, and boosts your immunity. The squash also changes this dish from the standard eggplant gray to an appealing yellow-orange.

1 **pound butternut squash**	3 **tablespoons extra-virgin olive oil**
5 **cloves garlic**	1 **tablespoon sesame tahini**
3 **tablespoons lemon juice**	1½ **teaspoons sea salt**

Preheat oven to 375°.

1. Cut butternut squash in half lengthwise. Place halves cut side down on a baking sheet. Bake 45 to 60 minutes, until soft when pierced with a fork.

2. With a large spoon, scoop seeds out of squash and discard. Scoop butternut flesh into the bowl of a processor or blender (see Note).

3. Add garlic, lemon juice, olive oil, tahini, and salt. Pureé mixture until smooth.

4. Chill at least ½ hour and serve with crackers and vegetable sticks.

NOTE: If using a blender, combine squash and other ingredients in a bowl and blend in batches.

SUGGESTED ACCOMPANIMENTS: Serve with whole grain pita triangles, bread sticks, or as a sandwich with sliced tomato and sprouts.

★★★　VITAMIN A, VITAMIN C
　★　　VITAMIN K, MAGNESIUM, MANGANESE, FOLIC ACID

❧ Greek Cucumber and Yogurt Dip ❧

Yield: 2½ cups

Here's a menopause food—cooling cucumbers and refreshing yogurt. Chop, mix, and you have a mini-meal.

2 cucumbers, peeled and seeded
2 cups plain bacteria-active yogurt
   (see Note)
1 clove garlic, minced or pressed
2 tablespoons extra-virgin
   olive oil

1 tablespoon lemon juice or cider
   vinegar
½ teaspoon sea salt
   Several grinds fresh black pepper
1 loaf crusty whole wheat bread, or one
   package whole wheat pita

1. Grate or chop cucumbers fine. Place in a bowl and add yogurt, garlic, olive oil, lemon juice, salt, and pepper. Stir well.

2. Serve with warmed bread slices or pita triangles.

Note: For a thicker dip, start with drained yogurt (see page 280).

Suggested accompaniments: Whole Grain Bread with Escarole and Kidney Bean Soup.

★★★   SELENIUM, MANGANESE, VITAMIN K, LINOLEIC ACID

Tips for using this salad:

- Use instead of butter on baked potatoes.
- Use instead of mayonnaise on sandwiches.
- Garnish soups, such as black bean, vegetable, or borscht.
- Replace sour cream in a stew.

❧ Chick-pea Béchamel ❧

Yield: 2½ cups   (4 generous servings)

This recipe gives you a way to have legumes as a sauce. Our Chick-pea Béchamel is low in calories and high in minerals and still lets you enjoy its creamy texture.

Have on hand: 1 cup each cooked chick-peas and cooking liquid (see page 120).

1 onion, minced
¼ cup filtered water
3 cloves garlic, minced
1 cup cooked chick-peas
1 cup chick-pea cooking liquid or filtered water

1 tablespoon prepared mustard
½ teaspoon sea salt
⅛ teaspoon black pepper
1 tablespoon extra-virgin olive oil
¼ teaspoon brown rice vinegar or cider vinegar

1. In a small skillet, steam onion in water for 2 minutes. Add 2 cloves garlic, cover, and cook over medium heat until onion and garlic are almost translucent, 5 to 7 minutes.
2. In a blender, put cooked onion, garlic, chick-peas, ½ cup chick-pea cooking liquid, mustard, salt, pepper, olive oil, vinegar, and remaining clove of raw garlic. Blend until smooth, adding more liquid as needed.
3. Heat in a small saucepan before using.

VARIATIONS: This sauce is a basic format for any bean sauce. Other varieties of beans can be substituted, although the chick-peas are our favorite.

SUGGESTED USES: Spoon over grain, vegetables, or fish. Spread on bread or crackers.

★★★   FOLIC ACID
★   MANGANESE, IRON, VITAMIN B_6, MAGNESIUM, COPPER

❦ Basil-Parsley Pesto ❦

Yield: 2 cups

This pesto is a great way to sneak more nuts into your meals, classic Italian pesto made with the usual pine nuts or, even better, menopause-friendly walnuts. Here's where fat belongs, sparking the flavors of a nutritious bowl of pasta or brown rice. Satisfy your hunger for calories and know that you are still taking good care of yourself.

To store extra pesto, place it in a container and cover with ⅛ inch olive oil to seal it from the air. This will allow the pesto to last several weeks in the refrigerator. Spread it on bread, stir it into soup, and place it on top of whole grain pasta.

1 cup walnuts or pine nuts
3 cloves garlic, peeled
2 tablespoons chick-pea miso
½ teaspoon sea salt

1 bunch basil, leaves only (about 1 cup)
1 bunch parsley, leaves only (about 1 cup)
½ cup extra-virgin olive oil

1. Put walnuts in a processor with garlic and pulse a few times. Add miso, salt, basil, and parsley. Pulse until well chopped.

2. Add ¼ cup olive oil, and purée. Drizzle in remaining olive oil.

SUGGESTED USES: Spread this on top of fish fillets, chicken, or tempeh and bake, serving it with lemon. Spread it on bread and broil to make a bruschetta appetizer, or stir it into a bowl of soup or beans to make a hearty and flavorful meal. Instead of salt, use 2 teaspoons to flavor a vegetable soup, and it's great on top of whole grain pasta.

★★★   OMEGA-3 FATTY ACIDS, VITAMIN K, LINOLENIC ACID
  ★   VITAMIN C, MANGANESE, FOLIC ACID, MAGNESIUM

❧ Wild Mushroom Sauce ❧

Yield: 2 cups   (4 generous servings)

At menopause many women find they crave watery foods. Mushrooms are in this category.

4 tablespoons unsalted butter
2 shallots or 3 cloves garlic, minced
½ pound button mushrooms, sliced
½ pound fresh wild mushrooms, such as cremini, portobello, shiitake, morel, chanterelle, sliced

1 teaspoon herbal sea salt
1¼ cups filtered water or vegetable stock (see recipe)
2 tablespoons whole wheat flour
Freshly ground black pepper

1. In a medium pot, heat 2 tablespoons butter and add shallots. Cook on medium heat about 2 minutes. Add mushrooms and herbal salt, stirring well. Add ¼ cup water, cover, and cook 5 minutes on low heat.

2. In a small sauté pan, heat flour and remaining 2 tablespoons butter. Cook on medium heat until it begins to smell roasted, about 3 to 4 minutes.

3. Add several tablespoons of water at a time to flour mixture, stirring well to form a paste at first and, as more water is added, to form a sauce consistency, using at least ¾ cup.

4. Pour any remaining water plus enough to make 1 cup into mushrooms and bring to a boil. Stir sauce from frying pan into mushrooms and liquid. Return to a boil, lower flame, and cook 3 to 5 minutes. Add pepper to taste and serve.

VARIATIONS: For a delicious soup, add water to leftover sauce, and season to taste while heating.

SUGGESTED USES: Over grain, spread on bread or toast (crostini), or mixed with beans.

★★★ PANTOTHENIC ACID, COPPER, RIBOFLAVIN, NIACIN, VITAMIN A
  ★ SELENIUM, VITAMIN D, VITAMIN B$_6$

❧ Latin Cilantro-Garlic Sauce ❧

Yield: 1½ cups   (4 generous servings plus extra)

Sauces can be as healthy as main courses, and they don't need to be saturated with salt and sugar or unhealthy oils. This sauce gives you an array of ingredients that are good for your heart—cilantro, garlic, and extra-virgin olive oil, with just a little salt.

1 **bunch cilantro, leaves only, minced**
1 **bunch parsley, leaves only, minced**
4 **cloves garlic, minced**
⅓ **cup extra-virgin olive oil**

⅓ **cup flax seed oil**
2 **tablespoons brown rice vinegar**
1 **tablespoon chick-pea or red miso**
    Pinch sea salt

1. In a medium bowl, mix together cilantro, parsley, garlic, olive and flax seed oils, vinegar, miso, and salt. (For a smoother texture, purée in a processor.)
2. Serve cold or at room temperature.

VARIATIONS: Use dill or basil instead of cilantro, add scallions or onions to add a piquant flavor, or use either cilantro or parsley alone.

SUGGESTED USES: Serve 1 teaspoon on whole grain pasta or grains, or stir into beans or soup for flavoring.

★★★   VITAMIN K, VITAMIN C, OMEGA-3 FATTY ACIDS
  ★   VITAMIN E, FOLIC ACID, LINOLEIC ACID, IRON, VITAMIN A

❧ Quick Barbecue Sauce ❧

Yield: ½ cup

Healthy eating can include all the flavors you love. We make this Barbecue Sauce without refined sugar, but it's still sweet because of the blackstrap molasses.

2 tablespoons unsweetened ketchup (see Note)

2 tablespoons shoyu soy sauce

2 teaspoons unsulphured blackstrap molasses

¼ teaspoon chili powder

1 clove garlic, pressed

¼ small onion, grated

½ teaspoon sea salt

In a small bowl, combine ketchup, shoyu, molasses, chili powder, garlic, onion, and salt. Mix well.

NOTE: Commercial ketchup contains sugar.

SUGGESTED USES: Serve this with broiled fish, chicken, meat, tofu, or tempeh. It is also great mixed into beans and then baked 1 or 2 hours.

★★★ IRON

★ MANGANESE, COPPER, VITAMIN B$_6$, MAGNESIUM

❧ Almond Romesco Sauce ❧

Yield: 2 cups

Nuts have healthy oils, vitamins, and minerals, and you need to eat them regularly. Here's a classic Spanish sauce based on almonds, tomatoes, and garlic. Try some on a sandwich instead of mayonnaise.

½ cup extra-virgin olive oil
½ cup almonds
4 to 6 cloves garlic, peeled and left whole
5 ripe plum tomatoes, seeded and chopped coarsely

¼ teaspoon sea salt
Few grinds of fresh black pepper
¼ teaspoon cayenne pepper
¼ cup filtered water
1 tablespoon balsamic or cider vinegar

1. In a medium skillet, heat 2 tablespoons olive oil and add almonds and garlic. Cook on medium-low heat until garlic is golden, about 5 to 7 minutes, stirring occasionally.

2. Add tomatoes and cook for 3 or 4 minutes. Turn off heat and let sit 5 minutes to cool.

3. Place tomato mixture in a mortar, blender, or processor. Add salt, peppers, water, and vinegar. Pulverize or purée, adding a little oil at a time to make a thick sauce.

SUGGESTED USES: Spread on fish or meat before broiling or stewing; use on pasta or vegetables as a sauce. Spread on bread and broil for delightful and crunchy crostini.

★★★   VITAMIN E, LINOLEIC ACID, MAGNESIUM, MANGANESE
★   VITAMIN C, COPPER, OMEGA-3 FATTY ACIDS

❧ Cilantro Salsa ❧

Yield: 1½ cups

Salsa made with onions is heart healthy. Especially when eaten raw, onions raise your HDL, the good cholesterol, and help dissolve clots. Have them regularly, the stronger the flavor the better. These do the most good.

1 bunch cilantro, minced	1 cup filtered water
4 scallions, minced	Juice of 2 lemons
1 small yellow onion, minced	1 teaspoon sea salt
1 small red onion, minced	¼ teaspoon hot sauce

1. In a small bowl, put cilantro, scallions, and onions. Mix in water, lemon juice, salt, and hot sauce.

2. Let sit 15 minutes before using so that the flavors can develop, incorporating the strong onion flavor. If you like, purée in a blender.

VARIATIONS: Add any or all of the following ingredients: 2 chopped tomatoes; 2 to 3 tablespoons extra-virgin olive oil; ½ bunch finely chopped parsley; 1 chopped ripe avocado.

SUGGESTED USES: Serve with Twice-Cooked Beans Wrapped in Corn Tortillas for a perfect match.

★★★ VITAMIN K, VITAMIN C, FOLIC ACID
★ VITAMIN A, IRON, VITAMIN B$_6$, POTASSIUM, MAGNESIUM

❧ Persimmon Salsa ❧

Yield: 2 cups

Enjoy a variety of fruits, including the exotic ones. Japanese persimmons are a crisp and crunchy variety that can be eaten like an apple. They are a bright orange color and have a squat, round shape, somewhat similar to a miniature pumpkin. If this variety cannot be found, a fine substitute will be half a sweet apple or pear. California persimmons are ripe when soft and have a luxurious, slithery texture.

1 ripe California persimmon	¼ cup apple juice
½ Japanese persimmon	¼ cup filtered water
½ onion, chopped fine	Juice of ½ lemon
¼ cup cilantro leaves, chopped coarsely	2 tablespoons cider vinegar
3 to 4 cloves garlic, pressed	⅛ teaspoon sea salt
	⅛ teaspoon white pepper

1. Quarter California persimmon and, with a spoon, scoop out flesh, discarding skin and any seeds. Chop and place in a small bowl.
2. Skin Japanese persimmon, discard skin and any seeds, and mince fine. Add to bowl with onion, cilantro, garlic, apple juice, water, lemon juice, vinegar, salt, and pepper.
3. Stir well and refrigerate at least ½ hour.

VARIATIONS: Instead of persimmons, use mangoes, apricots, papaya, or pineapple. For spicier flavor, use ½ to 1 finely chopped jalapeño pepper or chili powder.

SUGGESTED USES: Serve with corn chips or Plantains Sautéed in Butter, or serve over grain or with cooked fish, poultry, or meat dishes.

★★★ VITAMIN C, VITAMIN A, MANGANESE
★ COPPER, MAGNESIUM, FOLIC ACID, VITAMIN B$_6$

❧ Fig Sauce with Basil ❧

Yield: 1 quart *(4 generous servings plus extra)*

We may think of figs as exotic fruits, but they deserve to be eaten as regularly as apples and bananas. They supply lots of nutrients including that important combination, calcium and magnesium, for heart and bone health. Enjoy them fresh in summer and dried the rest of the year.

1 cup dried unsulphured calmyrna or
  black mission figs
1 cup filtered water
1 teaspoon dried basil
  Pinch sea salt

½ cup unfiltered apple juice
2 tablespoons arrowroot or 1
  tablespoon kuzu
½ cup plain bacteria-active yogurt
4 small sprigs fresh basil

1. Using a paring knife, remove hard tips from fig stems.

2. In a small saucepan, bring figs, water, basil, and salt to a boil, covered. Reduce heat and cook for 10 minutes, until soft.

3. In a blender, purée several batches of figs with cooking liquid until smooth. Return to saucepan and heat on medium-low.

4. Pour apple juice into a measuring cup and add arrowroot, stirring until dissolved. Pour into saucepan, stirring constantly. Return to a boil and cook until clear, then cook 30 seconds more.

5. Pour sauce into a serving bowl, allowing to cool. Serve at room temperature, or refrigerate until cold, about 1 hour. Put yogurt in the center of the sauce. Garnish with basil sprigs and lay a serving spoon nearby, allowing each person to take some sauce and yogurt, as desired.

SUGGESTED USES: Serve with lamb, yogurt, or on grain or toast.

★★★ IRON, MAGNESIUM, CALCIUM, POTASSIUM
  ★ COPPER, MANGANESE, VITAMIN B$_6$

Figs are on the menopause menu because they are full of minerals (iron, potassium, and zinc) and contain lots of fiber. Insoluble fiber reduces colon cancer, and soluble fiber lowers cholesterol and the risk of heart disease. In experiments, extracts of figs have been used to shrink tumors. Chinese medicine recommends figs to cleanse the intestines and counteract toxins.

❧ Tomato Sauce ❧

Yield: 2 quarts

Here's a year-round tomato sauce that uses boxed tomatoes—yes they do come in boxes—and they're wonderfully flavorful.

3 tablespoons extra-virgin olive oil	2 bay leaves
1 onion, minced	2 cups filtered water
6 cloves garlic, chopped	2 teaspoons basil
1 35-ounce box strained tomatoes (see Note page 173)	1 to 2 teaspoons sea salt
	½ teaspoon sage
5 raisins or ½ carrot	Pinch oregano

1. Heat olive oil in a large saucepan and add onion and garlic.
2. Add strained tomatoes, raisins, bay leaves, water, basil, salt, sage, and oregano. Bring to a boil, covered, lower to a simmer, and cook 30 minutes, stirring several times.
3. Remove bay leaves, and serve hot.

SUGGESTED USES: Serve over pasta or any grain, with meat loaf, fish, or chicken.

★★★   VITAMIN A, VITAMIN C
★   VITAMIN K, VITAMIN E, VITAMIN B$_6$, FOLIC ACID

❧ Tofu Alfredo Sauce ❧

Yield: 4 cups   (8 ½-cup servings)

Enjoy the rich texture of Alfredo Sauce without the fat, if you've added a few pounds at menopause (most women do). This sauce is good on any whole grain or pasta.

1 **pound firm or soft tofu**	2 **teaspoons oregano**
1 **cup filtered water**	1 **bay leaf**
¼ **cup light miso, such as chick-pea**	1 **onion, minced fine**
¼ **cup extra-virgin olive oil**	½ **teaspoon herbal sea salt**
2 **teaspoons basil**	

1. In a blender or processor, purée tofu, water, and miso.
2. In a medium-size saucepan, heat olive oil and add basil, oregano, bay leaf, and onion. Cook on moderate heat, uncovered, 4 to 5 minutes. Lower heat, add salt, cover, and cook another 10 minutes.
3. Add blended tofu mixture to saucepan and stir well. Bring mixture to a boil—be careful, since it tends to splatter. Lower heat and simmer, uncovered, 3 to 4 minutes. Remove bay leaf.

SUGGESTED USES: Serve over pasta, rice, millet, or steamed vegetables, or spread on toast.

★★★   IRON, OMEGA-3 FATTY ACIDS, LINOLENIC ACID
  ★   MANGANESE, MAGNESIUM, FOLIC ACID, CALCIUM

❧ Lemon-Lime-Orange Marinade ❧

Yield: 2 cups

Even if you are not strictly vegetarian, it's not a bad idea to eat vegetarian a couple days a week, filling yourself with vegetables and low-fat sources of protein. This marinade is great over tofu or meat and features citrus high in Vitamin C and bioflavonoids.

2 lemons	1 pound tofu, tempeh, fish, chicken, or meat
2 limes	½ cup unfiltered apple juice
2 oranges	½ cup filtered water
2 cloves garlic	
½ teaspoon herbal sea salt	

1. Peel lemons, limes, and oranges, and cut them into halves. Using the tip of a paring knife, remove any seeds. Put fruit into a blender or processor with garlic and salt. Purée until smooth.

2. Place any protein food of your choice in a baking dish. Pour the marinade over this spreading to an even layer, and allow to marinate, refrigerated, ½ hour for every ½ inch of thickness.

3. Preheat oven to 350°.

4. Mix apple juice and water together and add to baking dish. Bake 15 to 40 minutes, depending on the protein food's usual baking time.

5. Serve leftover marinade mixed with pan juices as a sauce.

VARIATION: To make a thicker sauce, combine any leftover marinade, the pan juices, and 2 teaspoons arrowroot dissolved in 2 tablespoons water in a saucepan. Heat until thickened and clear.

SUGGESTED USES: Marinate fish steaks or fillets, ribs, chicken, or tempeh.

★★★   VITAMIN C, FOLIC ACID, BIOFLAVONOIDS
  ★   VITAMIN B_6, THIAMIN, PANTOTHENIC ACID, RIBOFLAVIN, POTASSIUM, IRON

❧ Teriyaki Marinade ❧

Yield: 1 cup

Teriyaki is usually just a savory sugar sauce. We substitute more nutritious sugars but retain the Asian flavoring.

½ cup filtered water
3 cloves garlic, pressed
    3-inch piece fresh ginger, grated
    (about 2 tablespoons)
3 tablespoons shoyu soy sauce
2 teaspoons unsulphured blackstrap
    molasses

1 teaspoon maple syrup
½ teaspoon salted plum paste
    (umeboshi) or 1 tablespoon salted
    plum vinegar (umeboshi)
Pinch sea salt

1. In a blender, put water, garlic, ginger, soy sauce, molasses, maple syrup, plum paste, and salt. Blend until smooth.

2. Place any protein food of your choice (tofu, tempeh, fish, chicken, or meat) in a baking dish. Pour the marinade over this and allow to marinate, refrigerated, ½ hour for every ½ inch of thickness.

TO THICKEN: Use marinade as a sauce as is, or mix together ¼ cup cold filtered water and 2 tablespoons arrowroot and add to marinade. Bring to a boil, stirring, until thickened and clear.

SUGGESTED USES: Steam vegetables and drizzle with sauce, or stew chicken, fish, and tempeh in marinade, cooking until tender.

★★★ IRON, MANGANESE
  ★ VITAMIN B$_6$, COPPER, MAGNESIUM

❧ 16 ❧
Nuts and Seeds

Almond Milk
Tahini Milk
Sunflower Seed Pâté
Green Bean and Walnut Pâté
Chestnut, Pine Nut, and Currant Stuffing
Whole Grain Crackers with Four Seeds
Almond and Apple Butter Spread
Sunflower-Nori Snack
Crispy Walnut and Seed Bars
Toasted Nuts with Raisins and Apricots
Savory and Spicy Cocktail Mix
Walnut Cream

❧ ❧ ❧

❦

If your concern with weight gain stops you from eating nuts because they are high in fat, please reconsider. They are wonderful sources of vitamins, minerals, and healthy fats—all good for female health. The majority of oils in almonds are monounsaturates and walnuts are high in omega-3 fatty acids. And of course oils made from them are cholesterol free, as are oils made from seeds.

Seeds, too, are a staple "on the menu"—sunflower, sesame, and pumpkin seeds for the calcium, magnesium, and potassium they contain. Along with nuts, we've included these in chicken, grain, and vegetable dishes and have woven their flavors into soups and salads. We even give recipes for almond and tahini milks, rich liquids that can easily substitute for dairy milk.

Shopping: The valuable fats in nuts and seeds require that you take extra care with the purchase and storage of these foods, since rancid fats are toxic. When nuts are shelled and removed from their protective covering there is a greater risk of rancidity, and if rancid, the nuts will taste bitter.

Storage: Always store nuts and seeds in airtight containers.

Nuts and Seeds	Store in	Storage Time
Nuts and seeds in shell	cool and dry place	1 year
Shelled nuts and seeds	refrigerator	4 months
Shelled nuts and seeds	freezer	1 year

❧ Almond Milk ❧

Yield: 2½ to 3 cups   (4 servings)

Any nuts can easily be turned into milk, giving you a unique way to benefit from these nutritive foods. Almonds are a good source of protein and high in monounsaturated fats, the same that are in olive oil, which is famous for being heart-friendly. They are also high in vitamin E. And nut milks don't have the synthetic hormones and antibiotics that are added to commercial milk.

Before you begin, soak 1 cup whole almonds 6 to 8 hours or overnight in filtered water.

1 to 1½ cups soaked whole almonds   **3 cups filtered water**
   (from 1 cup dried)   **½ teaspoon pure vanilla extract**

   1. In a blender, grind almonds into a coarse meal. Add 2 cups water, ½ cup at a time, as the almond liquid thickens. It will be thin and milky.
   2. Place a medium wire-mesh strainer over a bowl. In batches, pour the almond liquid into the strainer. With a metal spoon, lift almond meal from strainer, allowing the liquid to flow out of the meal. Do not press on the meal, as it will push grainy particles into the milk.
   3. Return almond meal to blender and add ½ cup water. Repeat step 2. Then repeat these steps once more with the remaining ½ cup of water.
   4. Discard almond meal. Stir vanilla into almond milk.
   5. Use immediately or store up to 5 days, refrigerated. For a smoother milk, pour the liquid through a second and finer-meshed strainer. Discard any further pulp.

VARIATIONS: To make other nut or seed milks, use cashew pieces, sesame seeds, sunflower seeds, walnuts or pecans.

★★★ VITAMIN E, NIACIN
   ★ MAGNESIUM, LINOLEIC ACID, MANGANESE, RIBOFLAVIN, CALCIUM, SELENIUM, BORON

Some recipes for nut milks start with unsoaked almonds and others use blanched almonds. To save time blanching and skinning almonds, soak them first to soften. This produces a greater yield and smoother milk.

❧ Tahini Milk ❧

Yield: 1 cup   (1 serving)

If you want some nondairy milk quickly, make this sesame-seed version. It's high in thiamin; too little of this vitamin and memory fuzzes and nerves fray.

2 **tablespoons sesame tahini, or almond   or cashew butter**
1 **cup filtered water**

¼ **teaspoon pure vanilla extract   (optional)**

1. Place tahini, water, and vanilla in a blender, or whisk in a bowl. Blend until smooth.
2. Use immediately or refrigerate in a covered container for 4 to 5 days.

★★★   LINOLEIC ACID, THIAMIN, COPPER, IRON, FOLIC ACID, CALCIUM

Nut milks can be successfully substituted for commercial cow's milk in puddings, and poured over hot or cold cereal.

❧ Sunflower Seed Pâté ❧

Yield: 1 loaf   (30 to 40 servings of 2 tablespoons each)

When your blood sugar soars and dips, the signs can masquerade as the symptoms of menopause—irritability, fatigue, and mental confusion. To the rescue sunflower seeds, as in this pâté; the seeds are up to 50 percent protein coupled with fats and carbohydrates, sources of steady energy.

1 tablespoon extra-virgin olive oil	1 teaspoon thyme
2 onions, diced	1 teaspoon marjoram
½ pound button mushrooms, sliced	½ teaspoon black pepper
¼ cup sun-dried tomatoes	2 cups sunflower seeds
2 teaspoons basil	½ cup filtered water or vegetable stock
1½ teaspoons herbal sea salt	(see recipe)

1. In a medium sauté pan, heat oil over medium heat. Add onions and cook until caramelized, about 15 minutes.

2. Add mushrooms, sun-dried tomatoes, basil, herbal salt, thyme, marjoram, and pepper. Cover and cook on low 5 minutes.

3. Stir in sunflower seeds and water or stock, cover, and reduce heat to low. Cook 10 minutes. Turn off heat and let sit in covered pan 15 minutes.

4. In a processor or blender, purée the seed mixture until smooth.

5. Press into a 4-cup loaf pan, ramekins, or small bowls. Refrigerate, covered, 1 hour.

VARIATIONS: Substitute walnuts or pecans for sunflower seeds.

SUGGESTED ACCOMPANIMENTS: Spring Greens Potage with Asparagus and whole wheat rolls.

★★★   LINOLEIC ACID, THIAMIN, PANTOTHENIC ACID, FOLIC ACID, MAGNESIUM
  ★   COPPER, SELENIUM, PHOSPHORUS, VITAMIN B$_6$

> For a party, the pâté can be served as a loaf or as individual hors d'oeuvres, spread on endive leaves or thin wedges of apple. But pâtés are for more than special events. Use several tablespoons on sandwiches or crackers and stuffed in celery for a snack.

❧ Green Bean and Walnut Pâté ❧

Yield: 3 cups   (4 generous servings plus extra)

Lederman Caterers in New York created the original version of this unique pâté, which closely resembles the taste and texture of chopped chicken liver. Its luxurious taste and texture come from walnuts, which are the only nut that has large amounts of omega-3 fatty acids, the EFA that is good for the heart. We recommend eating a few almost every day.

This can also be served spread on rice cakes or crackers.

¼ pound green beans, tips removed
½ cup filtered water
1 tablespoon extra-virgin olive oil
1 onion, sliced
¼ teaspoon sea salt
½ cup walnuts

2 teaspoons chick-pea miso
Freshly ground black pepper
4 stalks celery, cut into 2-inch lengths
4 black oil-cured or Greek olives, pitted and chopped

1. In a small saucepan, put green beans and water. Cover and steam until tender, about 12 to 15 minutes. The beans will no longer be bright green.
2. In a small sauté pan, heat oil and add onion. Cook, uncovered, over medium-high heat until a rich golden color, about 10 minutes.
3. In a food processor, put green beans and onions with salt, walnuts, miso, and pepper. Pulse until smooth.
4. Serve pâté stuffed in celery. Top with several pieces of chopped olive.

SUGGESTED ACCOMPANIMENTS: Bowl of Antipasto, Steamed Scallops Seviche Style, and whole grain Italian bread.

★★★   OMEGA-3 FATTY ACIDS, COPPER

❧

Chinese diet therapy ranks walnuts high as a food for menopause. They are thought to resemble and thus nourish the kidneys, the Chinese term for which is used in Chinese medicine to indicate many functions of the body that are affected by menopause.

❧

❧ Chestnut, Pine Nut, ❧ and Currant Stuffing

Yield: 3 quarts   (enough for a 14- to 18-pound turkey or 2 large chickens)

This is a hearty Greek stuffing, a meal in itself with turkey, nuts, and herbs. For diversity we add chestnuts, which are very low in fat—only about 1 to 3 percent, compared with 50 percent or more for most other nuts. Chestnuts contain vitamin C, an essential for healthy adrenals and an antioxidant that prevents aging.

Before beginning, reconstitute 1 cup dried chestnuts (see Notes).

2 tablespoons extra-virgin olive oil
2 medium onions, minced
1½ pounds organic turkey, ground (see Notes)
1 turkey liver, organic only (see Note page 257; optional)
½ bunch parsley, chopped
1 teaspoon cinnamon
1 teaspoon sage
1 teaspoon sea salt
½ teaspoon black pepper
1 cup dried currants
1 cup walnuts, chopped coarsely
2 cups dried chestnuts, reconstituted and chopped (see Notes)
1 cup pine nuts
6 slices hearty whole wheat bread
4 cups chicken, turkey, or vegetable stock (see index), organic preferred

1. In a large skillet, heat oil and add onions. Cook on a medium-high flame until they begin to caramelize and turn golden, about 15 minutes.
2. Add ground turkey to skillet, breaking it into small pieces. Chop liver and add with parsley, reserving 2 or 3 tablespoons of the parsley. Add cinnamon, sage, salt, pepper, and currants. Stir well.
3. Add walnuts, chestnuts, and pine nuts to meat. Cover and let cook 5 to 10 minutes.
4. Preheat oven to 350°.
5. Cut bread into small cubes. Add cubes to turkey mixture and stir well.
6. Transfer to a large rectangular roasting pan. Pour stock over stuffing, cover with parchment paper and then foil, and place in oven to bake. (Or use to stuff the cavity of a turkey or chicken.)
7. After 30 minutes, remove parchment paper and foil, and gently stir, turning over the stuffing but being careful not to mash it. Return stuffing to oven without the cover and cook another 30 minutes, stirring once or twice to keep the outside edges

from burning. When done, the stuffing will have absorbed the stock and turned darker brown, and some of the nuts will be nicely roasted.

8. To serve, turn into a serving bowl and garnish with reserved chopped parsley.

NOTES: 1. To reconstitute dried chestnuts, cover 2 cups chestnuts with 4 cups filtered water, bring to a boil covered, and simmer 20 minutes. Cool and remove any shell that remains in the chestnut creases. Or use fresh chestnuts, roasting or boiling first, then removing the shell.

2. If you prefer this stuffing vegetarian, use 4 or 5 cups of cooked grain, beans, tempeh, or bread cubes instead of the ground turkey and liver.

★★★   VITAMIN B$_{12}$, OMEGA-3 FATTY ACIDS, LINOLEIC ACID
  ★   MANGANESE, VITAMIN C, FOLIC ACID, IRON, MAGNESIUM

Do what Lissa's family does—cook the stuffing in a separate pan, and save the work of stuffing the turkey! Once the turkey is done, pour the delicious juices or stock over the stuffing and bake. Besides, this way it takes less time to cook the turkey and you can be sure the internal temperature rises sufficiently.

❧ Whole Grain Crackers with Four Seeds ❧

Yield: 24 crackers

Seeds are small, but don't underestimate them. They are the fuel-packed source of future plants and are especially rich in the B-vitamins, vitamins A, D, and E, and potassium, magnesium, zinc, and calcium, plus unsaturated fats and protein. More than a garnish, they are quality foods and an important part of the menopause menu.

1 cup oatmeal
3 tablespoons flax seeds
½ cup unsalted butter, at room
temperature
½ cup whole wheat pastry flour

½ teaspoon sea salt
Filtered water
2 tablespoons unhulled sesame seeds
2 tablespoons cumin or caraway seeds
2 tablespoons poppy seeds

Preheat oven to 350°.

1. In a processor or blender, grind oatmeal and flax seeds. To processor, add butter and flour. (If using a blender, put ground oatmeal and seeds in a bowl and cut in butter, then add flour, mixing with a spoon.) Mix in salt.

2. Prepare a baking pan with parchment paper or butter. With wet hands, press cracker dough evenly on sheet to make a ⅛- to ¼-inch-thick layer. (The dough may not cover the entire pan.)

3. Using a pastry brush, moisten the top of the crackers with water. Mix seeds together and sprinkle evenly over the top of the dough. Lay a piece of parchment over the seeds and press firmly into the cracker dough.

4. With a knife, score dough into 2-inch square or diamond shapes.

5. Bake for 15 to 20 minutes, until golden. Cool 5 minutes, then cut and break crackers apart.

SUGGESTED ACCOMPANIMENTS: Spring Greens Potage with Asparagus, or Butternut Babaganoush.

★★★ OMEGA-3 FATTY ACIDS, MANGANESE, VITAMIN B$_6$
 ★ THIAMIN, MAGNESIUM, IRON

❧ Almond and Apple Butter Spread ❧

Yield: 1 cup   (16 tablespoon-size servings)

This intriguing salty-sweet spread can satisfy your hunger and curtail your cravings for less nutritious foods. Almonds and apples both contain boron, the mineral that helps estrogen do its job, and the miso aids digestion. Over time, eating quality foods such as this spread can help you lose weight by helping you avoid caloric foods that are missing nutrients and don't really feed you.

⅓ cup almond butter   ⅓ cup white or chick-pea miso
⅓ cup unsweetened apple butter

1. In a small bowl, blend almond butter, apple butter, and miso.
2. Spread on rice cakes or whole grain crackers and munch away! Or refrigerate for future use.

VARIATIONS: Replace almond butter with sesami tahini or cashew butter. Stir in enough stock or filtered water until it becomes sauce consistency. Serve on pasta or over grain.

SERVING ACCOMPANIMENTS: Breakfast Corn Muffins and Fresh Herb Frittata.

★★★   SODIUM, LINOLEIC ACID
★   MAGNESIUM, MANGANESE, OMEGA-3 FATTY ACIDS, BORON

❧

Rice cakes function like crackers. They are handy platforms for a variety of toppings: a little leftover seafood salad, twice-cooked beans, nut butter, or all-fruit preserves. They come in palm-sized rounds and smaller versions the size of poker chips.

❧

❧ Sunflower-Nori Snack ❧

Yield: 2½ cups   (4 generous servings plus extra)

Seaweed is an especially good source of minerals, because it grows in seawater, where the minerals are constantly being replenished. Here we use nori, the seaweed around sushi. When you nibble this snack you munch on minerals.

2 sheets nori, or 2 tablespoons
   flakes
1 cup sunflower seeds

½ cup dried currants
1 cup toasted sesame seeds
   (optional)

1. Toast nori sheets over an open flame (this can be done on an electric stove) by placing it directly over the burner without it touching the flame, moving the nori back and forth until it turns from green in color to dark purple. Turn it over from time to time and switch sides where it is held to toast fully.

2. In a small bowl, mix sunflower seeds with currants. Cut or tear nori into small pieces and add to bowl. Mix well. Add sesame seeds for extra calcium.

SUGGESTED USES: Enjoy as a snack, or sprinkle on grain or hot cereal.

★★★   VITAMIN A, VITAMIN E, THIAMIN, MAGNESIUM, COPPER, IRON, FOLIC ACID
  ★   PHOSPHORUS, PANTOTHENIC ACID, CALCIUM, SELENIUM

❧ Crispy Walnut and Seed Bars ❧

Yield: 20 1-inch-square bars

To bring their systems into balance at menopause, Chinese women traditionally eat a mixture of walnuts and sesame seeds made into a candy. We developed our own version, adding some ingredients to give you concentrated amounts of copper, B vitamins, boron, and bioflavonoids, plus the omega-3 fatty acids—all nourishment to counteract your symptoms. These high-energy and nutrient-packed bars store and travel well (good car food because they don't crumble). Keep some around for snacking and you'll be doing yourself a favor.

¾ cup rice syrup (see below)
2 tablespoons sesame tahini or cashew
  butter
  Pinch sea salt
1 teaspoon pure vanilla extract
½ cup dried currants or raisins

¼ cup walnuts, chopped coarsely
¼ cup sunflower seeds
¼ cup unhulled sesame seeds
¼ cup flax seeds (see Note)
2 cups puffed rice cereal
  (such as Brown Rice Crispies)

1. In a medium saucepan, heat rice syrup on medium-high heat. Stir in tahini and salt, and cook until syrup begins to caramelize slightly and drops in strings when lifted with a spoon, about 5 to 7 minutes. Stir constantly.

2. Add vanilla, stirring well, and cook another 30 seconds. Turn off flame and add currants.

3. In a medium bowl, mix together walnuts, all seeds, and rice cereal. Pour rice syrup mixture over cereal mix and stir until evenly blended.

4. Have handy a small bowl of water to keep hands wet, and form mixture into round balls. (Or press into an oiled rectangular pan and let set about 30 minutes; then cut into bars about 1 × 1 inch square.)

5. Place each ball or bar in a paper muffin cup. To store, put into a plastic container or wrap in plastic.

NOTE: The flax seeds are small; to help make them easier to chew, grind them into a meal. To do this, place them in a dry blender or spice grinder and whiz until powdery.

★★★ OMEGA-3 FATTY ACIDS
★ VITAMIN B_6, THIAMIN, MAGNESIUM, CALCIUM, NIACIN, COPPER, BORON

❧

Rice syrup retains about 40 percent of the complex carbohydrates found in the original grain, and is less sweet than table sugar. Being less refined than white sugar, it is absorbed into the bloodstream more slowly, helping to keep steady your blood-sugar levels, energy, and spirits.

❧

❧ Toasted Nuts with Raisins and Apricots ❧

Yield: 6 cups   (12 servings)

Coffee, tea, and the phosphorous in soda depletes your body of magnesium. Here's a better snack break—a magnesium-high mix of nuts, seeds, and dried fruit. Keep a stash in your car and in your desk drawer.

½ **cup almonds**
½ **cup cashews**
½ **cup pecans**
½ **cup sunflower seeds**
½ **cup walnuts**
½ **cup pumpkin seeds**

2 **cups monukka raisins, organic preferred (see Note)**
½ **cup dried unsulphured apricots, chopped coarsely**
⅛ **teaspoon sea salt (optional)**

Preheat oven to 350°.

1. In a baking pan, place each kind of nut and seed in an individual pile across the baking sheet, and flatten into a single layer. Put baking pan into oven. The nuts and seeds will toast at individual cooking times, ranging from 6 to 12 minutes. They will be very fragrant and slightly golden in color. Check after 5 minutes and remove individual piles with a spatula as they are done, returning the baking pan to the oven each time to allow the others to finish cooking. (The first to be done will be the sunflower seeds.) Thereafter, check every 2 minutes and use a spatula to remove any toasted nuts and seeds, placing them in a mixing bowl to cool.

2. Add raisins, apricots, and salt to nuts and seeds.

3. Cover bowl with a pot lid or plastic wrap until the nuts have cooled. This will add some plumpness to the dried fruit.

NOTE: Popular raisin varieties come from sun-dried Thompson seedless and monukka grapes. Thompson raisins are the common variety found in the stores. We prefer monukka raisins, which are large and plump, have small edible seeds, and have a rich, deep taste. Thompson raisins can be substituted for these.

★★★ LINOLEIC ACID, OMEGA-3 FATTY ACIDS, MAGNESIUM
 ★ MANGANESE, COPPER, PHOSPHORUS, THIAMIN, IRON, BORON

❧ Savory and Spicy Cocktail Mix ❧

Yield: 4 cups

The EFAs, while they are super for your health, break down more easily than do the more stable saturated fats. Having higher amounts in your diet requires that you also increase your intake of anti-oxidant vitamins. This cocktail mix provides both the EFAs and the anti-oxidant vitamin E.

1½ cups almonds
 1 cup walnuts
 1 cup pecans
 2 tablespoons unsalted butter
 2 teaspoons chili powder

¼ teaspoon cinnamon
¼ teaspoon ground ginger
½ teaspoon sea salt (optional)
¼ teaspoon black pepper

1. In a medium bowl, mix almonds, walnuts, and pecans.

2. In a medium sauté pan, melt butter over medium heat. Add chili powder, cinnamon, ginger, salt, and pepper. Stir, allowing the spice-butter mixture to bubble very lightly, about 30 seconds. Immediately add the nuts. Stir to coat nuts completely with the spices. Cook over medium heat 5 to 7 minutes, stirring continuously until the aroma is fragrant and nuts are toasted and slightly golden.

3. Remove from heat and immediately pour the hot nuts into a wide bowl. Allow to cool. (Toss occasionally to allow moisture to escape.)

4. Store when cool in an airtight glass jar.

VARIATIONS: Add pumpkin seeds, raisins, or dried currants.

SUGGESTED USES: Party food and snacking.

★★★   OMEGA-3 FATTY ACIDS, VITAMIN E
  ★   CALCIUM, MANGANESE, MAGNESIUM, COPPER

❧ **Walnut Cream** ❧

Yield: 1½ cups

Instead of whipped cream, try a dollop of this on top of fruit compote or over sliced strawberries. The fat in the walnuts, mostly unsaturated, provides a voluptuous texture, and these nuts give you copper, important in the formation of collagen, the supporting substance in your skin. These are calories well spent.

1 cup walnuts	Pinch sea salt
3 tablespoons maple syrup	2 to 4 tablespoons unfiltered apple
¼ cup unsweetened coconut (optional)	juice
1 teaspoon pure vanilla extract	

In a processor or blender, grind the walnuts. Add maple syrup, coconut, vanilla, salt, and 2 tablespoons apple juice. Blend well, adding more juice as needed to blend and make smooth. Serve on your favorite dessert.

VARIATIONS: Substitute cashews, almonds, pecans, Brazil nuts, or sunflower seeds. Nut butters can also be substituted, using ¾ cup of butter for every cup of nuts.

SUGGESTED ACCOMPANIMENTS: Serve as a topping for fruit cobblers, poached fruit, sliced berries, and even as a cake filling or frosting.

★★★ OMEGA-3 FATTY ACIDS, MANGANESE
  ★ COPPER, MAGNESIUM, IRON

❧

When purchasing shelled walnuts, break one to see if it is fresh; it should be brittle and snap. If the nuts are shriveled or rubbery, they are old and may be rancid. Avoid these.

❧

❧ 17 ❧

Desserts and Nourishing Sweets

A Quick Cake
Italian Almond Cake
Carob Cake with Walnuts
Yogurt Cheesecake with Loganberry Glaze
Strawberry Tart with Walnut Crust
Fresh Blueberry Cobbler
Peach Crumble
Banana Refrigerator Cake
Apricot-Cashew "Mousse"
Light Lemon Pudding Parfait with Kiwi Slices
Fresh Summer Fruit Compote
Poached Pears in Ginger-Kuzu Sauce
Frozen Banana Maple-Walnut Whip
Beverly's Cantaloupe with Freshly Grated Ginger
Baked Apples Stuffed with Raisin-Ginger Chutney
Old-Fashioned Oatmeal Raisin Cookies
Broiled Dates Stuffed with Almonds
Broiled Maple Apples
Apricot-Date-Pecan Bonbons
Dark Chocolate Candy ('90s "Chunkies")

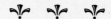

In our desserts, we use whole grain flours and the best quality ingredients to make every calorie count, so enjoy these wonderful guilt-free delights.

Dessert-making usually requires a source of fat and a source of sweet, and there are healthy options for both. Unsalted butter is our choice for baked goods because this saturated fat is stable at high temperatures and it doesn't readily break down into toxic substances. We also use flax seed oil for the essential fatty acids it supplies and its buttery taste. We don't use canola oil, which is partially refined to take away its bitter flavor, or unrefined safflower oil, which has a heavy texture when baked.

Our preferred sweetener for dessert-making is maple syrup for both flavor and the minerals it contains. It is also a less concentrated sweet than honey or refined white sugar. We avoid white sugar because it contains no vitamins or minerals, and once absorbed, it breaks down so quickly that the body can use only some of it for energy and stores the rest as fat. See our Appendix for some basic tips on sweetness conversion to assist you if you're inclined to adapt your old-time favorite dessert recipes to better-quality ingredients.

The recipes call for whole wheat pastry flour, which yields a lighter baked product than the whole wheat flour (also known as bread flour) that you normally find in the grocery store. Whole wheat pastry flour can be found in natural food stores, often in the refrigerator section to keep chilled and prevent its germ from going rancid. (Please keep all flours refrigerated.) We recommend aluminum-free baking powder (most commercial baking brands are not) since intake of minerals such as aluminum has been associated with osteoporosis. When using this type of baking powder, have your oven preheated and the pans greased before mixing the wet ingredients into the dry, since this type of baking powder has less action time.

To wash fruit: If the fruit is not organic, wash gently with a mild soap and water even if you plan to peel it. Rinse well and set on a cotton towel to dry. Berries are best washed in a large bowl of water. As you lift them out with your hands, check for twigs, leaves, and damaged fruit, then place in a colander to drain.

❧ A Quick Cake ❧

Yield: 8 × 8-inch cake   (8 servings)

Here's a short cut to homemade cake—whole grain pancake mix poured into a pan with fruit on top. No-effort nourishment for body and soul!

2 **to 3 cups chopped fresh fruit (apples, pears, peaches, plums, or bananas)**
1 **teaspoon cinnamon or powdered ginger**
  Pinch sea salt
¾ **cup maple syrup**
2 **tablespoons arrowroot (or use 2 additional tablespoons of pancake mix)**

2 **cups whole grain pancake or muffin mix (see Appendix, page 361)**
1 **to 1½ cups liquid (see Note)**
¼ **cup unsalted butter, melted, or flax seed oil**

Preheat oven to 350° degrees.
Prepare an 8 × 8-inch cake pan with butter or parchment paper.

1. In a medium bowl put fruit, cinnamon, salt, ¼ cup maple syrup, and arrowroot. Mix well and set aside.

2. In a second medium bowl put pancake mix. In a large measuring cup mix together 1 cup liquid, remaining ½ cup maple syrup, and butter. Pour into pancake mix, stirring just enough to moisten. Add more liquid as needed to make a thick batter.

3. Pour cake batter into prepared cake pan. Top with fruit and place in preheated oven. Bake for 30 to 35 minutes.

4. Remove from oven and cool. Cut into squares and serve warm.

Note: Depending upon the whole grain mix you are using, you can add filtered water, nut or seed milk, or apple juice.

VARIATIONS: To make an upside-down cake, place the fruit in the cake pan and then top with cake batter. For additional texture, add nuts or seeds to cake batter.

★★★ VITAMIN C, CALCIUM, THIAMIN
  ★ NIACIN, VITAMIN E, IRON

❧ Italian Almond Cake ❧

Yield: 10-inch cake   (8 to 12 servings)

We start with almonds, the nut that is highest in mono-unsaturated oils, the hallmark of the healthy Mediterranean diet. Other nuts with the same good oil include macadamia, cashew, pistachio, pecan, and filbert.

2 cups whole almonds
½ cup maple syrup
4 eggs, organic, free-range preferred, separated, at room temperature
Grated rind of 1 lemon or orange, organic preferred

1 teaspoon cream of tartar
½ teaspoon sea salt
6 tablespoons whole wheat pastry flour

Preheat oven to 350°.
1. Using a blender or processor, grind the almonds to a fine meal.
2. Add maple syrup, egg yolks, and grated lemon rind to almonds, mixing well.
3. In a separate bowl with a clean whisk or beaters, whip the egg whites with cream of tartar and salt until stiff peaks are formed.
4. Add almond mixture, a little at a time, and sift flour through a strainer over beaten egg whites. Fold carefully with a rubber spatula, mixing as little as possible to incorporate.
5. Thickly butter a 10-inch springform pan. Gently pour the batter into the pan, giving it a little shake to level it off.
6. Bake for 30 minutes, or until an inserted toothpick comes out dry.
7. Remove spring lock and let cake cool completely before serving.

Suggested accompaniments: Serve as is or with unsweetened real whipped cream—can you believe we're saying this?!

★★★ VITAMIN E, MAGNESIUM, MANGANESE, LINOLENIC ACID
 ★ FOLIC ACID, RIBOFLAVIN, PHOSPHORUS, COPPER, IRON, ZINC

The average American eats 145 pounds of refined sugar per year added to drinks like coffee and tea; sprinkled on breakfast cereal; in candy, ice cream, and soda; in commercial breads, bakery products, ready-made tomato sauces, "honey-cured" hams, and all manner of processed foods.

❧ Carob Cake with Walnuts ❧

Yield: 8 × 8-inch cake   (6 servings)

Though the color of carob is similar to chocolate, unlike its counterpart, carob contains no caffeine. Some people eat it in place of chocolate, but we personally don't think it's a substitute, and value carob for its own natural sweetness and rich taste. This nutritious whole foods cake is such good fuel that it's fine to enjoy some at breakfast.

1½ cups whole wheat pastry flour
3 tablespoons carob powder
2 teaspoons aluminum-free baking powder
½ teaspoon sea salt
6 tablespoons unsalted butter (see Note) or flax seed oil

⅔ cup maple syrup
1 teaspoon pure vanilla extract
¾ cup nut, rice, or soy milk
¾ cup walnuts, chopped coarsely

Preheat oven to 350°.

1. To a medium bowl, add flour, carob powder, baking powder, and salt. Mix well.

2. In a small saucepan, melt butter on low heat. Remove from stove. Add maple syrup and vanilla, mixing well. Stir in milk and mix well.

3. Pour butter mixture into carob mixture and stir until moistened.

4. Pour into buttered 8 × 8-inch pan. Sprinkle nuts on top and immediately place in preheated oven. Bake until cake begins to come away from the sides of the pan, about 30 to 35 minutes.

5. Cool and cut into squares.

NOTE: To measure butter, fill a 2-cup measuring cup with 1 cup cold water. Cut chunks of butter into water until it measures between 1¼ cups and 1½ cups. This will be 6 tablespoons.

VARIATION: To make a chocolate cake, substitute an equal amount of cocoa powder for carob. (If you make this cake with carob, please don't call it chocolate cake.)

SUGGESTED ACCOMPANIMENTS: Serve topped with thinned raspberry jam and a strawberry on the side.

★★★   OMEGA-3 FATTY ACIDS, MANGANESE, LINOLEIC ACID, CALCIUM
  ★   SELENIUM, ZINC, MANGANESE

❧ Yogurt Cheesecake with Loganberry Glaze ❧

Yield: 10-inch cake   (8 to 12 servings)

The way of eating we recommend includes rich and luxurious foods. Feeling well fed and satisfied is part of caring for yourself at menopause. Here's our version of cheesecake made with very nutritious ingredients.

Have on hand: 2 cups yogurt cheese (drained from 1 quart whole-milk yogurt; see page 280).

CRUST:

2½ cups whole wheat bread crumbs or crushed graham crackers (see Notes)
¼ cup sunflower seeds
2 tablespoons unsalted butter

2 tablespoons maple syrup
⅛ teaspoon cinnamon
Pinch sea salt

FILLING:

2 cups yogurt cheese
¼ cup maple syrup
¼ cup maple crystals
4 eggs, organic, fertile, and free-range preferred (see Notes)

1 teaspoon pure vanilla extract
Grated rind of 1 lemon
Pinch sea salt

GLAZE:

4 ounces loganberry all-fruit preserves (or other flavor)

2 to 3 tablespoons unfiltered apple juice

Preheat oven to 350°.

CRUST:

1. In a processor, put bread crumbs, sunflower seeds, butter, maple syrup, cinnamon, and salt. Blend until mixed, about 30 seconds.
2. Butter a springform pan. With wet fingers, press crumb mixture into pan. Bake until lightly golden, about 5 minutes. Set aside to cool.

FILLING:

1. In a medium bowl, mix drained yogurt with maple syrup and crystals, eggs, vanilla, lemon rind, and sea salt. Beat until smooth.
2. Pour yogurt mixture into partially baked crust. Place on a flat baking sheet and bake in preheated oven 1 hour. Turn off heat and allow to cool in oven with door closed, about 45 minutes to 1 hour.

GLAZE:

1. Pour preserves into a small bowl. Add 1 tablespoon of juice at a time, and mix until thinned enough to spread. Using a spatula, spread glaze on top of cake, which can either be at room temperature or cold.
2. Serve at room temperature or refrigerate at least 1 hour prior to serving.

TO SERVE: Using a sharp knife, run blade around edge of cake, loosening it from pan. Release spring and remove cake from the base to a cake platter.

NOTE: 1. It takes approximately 4 cups of whole graham crackers or cookies to make 2 cups. Pulverize in processor first, and then add remaining ingredients.
2. For a lighter cake, separate eggs and whip whites. Fold in at the end, just before baking.

★★★ SELENIUM, MANGANESE, VITAMIN B$_{12}$, VITAMIN K, LINOLENIC ACID, RIBOFLAVIN

Other Topping Suggestions

1. Fresh fruit topping: After cake has cooled, place sliced fruit on the cake top. In a small pot heat 1 cup apple juice with 2 tablespoons agar-agar flakes, cooking for 5 to 7 minutes. Spoon apple juice glaze over fruit, covering all fruit. Place cake in refrigerator to chill, about 45 minutes, and serve according to instructions.

2. Cream cheese glaze: In a small bowl mix together 1 cup yogurt cheese with 3 tablespoons maple syrup. Add ½ teaspoon vanilla extract, if desired. Spread on top of cooled cake before serving.

❧ Strawberry Tart with Walnut Crust ❧

Yield: 9-inch tart   (8 servings)

Here's a tart made with wise ingredients for teatime, dessert, or breakfast. We sweeten with maple syrup and fruit juice rather than white sugar, which can raise triglyceride levels and your risk of heart disease. And for fat in the crust we use butter, stable at the high temperatures of baking, and less likely to form into dangerous trans-fatty acids when heated.

CRUST:

1½ cups walnuts or sunflower seeds
 ½ cup oatmeal
 1 cup whole wheat bread crumbs
    (or 1 additional cup oatmeal)
 ¼ teaspoon cinnamon

¼ cup maple syrup
¼ cup unsalted butter, at room
    temperature, or flax seed oil
⅛ teaspoon sea salt

TOPPING:

1 cup apple juice, unfiltered preferred
2 pints strawberries
½ cup all-fruit strawberry jam
2 tablespoons kuzu or 4 tablespoons
   arrowroot powder

¼ cup filtered water or juice
1 teaspoon pure vanilla extract
2 tablespoons maple syrup (optional)
2 tablespoons unsweetened coconut

Preheat oven to 350°.

1. In a processor or blender, grind walnuts and oatmeal into a meal. Add bread crumbs, cinnamon, syrup, butter, and salt. Pulse until blended.

2. Butter or oil a 9- or 10-inch springform or tart pan. With wet fingers, press dough evenly into the pan, but only on the bottom. Bake in preheated oven until golden, about 20 to 25 minutes. Allow to cool completely.

3. In a small saucepan heat juice. Remove green tops from all strawberries; set aside 8 beautiful strawberries. Slice all but the 8 strawberries and add to heating juice. Add jam and stir. Cover and cook on low heat until strawberries have softened, about 10 minutes.

4. Dissolve kuzu in water and add to pot. Bring to a boil, stirring constantly, until color clears. Add vanilla and cook another 30 seconds. Carefully taste, as it will be hot, and stir in maple syrup if strawberry filling is not sweet enough.

5. Pour strawberry filling over top of cooked tart shell and spread evenly. Slice remaining strawberries thin and place in an overlapping fashion as a border around the outside of the tart. Dust center lightly with coconut and chill, about 30 minutes.

VARIATIONS: Use all the strawberries in the filling and top the tart with peeled, sliced kiwi.

★★★   VITAMIN C, OMEGA-3 FATTY ACIDS
★   LINOLEIC ACID, MANGANESE, VITAMIN K

In recipes for baked goods, nut butters can be substituted for butter. Since they are only about half oil, you may need to add twice as much to a recipe, or alter the recipe to use less. In truth, we find that in many standard cookbook recipes the fat can be cut down by half and the result is still good.

❧ Fresh Blueberry Cobbler ❧

Yield: 4 generous servings plus extra

Blueberries have been shown to be as effective as cranberries in treating bladder infections, more common in women after menopause. When in season, have a serving of this delicious cobbler.

BERRIES:

2 pints fresh blueberries (see Note)
2 tablespoons arrowroot
¼ cup maple syrup

1½ teaspoons cinnamon
½ teaspoon ground ginger
⅛ teaspoon sea salt, plus a pinch

TOPPING:

1½ cups whole wheat pastry flour
1 teaspoon baking powder, aluminum-free preferred
1 teaspoon cinnamon

¼ teaspoon sea salt
¼ cup unsalted butter, melted
1 cup nut, rice, or soy milk
¼ cup maple syrup

Preheat oven to 350°.

1. In a medium-size bowl, mix together blueberries, arrowroot, maple syrup, cinnamon, ginger, and pinch of salt. Stir well. Pour into a buttered 8 × 10-inch baking pan.

2. To make topping, in a medium-size bowl, mix together pastry flour, baking powder, cinnamon, and salt. In a small bowl, mix together butter, nut milk, and syrup. Pour milk mixture into flour mixture and stir until moistened. It should be the consistency of thick pancake batter.

3. Using a tablespoon, drop and drizzle spoonfuls of batter over blueberries. It does not have to cover the entire surface, but be sure that the batter gets into the corners and along sides.

4. Place in preheated oven and bake until top is golden, about 30 to 40 minutes.

5. Remove from oven and serve hot, or at room temperature.

NOTE: To wash blueberries or any berries, pour into a large bowl and fill with water. They will float. Lift some berries into your hand and remove any visible leaves and stems and discard. Placed cleaned berries in a colander, and continue process, until no berries remain in the water.

SUGGESTED ACCOMPANIMENTS: Serve with unsweetened yogurt, heavy cream, or Frozen Banana Maple-Walnut Whip, if desired.

VARIATION: Any fruit will be mouthwatering and delicious using this recipe. Try these fruit and spice combinations:

- Peaches with ginger and cinnamon
- Plums with cardamom and cloves
- Strawberries with nutmeg and ginger
- Apples with allspice and cinnamon

For instant topping, use 1½ cups of whole grain pancake or cake mix, following directions on the box. Add some spices, such as cinnamon and ground ginger, and a little maple syrup to sweeten.

★★★   MANGANESE, FOLIC ACID, SELENIUM, VITAMIN C, ZINC, THIAMIN

❧ Peach Crumble ❧

Yield: 4 generous servings plus extra

Here's a simple technique for making a scrumptious dish of fruit and crumbs. The topping is high in manganese, which helps maintain your hormone levels. Refrigerated, this dessert keeps for at least a week, and is great for breakfast.

FRUIT:

2 pounds fresh, ripe peaches
¼ cup maple syrup
1 tablespoon arrowroot
1 teaspoon ground ginger

1 teaspoon cinnamon
½ teaspoon allspice
   Pinch sea salt

CRUMBLE:

1 cup whole wheat pastry flour
1 cup oatmeal
1 teaspoon cinnamon
¼ teaspoon cardamom

¼ teaspoon sea salt
¼ cup unsalted butter, at room temperature
¼ cup maple syrup

Preheat oven to 350°.

FRUIT:

Cut peaches in half, remove pit, and cut each half into four or five slices. Put peach slices into a medium bowl and add maple syrup, arrowroot, ginger, cinnamon, allspice, and salt. Toss well. Pour into buttered 8 × 8-inch baking pan.

CRUMBLE:

1. In a small bowl, mix pastry flour, oatmeal, cinnamon, cardamom, and salt. Add butter and maple syrup to flour mixture, and mix until moistened.

2. Scatter crumble on top of fruit. Bake until the crumble is golden, about 30 to 40 minutes.

3. Serve warm or at room temperature.

VARIATIONS: Apples, blueberries, plums, pears, cherries, or a mixture of fruit will also taste delicious.

SUGGESTED ACCOMPANIMENTS: Serve with some Sweet Almond-Butter Dressing or a dollop of yogurt.

★★★　MANGANESE, SELENIUM
　★　IRON, OMEGA-3 FATTY ACIDS, VITAMIN A, VITAMIN K

Eat what nature has to offer, season by season. There's no substitute for the peaches that ripen in July and August.

❧ Banana Refrigerator Cake ❧

Yield: 8 × 12 cake   (8 to 12 servings)

This whole foods cake tastes like a treat but it's also a nutritious snack. You'll benefit from its store of vitamin B₆, which may be depleted by estrogen replacement therapy. The technique we use in this recipe is handy to know because this dessert requires no baking!

3 cups rice, soy, or almond milk
¼ cup agar-agar flakes or 2 teaspoons powder
½ cup rice syrup
3 tablespoons maple syrup
⅛ teaspoon sea salt
⅛ teaspoon coriander or cinnamon
2½ tablespoons arrowroot

¼ cup water
2 teaspoons pure vanilla extract
8 to 10 ounces of homemade or sugar-free store-bought cookies (graham crackers, gingersnaps, lemon wafers; see Appendix for suggestions)
4 ripe bananas
1 pint strawberries (optional)

1. In a medium-size saucepan, mix milk with the agar, rice and maple syrups, salt, and coriander. Bring to a boil, reduce heat to a simmer, and cook 5 to 7 minutes partially covered to dissolve agar. Stir occasionally.

2. In a small bowl, mix arrowroot, water, and vanilla together. Add to milk mixture, bring to a boil again, stirring constantly, and then cook 30 more seconds. Set aside and begin to cool.

3. Place cookies in a paper or plastic bag and crush into small pieces with a rolling pin or mallet. (Or crush the cookies in a processor using the pulse action.) Do not pulverize.

4. Butter or oil a baking dish with sides at least 2 inches high. Place all but ½ cup of the cookie crumbs on the bottom of the dish. Peel bananas and slice on top of crumbs.

5. Carefully pour the milk mixture on top of bananas. Top with remaining cookie crumbs. Place in refrigerator until set, about 1 hour.

6. Serve cold. For additional sweetness, dissolve ¼ cup of your favorite all-fruit jam with 3 tablespoons apple juice and use as a sauce. Place a strawberry on the plate for additional color.

★★★ VITAMIN B₆, MAGNESIUM, MANGANESE, NIACIN
  ★ POTASSIUM, VITAMIN C, FOLIC ACID, RIBOFLAVIN, PHOSPHORUS

❧ Apricot-Cashew "Mousse" ❧

Yield: 4 generous servings

Sweet desserts can upset your blood-sugar level but this one's high in magnesium, which plays a role in stabilizing blood glucose. Our "mousse" is a whipped dessert made from a vegetarian gelatin of the seaweed agar-agar.

½ cup dried apricots, unsulphured preferred
2 cups apricot juice or unrefined apple juice
1 cup filtered water
1 bar agar-agar or ¼ cup flakes (see Note)

2 teaspoons pure vanilla extract
2 teaspoons cashew butter or tahini
¼ cup almonds, toasted and chopped coarsely

1. In a medium saucepan, heat apricots, juice, water, and agar-agar. Bring to a boil, uncovered. Lower flame and simmer, covered, until agar is melted, about 10 to 12 minutes for bars and 5 to 7 minutes for flakes.
2. Add vanilla, stir, and cook 1 more minute.
3. Pour into a shallow pan or bowl. Cool until gel sets, about 1 hour at room temperature or 20 minutes in freezer.
4. Cut gel into cubes and purée in blender or processor until smooth, adding cashew butter or tahini. Pour into goblets or bowls and garnish with almonds.

NOTE: When using agar-agar bars, wash under cold water until softened, squeeze water out of bar, and then add to pot with juice. Flakes do not need to be washed.

VARIATIONS:
1. Make gel with juice only (any flavor), omitting the apricots.
2. Make gel with fresh fruit instead of dried fruit.
3. Blend one third of the gel. Cut remainder into cubes. Use blended whip as a sauce over cubes.

SUGGESTED ACCOMPANIMENTS: Serve with crunchy cookies and iced herbal tea.

★★★   MAGNESIUM, FOLIC ACID, IRON, MANGANESE, BORON

❧ Light Lemon Pudding Parfait ❧ with Kiwi Slices

Yield: 5 cups (*4 servings*)

We top this parfait with kiwi, a fashionable fruit that's high in vitamin C, which our adrenals need to help us handle stress. Menopause symptoms worsen as our adrenals weaken, so it's a good idea to boost your kiwi consumption.

¼ **cup agar-agar flakes or 1 bar**
2 **cups unfiltered apple juice**
1½ **cups rice syrup**
¼ **cup maple syrup**
¼ **teaspoon turmeric**
⅛ **teaspoon sea salt**
4 **tablespoons kuzu**

½ **cup filtered water**
2 **teaspoons pure vanilla extract**
1½ **teaspoons grated lemon rind, organic preferred**
¾ **cup lemon juice**
¼ **cup unsweetened coconut**
2 **kiwis, peeled and sliced**

1. In a medium saucepan, mix agar (if using bar, rinse in cold water until softened and squeeze dry before adding), apple juice, rice and maple syrups, turmeric, and salt. Bring to a boil, lower flame to medium, and cook until agar has melted, about 10 minutes, stirring occasionally.

2. In a small bowl, mix kuzu, water, and vanilla. Add to saucepan, stirring well, and cook until kuzu clears; cook 30 seconds more. The liquid will thicken slightly.

3. Remove juice mixture from heat, add lemon rind and juice. Stir well.

4. Pour ½ cup of pudding into each of four parfait glasses. Sprinkle with 1 or 2 teaspoons coconut. Add another ½ cup pudding and another layer of coconut. Pour in final layer of pudding and let cool, about 1 hour. (To speed the process, place glasses filled with warm pudding in the freezer for 15 to 20 minutes.)

5. Before serving, garnish each dish with kiwi slices.

VARIATION: To make a pie, pour filling into a prebaked pie shell and chill in the refrigerator 2 hours to set.

SUGGESTED ACCOMPANIMENTS: Hot mint tea.

★★★ VITAMIN C, NIACIN, MAGNESIUM
★ VITAMIN B$_6$, RIBOFLAVIN, MANGANESE, POTASSIUM, FOLIC ACID

Agar-Agar Equivalencies and Cooking Times

To gel 2½ cups liquid:

Agar-Agar	Amount	Cooking Time
Flakes	¼ cup	5 to 7 minutes
Bar	1 bar	12 to 15 minutes
Powder	2 teaspoons	Bring to a boil

NOTE: When using arrowroot or kuzu with agar-agar, reduce agar by half. Agar-agar will also replace gelatin in any recipe.

❧ Fresh Summer Fruit Compote ❧

Yield: 6 cups   (4 generous servings plus extra)

If you've never shopped at a farmer's market, let the summer harvest inspire you to make a visit. The fruit will most likely be freshly picked and especially full of many nutrients, because it comes to you direct from the fields.

2 **ripe peaches, quartered and pitted**
4 **apricots, halved and pitted**
2 **cups cherries, stems removed**
½ **pint blackberries or strawberries, hulled**

2 **cups unfiltered apple juice**
1 **teaspoon pure vanilla extract**
4 **sprigs fresh mint**

1. In a medium saucepan, in the following order layer peaches, apricots, cherries, and blackberries. Mix juice and vanilla and pour over fruit. Bring to a boil, covered, and turn off heat. Do not stir. Let fruit sit in covered pot for 1 or 2 minutes.

2. Serve in wine goblets with mint sprigs (remembering that cherries have pits).

Optional: To thicken juice, reserve ½ cup apple juice and mix with 3 tablespoons arrowroot or 2 tablespoons kuzu. Using a slotted spoon, remove fruit from pot to goblets. Heat juice in pot to a boil, add arrowroot or kuzu, cook until clear and then another 30 seconds. Let cool a few minutes and pour over fruit while warm.

VARIATIONS: Make this with mixed dried fruits and add raisins, fresh apples, and pears.

SUGGESTED ACCOMPANIMENTS: Top with several teaspoons of plain yogurt and serve with a cup of herbal tea.

★★★ VITAMIN C, VITAMIN A, RIBOFLAVIN, THIAMIN, POTASSIUM
★ COPPER, IRON, MANGANESE, OMEGA-3 FATTY ACIDS

❧ Poached Pears in Ginger-Kuzu Sauce ❧

Yield: 4 servings

Eating a variety of foods is a basic guideline for health, and this dessert includes different versions of the same food. Explore your way through the wonderful variety of pears that are available season by season—d'Anjou, Bosc, Seckel, and Red Bartlett.

4 **Bosc pears, with stems if possible**
1 **cup apple juice, unfiltered preferred**
2 **slices fresh ginger**
¼ **teaspoon allspice or cinnamon**
¼ **cup filtered water**

1 **tablespoon kuzu or arrowroot**
1 **teaspoon pure vanilla extract**
½ **recipe Sweet Almond-Butter Dressing (see recipe)**

1. In a medium saucepan, deep enough to fit pears in depth as well as width, stand pears up in pot and add juice, ginger (make sure ginger slices are covered by the juice), and allspice. Bring to a boil, lower heat, and simmer until pears are soft, about 10 to 15 minutes.

2. Using a slotted spoon, carefully remove pears to a plate. Remove and discard ginger slices.

3. Bring juice to a boil and cook uncovered for about 10 to 15 minutes, reducing juice by half.

4. In a small container, mix water and kuzu until dissolved. Pour into juice and bring to a boil, stirring constantly. Cook until liquid clears, add vanilla, and cook another 30 seconds.

5. Stand pears up on individual plates and spoon several tablespoons of sauce over each. Serve warm or at room temperature with Sweet Almond-Butter Dressing on the side in a small bowl.

VARIATIONS: Try any variety of fruit with this same technique, such as peaches, apples, and plums. Fruit can also be cored or pitted and sliced before poaching.

SUGGESTED ACCOMPANIMENTS: Offer some toasted almonds on the side.

★★★   VITAMIN E, VITAMIN C, FOLIC ACID, POTASSIUM, COPPER
★   MANGANESE, BORON

❧ Frozen Banana Maple-Walnut Whip ❧

Yield: 3 cups   (4 generous servings)

This is our version of ice cream—rich, luscious, and made with whole, unrefined foods. It contains vitamin B_6, manganese, magnesium, and copper, all important for strong, healthy bones. Serve in long-stemmed wine glasses and give your family and friends a healthy treat!

Have on hand: 4 ripe bananas (see Note), peeled and frozen in plastic for at least 12 hours.

4 frozen bananas
3 tablespoons maple syrup
1 tablespoon cashew butter or tahini

¼ cup unfiltered apple juice
½ cup walnuts, chopped coarsely, plus
   4 walnut halves

1. Cut bananas into pieces and put in blender or processor. Add maple syrup, cashew butter, and juice. Blend until smooth.

2. With a spoon, stir walnut pieces in, scoop banana whip into individual bowls or goblets, and serve with an attractive walnut half on top.

NOTE: Ripe bananas have yellow skins, little brown spots, and are without any green. We recommend purchasing the bananas several days in advance since they usually need ripening. Also, washing unpeeled bananas before peeling them is a good idea—it will clean off some of the chemicals (which can get on your hands and then on the banana itself as you peel it); or buy organic bananas.

★★★   OMEGA-3 FATTY ACIDS, VITAMIN B_6, MANGANESE
★   MAGNESIUM, COPPER, VITAMIN C, FOLIC ACID

Commercial ice cream is made from milk, which contains calcium, but it also has large amounts of refined sugar, and sugar is one of the substances that acidifies the body, causing calcium to be leached from the bones. You may put the right amount of calcium into your body, but when you are also eating sugar, you won't get the full benefit.

Beverly's Cantaloupe with Freshly Grated Ginger

Yield: 4 generous servings

A good way to rehydrate yourself after perspiring from hot flashes is to eat something juicy, such as a ripe melon. Grate some fresh ginger, sprinkle it over a slice, and transform the melon into an exotic dessert.

1 **ripe cantaloupe (see below)**	4 **mint sprigs or whole strawberries**
3 **inches fresh ginger**	

1. Cut cantaloupe into quarters.
2. Grate ginger over cantaloupe slices. Serve with a sprig of mint or a strawberry.

SUGGESTED ACCOMPANIMENTS: Serve as a snack or after a summer meal.

★★★ VITAMIN A, VITAMIN C
★ FOLIC ACID, VITAMIN B$_6$, POTASSIUM, NIACIN, THIAMIN, MAGNESIUM

To Pick a Cantaloupe

Look for a cantaloupe that is all beige with no green tinge on the rind. It will have a slightly soft touch when pressed on the ends. If the cantaloupe is not cold, a sweet aroma will be apparent when it is smelled closely. If it has none, then it will not be a very tasty cantaloupe.

❧ Baked Apples Stuffed with ❧ Raisin-Ginger Chutney

Yield: 4 servings

Baked apples and the standard ingredients used to stuff them are good sources of boron. Enjoy this version filled with raisins and ginger or try the variations using almonds and cinnamon—all good boron foods. A deficiency of boron interferes with calcium metabolism and clear thinking.

RAISIN-GINGER CHUTNEY:

½ **cup filtered water**   ½ **cup grated fresh ginger**
½ **cup raisins, organic preferred**

APPLES:

4 **baking apples, such as Rome Beauty**   **Apple juice, unfiltered preferred**
   or Cortland

Preheat oven to 375°.

1. In a small saucepan, bring the water to a boil. Turn off heat and add raisins, cover pot, and let sit 5 minutes, until raisins swell.

2. Drain and reserve water from raisins; put raisins in a processor or blender with ginger (if using a blender, grate ginger first) and blend until raisins look chopped. Add a few tablespoons of soaking liquid to thin slightly.

3. Core apples, removing seeds without going through the bottom (a melon-ball scoop works great). Make a slit around the diameter of the apple (keeps apple from bursting while baking) and stuff it with chutney.

4. Place stuffed apples into a baking dish, and pour in ½ inch of juice. Put in oven and bake 45 minutes.

5. Serve warm for dessert or at room temperature for breakfast.

VARIATIONS: Instead of raisins, use dried figs, apricots, or dates, or stuff with whole raisins, almonds or almond butter, and sprinkle with cinnamon. The chutney can accompany curry dishes and be spread on toast or used on grain.

SUGGESTED ACCOMPANIMENTS: Broccoli with Currants and Flounder Rolls Stuffed with Salmon and Lemon.

★★★ VITAMIN B$_6$, POTASSIUM, MAGNESIUM
★ COPPER, IRON

We recommend buying organic raisins for several reasons. Grapes are one of the most heavily sprayed crops and commercial raisins are sprayed with oil to keep in the moisture—that's what makes them shiny. Golden raisins are Thompson seedless grapes that have been treated with the chemical sulphur dioxide.

❧ Old-Fashioned Oatmeal Raisin Cookies ❧

Yield: about 30 cookies

Cookies made with healthy ingredients qualify as good food for snacks. Pack some in your purse for times away from home and you'll keep yourself from snacking on the refined flour and sugar versions that in the long run deplete your energy.

½ cup unsalted butter, at room temperature
1 cup maple syrup
2 eggs, organic, free-range preferred
1 teaspoon pure vanilla extract
1½ cups oatmeal (not quick-cooking)
¾ cup whole wheat pastry flour

½ cup raisins or dried currants, unsulphured preferred
1 cup walnuts or pecans, chopped coarsely
½ cup unsweetened coconut (optional)
1 teaspoon sea salt
1 teaspoon cinnamon

Preheat oven to 350°.

1. In a medium bowl or processor, whip butter. Add maple syrup, eggs, and vanilla, beating well.

2. In a second medium bowl mix together oatmeal, flour, raisins, walnuts, coconut, salt, and cinnamon. With a wooden spoon, stir the oatmeal mixture into the butter combination until moistened.

3. Prepare two baking sheets with parchment paper. Using two teaspoons, drop dough onto baking sheets in mounds 1 inch apart.

4. Place sheets in preheated oven and bake 12 to 15 minutes, until golden. After 7 minutes, switch the top sheet with the bottom sheet to ensure even cooking.

5. Let cookies cool on baking sheet for a few minutes, then remove to a cooling rack or plates. (If using plates, do not stack cookies more than two high until fully cooled.)

VARIATION: For crunchier cookies, reduce the flour by 3 to 6 tablespoons, which will allow the cookies to spread more.

SUGGESTED ACCOMPANIMENTS: Herbal tea or grain coffee.

★★★   OMEGA-3 FATTY ACIDS, MANGANESE, LINOLEIC ACID
★   MAGNESIUM, SELENIUM, ZINC

Egg Replacement

Eggs make cookies cakier. If you prefer not to use eggs, substitute 1 teaspoon baking powder and ⅛ cup water, or grind 1 tablespoon flax seeds and add this plus ⅛ cup water per egg.

❧ Broiled Dates Stuffed with Almonds ❧

Yield: 12 dates   (4 servings)

These succulent dates are wonderful sources of several star menopause nutrients—vitamin E, magnesium, essential fatty acids, and boron. Notice that even the hint of butter that coats each date can impart its wonderful flavor and richness—enjoy the taste!

12 almonds	¼ teaspoon ground ginger
12 pitted dates (see Note)	⅛ teaspoon nutmeg
1 tablespoon unsalted butter	⅛ teaspoon sea salt
¼ teaspoon cinnamon	12 toothpicks, without frills

1. Stuff almonds into open ends of dates. They will slip in easily.
2. In a small saucepan, melt butter on low heat. Add cinnamon, ginger, nutmeg, and salt. Drop stuffed dates into melted butter mixture, stirring well to make sure the butter covers the dates completely.
3. Remove coated dates with a slotted spoon and place on a metal or enamel pan. Broil under heat for 10 minutes, turning once halfway through.
4. Insert a toothpick into each date, and place on a serving plate. Eat hot or warm.

NOTE: We find Medjool dates to be the tastiest, but these usually do not come pitted. To remove pit, carefully tear open top of date, partially exposing pit. Pull pit out with your fingers, stuff almond in, and push closed.

VARIATION: As an appetizer, serve on individual plates in a pool of 1 tablespoon warm tomato sauce mixed with ½ teaspoon yogurt per plate.

SUGGESTED ACCOMPANIMENTS: Hot mint tea and a good book to read.

★★★   VITAMIN E, MAGNESIUM, OMEGA-3 FATTY ACIDS, LINOLEIC ACID, BORON

❧ Broiled Maple Apples ❧

Yield: 4 servings

It takes 40 gallons of maple sap to make 1 gallon of maple syrup. There's 2 to 3 percent sucrose in the sap and 65 percent in the syrup. Although it is a concentrated sweet which, for the sake of your blood sugar you should only eat in small quantities, it is a better quality sugar and has a range of minerals—calcium, potassium, manganese, magnesium, phosphorus, and iron.

3 **apples, cored**
½ **cup apple juice or orange juice**
2 **teaspoons maple or date crystals**

½ **teaspoon cinnamon or ground ginger**
½ **cup walnuts, chopped coarsely (optional)**

1. Cut apples into rings. Place in a metal or enamel baking dish (see Note).
2. Pour juice over apples, making sure that all the fruit is covered. Dust with maple crystals and cinnamon.
3. Broil 6 inches from the flame, until golden on top, about 5 minutes. Turn over and broil another 3 to 4 minutes.
4. Arrange on plates and sprinkle with walnuts; serve hot.

VARIATIONS: Try this same technique with bananas, pears, peaches, plums, grapefruit (especially pink), oranges, and nectarines.

NOTE: Do not broil in glass, since it can crack from the high heat.

★★★   OMEGA-3 FATTY ACIDS, LINOLEIC ACID
★   MANGANESE, COPPER, MAGNESIUM, VITAMIN B$_6$, CALCIUM, POTASSIUM, PHOSPHORUS, IRON

When maple syrup is harvested from maple trees, to prevent the tap holes from closing, some producers use formaldehyde pellets in the process. Vermont has banned this practice. If formaldehyde has not been used, this may be stated on the label.

❧

❦ Apricot-Date-Pecan Bonbons ❦

Yield: 12 to 15 walnut-sized bonbons

Drying fruit concentrates the nutrients and for this reason we like them as a snack. In these bonbons, there's lots of manganese, a mineral that nourishes nerves and brain, and complements the stress vitamins, B-complex and C.

½ cup pitted dates (about 5 large)
1 cup unsulphured dried apricots
(about 25 to 30 whole; see Note)
1 cup pecans, toasted

½ teaspoon ground ginger
¼ teaspoon cinnamon
½ cup unsweetened coconut

1. In a processor, put dates, apricots, pecans, ginger, and cinnamon. Pulse until chopped and well mixed.
2. Put coconut in a wide bowl. Have a small bowl of water for your hands.
3. Dampen hands and make walnut-size balls of fruit and nut mixture. Roll balls in coconut until completely covered.
4. These bonbons can be stored in either a glass jar or a metal can with a tight-fitting lid. If all bonbons are not eaten in four to five days store in the refrigerator to keep coconut from going rancid.

NOTE: If apricots are very dry, place in ½ cup boiling filtered water and cover for 10 minutes. Remove from water and proceed.

VARIATIONS: Try making these with toasted walnuts or almonds instead of pecans and rolling them in carob or cocoa powder.

★★★   MANGANESE, LINOLEIC ACID, COPPER, VITAMIN A
★   OMEGA-3 FATTY ACIDS, PANTOTHENIC ACID, THIAMIN, POTASSIUM, IRON

There are two kinds of dried apricots that are common. There's the California apricot which is cut in half due to its large size and which has a sweet and tangy flavor. Turkish apricots are whole, a little plumper, and have a delicate muscatel grape flavor.

❧ Dark Chocolate Candy ('90s "Chunkies") ❧

Yield: 18 chocolates

This recipe gives you a way to have chocolate, without eating refined sugar. The sweet comes from maple syrup and raisins instead.

4 ounces unsweetened baking
   chocolate
½ cup maple syrup

1 teaspoon pure vanilla extract
¼ cup raisins
½ cup almonds or pecans, toasted

1. In a double boiler, heat chocolate until melted. Add syrup, vanilla, raisins, and almonds. Stir well.

2. Using two teaspoons, drop mixture onto parchment paper in 18 mounds. Allow to cool and harden.

3. Store in an airtight container. These candies will last a long, long time—unless you eat them all!

★★★ MANGANESE, VITAMIN E, MAGNESIUM, VITAMIN C, COPPER, IRON

❧

Our advice on candy is, if you are going to eat it, eat the best quality you can find. And the good news is that now you can find wonderful varieties, made with sweeteners other than refined sugar.

❧

❧ 18 ❧
Beverages and Tonics

Zen Punch
Frothy Mango Lassi
Hot Spiced Cider
Fresh Carrot-Apple Juice with Parsley
Liver Tonic (Lemon Tea)
Kidney-Balancing Tea (Ginger Tea)
Nappy-Time Drink (Kuzu Drink)
Digestive Beverage (Mint Tea)
Rose Hip Cooler

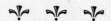

❧

There are many beverages you can use to quench your thirst and give yourself a relaxing break that can ease the symptoms of PMS and menopause and menstrual symptoms. Try a tasty mixture of fruit juice and herbal tea, juiced vegetables, or yogurt puréed with fruit. There are also teas with medicinal properties to give you energy or calm you down.

Water: Drink at least six to eight glasses a day. With the hot flashes and sweating of menopause, you may become a little dehydrated. And having enough water helps you maintain an even body temperature.

Water is the best liquid to replace fluids because it requires minimal processing by the body and can be a source of minerals. We highly recommend filtered water because today's water often contains toxins. And if you don't filter, in the morning before you fill your first glass, at least let the water run several minutes to clean out the toxins that may have settled in the pipes during the night. (Our Appendix guides you to the best of bottled water and filters.)

Caffeine: Beverages that contain caffeine—coffee, tea, and soda—are "off the menu." Caffeine is a stimulant that can overwork the adrenals, which you need in good condition throughout your life. They are essential for tolerating stress and they are also important to your body's production of estrogen postmenopause. And if you are premenopausal and still menstruating, caffeine can aggravate the mood swings and breast tenderness associated with premenstrual syndrome.

If you have difficulty stopping caffeine all at once, wean yourself with Swiss water-process decaffeinated coffee, which removes most of the caffeine with water rather than chemical solvents, or try a mix of coffee and coffee substitute. (See our list in the Appendix.) Even switching to green tea, which contains half the caffeine of coffee and less caffeine than black tea, is a good beginning. It also contains phytohormones and is associated with lower cancer risk and lower cholesterol.

Alcoholic beverages: With menopause, many women find they have much less tolerance of alcohol, getting higher quicker and feeling worse later. Alcohol can also bring on hot flashes. Red wine does contain estrogenic bioflavonoids (so does red grape juice), but it can still bring on flashes and we don't recommend using it if you're having these.

Iced beverages: Iced water with meals is counterproductive. It interferes with digestion, an essential for good health. Beyond this, some people have systems that are fundamentally cool and iced drinks are particularly not recommended for this body type. If you're sweltering from hot flashes, yet on the cool side in your body and cold drinks don't appeal, go with your instincts and refrain from icy beverages. Your body may be trying to harbor its internal warmth.

❧ Zen Punch ❧

Yield: 1½ cups   (1 serving)

Here's a healthy version of soda that a friend of ours invented. We use unfiltered juice because it has no added water, and there's enough intense flavor in this kind of juice that mixing it with sparkling mineral water will result in a drink that still has plenty of taste. Unlike commercial sodas, this is free of refined sugar, caffeine, and high amounts of phosphorus, all of which you need to avoid for the health of your bones.

1 **cup cold apple juice, unfiltered preferred**
½ **cup cold sparkling mineral water**

1 **lemon wedge**
   Whole strawberry (optional)

Pour juice into a tall glass. Add sparkling water and stir. Add ice, if desired. Slip lemon wedge onto rim of glass, drop in a strawberry and a straw.

VARIATIONS: Use other juice flavors such as apple-strawberry, apricot, or pear with sparkling mineral water. Add a lime or orange wedge for color and added zip.

★★★   VITAMIN C, VITAMIN K, IRON, MANGANESE

❧ Frothy Mango Lassi ❧

Yield: 4 cups   (4 servings)

A classic drink of India, this yogurt beverage is a good source of B_{12}, a vitamin good for your nerves. We also make B_{12} in our intestines, and bacteria-active yogurt, which contributes fresh flora, helps us to make our own supply.

2 **cups plain bacteria-active yogurt**   **Pinch cumin (optional)**
1 **or 2 mangoes, peeled (about 1 cup)**   4 **ice cubes, more as desired**

In a blender, put yogurt, fruit, cumin, and ice. Purée until smooth, and pour into tall glasses.

VARIATIONS: When they're in season, try this drink with papaya, banana, strawberries, pineapple, or fresh ginger for real zing! We also like it with some added Fig Sauce with Basil (see recipe).

★★★   VITAMIN B$_{12}$, VITAMIN A, RIBOFLAVIN
  ★   CALCIUM, PHOSPHOROUS, SELENIUM

❧ Hot Spiced Cider ❧

Yield: 4 cups   (4 servings)

If you want a hot drink besides tea, there's always the option of having some warmed cider. It's high in thiamin, which helps you avoid the memory lapses that can occur in menopause.

4 **cups apple cider or unfiltered**   1 **herbal tea bag, such as Harvest Spice**
  apple juice   **or Mu Tea**
1 **cinnamon stick**   1 **orange, organic preferred, sliced,**
                                               or ½ cup orange juice

1. In a small saucepan, bring apple cider and cinnamon stick to a boil. Turn off flame and add tea bag. Cover and steep for 3 to 4 minutes.
2. Remove tea bag and discard. Add orange slices or juice and serve hot in big mugs.

VARIATIONS: If you find you're out of spicy-tasting tea bags, while the cider is heating just add 4 whole cloves, 3 cardamom pods, 2 star anise or allspice berries, and several dashes of nutmeg.

★★★   VITAMIN C
  ★   THIAMIN, IRON, POTASSIUM, MANGANESE, BORON

Fruit Juices	
Best:	fresh; unfiltered; organic
Good:	made from fruit juice only
Avoid:	juice drinks made from concentrates; juice drinks containing added sugar

❧ Fresh Carrot-Apple Juice with Parsley ❧

Yield: 2 cups   (2 servings)

The American diet is low in beta-carotene, but this tasty drink will help correct that. Carrots are full of this vitamin, and when they are made into juice, it's more easily absorbed. We included parsley because it helps the liver remove toxins that can be a burden to your body at menopause.

4 carrots, cut in half lengthwise
2 apples, quartered, with seeds

½ bunch parsley, stems and leaves

1. Press 3 carrots, apples, and parsley through the juicer. Press remaining carrot through juicer.
2. Serve immediately in a tall glass. (Do not store freshly made juices since they lose many of their vitamins within a very short period of time.)

VARIATIONS: Try adding a 2-inch piece of fresh ginger for extra zing, or use beets instead of apples, and even add celery for a delightful flavor

★★★   VITAMIN A, VITAMIN K, VITAMIN C
  ★   FOLIC ACID, VITAMIN E, VITAMIN B_6, POTASSIUM, IRON, THIAMIN

❧

To make fresh fruit and vegetable juices you need an electric juicer. (Stomping on grapes is the only exception!) There are two basic types of juicing appliances: machines that centrifuge spin most of the pulp away from the juice, producing a smooth and pulp-free juice, and those that masticate, breaking up the cells and fibers, leaving more pulp in the juice.

❧

❧ Liver Tonic (Lemon Tea) ❧

Yield: 1 cup   (1 serving)

Your liver makes cholesterol, which is then converted into the many hormones in your body, including estrogen, progesterone, and testosterone. Giving your liver a tonic helps it do this important work.

1 cup filtered water, heated	**½ teaspoon maple syrup or**
Juice of ½ lemon	**unsulphured blackstrap molasses**
Pinch cayenne	

Mix together and drink while warm, on an empty stomach.

★★★   VITAMIN C, MANGANESE, FOLIC ACID
  ★   ZINC, VITAMIN B$_6$, MAGNESIUM, POTASSIUM

A Simple Liver Flush

These ingredients are the start of salad dressing, but used this way they can cleanse your liver. Use this as often as you like. It is best taken in the morning. Blend the ingredients and drink on an empty stomach.

1 clove garlic	1 tablespoon extra-virgin olive oil
Juice of ½ lemon	1 tablespoon filtered water

❧ Kidney-Balancing Tea (Ginger Tea) ❧

Yield: 1 cup   (1 serving)

Ginger is an herbal stimulant which is useful medicinally in the perimenopausal years to warm the entire pelvis and ease menstrual cramps. Because it is warming to the body, ginger might also trigger a hot flash. Experiment and see how it suits you.

1 cup filtered water   **3 fresh ginger slices**

1. In a small saucepan, heat water and ginger just to a boil. Lower flame and simmer uncovered 2 to 3 minutes. Water will become slightly yellow and no longer clear.
2. Sip while hot, preferably on an empty stomach or after a meal.

VARIATION: For a sweeter tea, add some warm apple juice.

★★★   MAGNESIUM, COPPER, POTASSIUM, VITAMIN B$_6$
★   VITAMIN C, MANGANESE

Coffee is a diuretic, stimulating the excretion of fluid and the vitamins and minerals it contains. This is true whether the coffee is caffeinated or decaffeinated. It also acidifies the system and more than 2 cups a day can trigger calcium to leave the bones.

❧ Nappy-Time Drink (Kuzu Drink) ❧

Yield: 1 cup   (1 serving)

If your sleep has been interrupted by night sweats, an afternoon nap may be in order. The kuzu in this drink is a relaxant and can help you drift off to sleep any time of the day or night.

**1 cup apple juice, unfiltered
    preferred**

**1 tablespoon kuzu (do not substitute
    arrowroot; see Note)**

1. In a small saucepan, stir together juice and kuzu until kuzu is completely dissolved.

2. Bring to a boil, stirring constantly, until thickened and clear. Cook another 30 seconds. Pour into a mug and sip, using a spoon if you like. (Liquid will be thick and hot.) Drink while warm.

NOTE: To measure kuzu, either pulverize it into powder and measure or generously fill (not heaping) a tablespoon, estimating that the open spaces will be filled by the kuzu that sticks up past the level measure and will about equal out.

VARIATIONS: You can stir a half teaspoon of tahini or almond butter into the hot kuzu drink or, if you prefer a salty version, mix together ½ teaspoon salted plum paste (umeboshi) with 1 cup heated filtered water and a few drops of shoyu soy sauce, instead of the apple juice.

★★★   IRON, MANGANESE, POTASSIUM

Many herbal teas such as chamomile are also used as relaxants. You can make a cupful and drink it or pour the strained tea into your bath water. Enjoy a relaxing soak and you'll absorb the tea solution through your skin.

In China and Japan kuzu drinks are used for many minor ailments, including headaches, indigestion, colds, digestive disorders, stress, tension, tight muscles, and, as we use it here, as a relaxant to help you fall asleep. Try some of this very unique food.

❧ Digestive Beverage (Mint Tea) ❧

Yield: 1 cup   (1 serving)

Peppermint is a cooling herb for hot flashes, and if you're in perimenopause and having uncomfortable menstrual cycles, peppermint can ease the pain of cramps. It's also great for digestion.

1 **peppermint tea bag**
1 **cup filtered water, boiling**

1 **teaspoon unsulphured blackstrap molasses**

1. Place tea bag in a mug and pour boiling water over. Steep for 2 to 3 minutes.
2. Remove and discard bag (it is not recommended to use herbal tea bags twice). Stir in molasses and sip slowly.

VARIATIONS: Try this as a refreshing iced tea. Make the tea double strength, and add ice to cool and dilute.

★★★ IRON, COPPER
  ★ CALCIUM, MANGANESE, MAGNESIUM, VITAMIN K, VITAMIN B$_6$

❧ Rose Hip Cooler ❧

Yield: 2 cups   (2 servings)

Fatigue is one of the most common symptoms of menopause and rose hip tea is a common tonic for exhaustion. It's full of vitamin C, which is used up quickly by stress.

1 rose hip tea bag
1 cup filtered water, boiling
1 cup apple juice

2 orange slices, organic preferred
   Ice cubes (optional)

1. Add tea bag to boiling water and let steep covered for 3 to 5 minutes.
2. Pour apple juice into two tall glasses, add tea and orange slices. Add ice cubes, if desired.

VARIATIONS: As a hot drink, steep 1 tea bag per cup and add ¼ cup apple juice to sweeten and cool.

★★★   VITAMIN C

APPENDIX

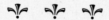

Foods We Recommend
Organic Certifying Organizations
Tips for Snacks and Mini-Meals
Eating Out
Ethnic Menu Choices
New Ingredients
Sweetness Conversion
Fats and Oils
Water and Filtering Units
Resources We Recommend
Foods That Contain . . .

Foods We Recommend

Whole Grain Pasta (the ones that are tasty):

De Boles (wheat-free corn)
DeCecco (whole wheat)
Delverde (whole wheat)
Eden (kamut)
Vita Spelt (spelt)
Westbrae (ramen—instant noodles and broth)
Several name brands also offer udon (whole wheat) and soba (buckwheat).

Boxed Grain, Bean, Cake, and Pancake Mixes

Arrowhead Mills (red lentils, whole grain pancake mixes, soup and grain mixes, whole grain cereals)
Fantastic Foods (instant soup cups, pilaf, hummus, and other instant bean dishes)
Lundberg Farms (the best brown rice, one-step pilaf and chili mixes, gourmet rice blends)
San Gennaro Polenta (ready-made polenta in a tube)

Meat and Poultry

Suppliers without hormones and antibiotics found in supermarkets.

Coleman Natural Meats: Natural and organic beef and lamb. Supplies western and eastern states.

Foster Farms: Poultry. Supplies western states.

Holly Farms: Poultry. Supplies eastern and midwestern states.

Kohler Farms: Beef. Wisconsin and Chicago area. Trademark name is PURElean BEEF.

Larsen Beef: Atlanta, GA; Long Island, NY; Tampa and Orlando, FL; Chicago area.

Laura's Lean Beef: Kentucky and southern Indiana.

Maverick Ranch Lite Beef: Denver, CO; Saint Louis, MO; New Jersey; Pennsylvania; New York City area.

Organic Cattle Co.: New York City area.

Quality Steaks: Massachusetts; New England area; Phoenix, AZ.

Fats and Oils

Alta Dena Certified Dairy. 800/645-5123. Hormone-free butter.

Barleans Organic Oils. 800/445-3529. Flaxseed and borage oils, expeller pressed and packaged in opaque containers.

Colavita extra-virgin olive oil.

Flora. 800/498-3610. Flax seed and other oils in brown glass bottles.

Greek Gourmet organic extra-virgin olive oil. 617/749-1866.

Omega Nutrition, USA. 800/661-3529. Organic flax seed oil and other fine-quality cold-pressed oils in black bottles.

Organic Valley Butter. 608/625-2602. Organic butter.

Herbal Teas and Grain Beverages

Bambu (grain coffee substitute)

Cafix (grain coffee substitute)

Celestial Seasonings (Sleepy Time and other caffeine-free herbal and iced teas)

Traditional Medicinals (herbal teas designed for various ailments)

Cookies

Amaranth graham crackers

Barbara's Small Indulgence Cookie

Mi-Del graham crackers

Westbrae Snaps (rice malt snaps—ginger, lemon, oatmeal)

Mail-Order Organic Foods

The book *Green Groceries—A Mail Order Guide to Organic Foods*, by Jeanne Heifetz (HarperCollins, 1992), has taken all of the guesswork out of purchasing mail-order organic foods including produce, fish, meats, and more.

Beano Hotline and free sample. 800/257-8650. (We prefer the drops.)

Bioforce of America. 800/445-8802. Herbamare (herbal sea salt) and Bambu (grain coffee substitute).

Brae Beef. 203/869-0106. Hormone-free beef and poultry.

D'Artagnan. 800/DAR-TAGN (327-8246). Antibiotic-free, hormone-free, pesticide-free, poultry, lamb, pig, goat, and wild game.

Food Animals Concerns Trusts. 773/525-4952. Contact for sources of humanely raised veal.

Mountain Rose Herbs. 800/879-3337. Certified organic herbs, teas, oils, cosmetics, and more.

Vermont Country Maple Products. 800/528-7021. Maple syrup, maple frosting, and granulated maple sprinkles.

Other Food Items

Ak-Mak (whole wheat sesame crackers)

Aunt Patsy's (organic soup mixes)

Barbara's (boxed breakfast cereals without refined sugar)

Cascadian Farms (organic all-fruit jams)

Enrico's (tomato sauce and salsa)

Hawthorne Valley Farm (organic biodynamic yogurt)

Jaclyn's (whole wheat bread crumbs)

R. W. Knudsen (organic and natural juices and soda without sugar and phosphates)

Lundberg Farms (rice cakes in assorted flavors, with or without salt)

Maine Coast (seaweeds pulverized and in convenient shakers)

Maranatha Natural Foods (organic raw and roasted nut butters, especially almond)

Muir Glen (unsweetened tomato products)

Pomì (shelf-stable boxed tomatoes—chopped or strained)

Seven Stars Farm (organic biodynamic yogurt)

Sunspire (malted chocolate and chips without refined sugar)

Timbercrest Farms (organic dried fruit in packages)

Vermont Country (maple sprinkles and maple frosting mixes)

Westbrae Natural Foods (cookies, mustard, unsweetened catsup, ramen and other foodstuffs)

Organic Certifying Organizations

Look for these names on labels of organic foods to ensure that quality standards have
been maintained.

The Organic Foods Production Association of North America (OFPANA): P. O. Box 1078,
Greenfield, MA 01301. 413/774-7511. Certifiers of organic produce. Publications and
memberships available.

Demeter Association, Inc.: 818/843-5521. Certifiers of organically grown and produced
yogurt from humanely treated animals.

Northeast Organic Farming Association: Connecticut 203/484-2445; Massachusetts
508/355-2853; New Hampshire 603/648-2521; New Jersey 609/737-6848; New York
607/648-5557; Vermont 802/223-7222. Certifiers of organic produce.

Tips for Snacks and Mini-Meals

There are lots of good foods to eat on the run. Between-meal eating can keep your
blood sugar steady and give you energy when you need it.

SNACKS

- Crunchy, raw vegetables
- Pickles
- Unsulphured dried fruit, especially figs
- Nuts and seeds
- Baked yams or sweet potatoes
- Plain bacteria-active yogurt
- Rice cakes with nut butter
- Fresh fruit including mangoes, tangerines, berries, figs, and pears of all kinds
- Miso soup
- And try these recipes: Crispy Walnut and Seed Bars, Sunflower-Nori Snack,
Toasted Nuts with Raisins and Apricots

MINI-MEALS

- Tortilla and scrambled egg
- Bowl of homemade soup
- Sardines in water
- Slice of bean loaf or pâté on whole grain bread

- Seasoned tempeh with mustard
- Whole grain bread and nut butter sandwich
- Healthy homemade muffins

INSTANT SALADS

- Cooked grain plus tomato and scallions with dressing
- Last night's cooked vegetables with vinaigrette
- Bag of prewashed and cut gourmet salad mix with dressing

CROSTINI AND BRUSCHETTA SUGGESTIONS

Slices of toast with a topping—as is or broiled.

- Sauce Romesco
- Garlic bruschetta (see Garlic Soup with Bruschetta)
- Roasted garlic and warm goat cheese on bread with black pepper
- Tomato, hard-boiled egg slices with tarragon, flax seed oil, and sea salt
- Crumbled feta with oregano
- Chopped shrimp and scallops
- Slices of avocado with caviar

Eating Out

When you don't feel like cooking, you can always nourish yourself by eating out. Here are some good food choices that you can find on many restaurant menus.

Breakfast	Lunch	Dinner
Oatmeal	Sardines in water	Bean or vegetable soup
Eggs and omelettes	Canned salmon	Broiled fish
Home-fried potatoes	Green salads	Fresh vegetable platter
Fresh melon slices	Fresh fruit salad	Oysters
	"Homemade" soup	Baked or roasted potatoes
	Fresh turkey or chicken sandwich	Roasted chicken
		Brown or wild rice
		Game meats

Ethnic Menu Choices

Many ethnic restaurants offer nutritious food choices. Each kind has its own specialty. Here is a guide to foods you can order that are on the menopause menu.

Italian: escarole, broccoli rabe, fish, shellfish
Indian: dhal (lentils), fresh vegetables, vegetarian dishes
Japanese: seaweed, miso, fish, shellfish, tofu
Chinese and other Asian countries: steamed fish, vegetables, brown rice, snails, shellfish, tofu
Middle Eastern: bean hummus, babaganoush, whole-wheat pita
Greek: octopus, taramasalata (roe), fish, shellfish, fresh vegetables, beans, stuffed vegetables
Latin: beans, salsa, plantains, salted cod, root vegetables
Mexican: corn tortillas, beans, fish, shellfish—and hold the cheese!

New Ingredients

Arrowroot—a thickening starch, in powder form, made from the cassava root. It can replace cornstarch and is used in recipes in equal amounts. To substitute for kuzu, twice as much is needed. Always dissolve in cold water first and then cook until clear.

Brown rice vinegar—a mild-tasting, less acidic vinegar than cider or wine vinegar.

Kuzu—a thickening starch made from the root of the kudzu plant. It is known to have medicinal properties for the treatment of insomnia, nausea, diarrhea, and indigestion. It replaces arrowroot and cornstarch in recipes; half the quantity of kuzu is needed when converting. Always dissolve in cold water first and then cook until clear.

Miso—fermented rice and soybean paste made with sea salt and used for flavoring soup, salad dressing, and sauce. It has healthful bacteria and enzymes that can be beneficial for the intestines. Miso is also made from barley, chick-peas, and brown rice, and is available soy free.

Sea salt—salt from evaporated sea water that has no added free-flowing agents, added iodine, or dextrose.

Herbal sea salt—sea salt with herbs free of hydrogenated fat and hydrolyzed vegetable protein. The brand we use is Herbamare.

Salted plum paste and salted plum vinegar—also known as umeboshi, these Japanese plums have been aged in sea salt for two years. Salted plums have both a salty and sour, lemony taste. They are used instead of salt and vinegar or salt and lemon. The plums and vinegar have not been fermented, and they both contain picric acid, which helps to remove toxins from the bloodstream.

Seaweed—contains iodine and calcium as well as other important minerals. Seaweed can be helpful in protecting from and removing radiation from the body. The more common varieties are: nori, kombu, kelp, agar-agar, dulse, wakame, arame, and hijiki.

Shoyu soy sauce—naturally brewed soy sauce made from soybeans, wheat, and sea salt. It has no chemicals or sugars added in its production. The wheat free variety is called tamari.

Sweetness Conversion

You can successfully convert your favorite recipes from white sugar to quality sweeteners by following these guidelines:

1. The sweetness of 1 cup of white sugar approximately equals 1 cup of maple syrup. But when you replace a dry ingredient with a liquid one, you need to remove 1 cup of liquid from the recipe or you need to add another 1 cup flour.
2. We find that most standard recipes are too sweet, so to compensate we cut the original amount of sugar by about half. Starting with 1 cup of sugar, we usually reduce this by half. We then convert this to ½ cup maple syrup, remembering to also reduce the liquid by ½ cup (or add another ½ cup flour). Whole grain flours absorb a little more liquid than white flour does, because of the bran, so it is good to know what the consistency of the original recipe is supposed to be, to decide whether to delete liquid or add more flour. (And sometimes there is no liquid in the recipe to delete, so only the addition of flour will be able to correct the addition of the liquid sugar.)

Please note that we find *it typically takes* one or two tries to get the recipe right, keeping notes for the next try—and that each trial is usually delicious!

Fats and Oils

The oils to buy are those that state on the label "unrefined" or for olive oil, "extra virgin." If you find oils with these designations, and also labeled organic, so much the better. The term "cold-pressed" means that no heat was applied while the seeds, nuts, or grains were being pressed into oil, but cold-pressed does not necessarily mean unprocessed. After pressing, the oils can still be exposed to high temperatures and chemicals during the other aspects of refining.

Fats and oils can be damaged by light, so it is best to purchase oils from the back of the shelf, in cans, or in black or dark bottles. Flax seed oil is available in the refrigerator sections of natural food stores. Once opened, the oil in bottles further deteriorates from exposure to the oxygen in the air, but light is the most damaging. We recommend buying fats and oils in small quantities. Store containers, whether opened or not, in a location that is both cool and dark. Opened containers should be kept in the refrigerator. To make sure an oil is not exposed to light, if it's in a transparent bottle, you can cover the container with a paper bag. We do keep a small amount of extra-virgin olive oil on the counter in easy reach for cooking and kept away from the heat of the stove. We use a classic Greek metal oil container that has a narrow spout and neck.

Most important for your health is to understand that there are different kinds of fats. While we need to reduce the amount of saturated fat in our diet, it's also vital to find a variety of food sources for the healthy fats that our bodies need. This "fat family tree" should clear up some of the confusion.

Water and Filtering Units

We've recommended filtered water throughout the book because clean water is important to our everyday lives and we have found that most tap and bottled waters do not meet our standards. We recommend filtering the municipal water that comes into your home, or if your water comes from a well, have it tested. If it's polluted, we recommend Mountain Valley bottled water.

Filtering Systems

There are three basic types of filtering units; all filters fit into at least one of these. Many are designed for countertop use, attaching to the faucet of your kitchen sink. Others can be installed under the sink and have a separate spigot for the filtered water, and some units have a holding tank. Here is an overview.

Granulated carbon. These filters usually attach to the faucet or fit on top of a container. The water goes through the charcoal in the unit (similar to a fish-tank filter) and when collected on the other side, does taste better. Granular carbon filters mainly eliminate the chlorine, which is what you're usually tasting. The carbon should be changed every three weeks, since it can only absorb a certain amount of chlorine and bacteria may grow while not in use. The prices of these units range from $30 to $50.

Reverse osmosis (RO). These have a pre-filter to remove rust and other large particles; a solid carbon block that removes many chemicals, pesticides, and residues; and a reverse osmosis membrane that removes these same toxins in a somewhat greater percentage but at a very slow pace. RO are either installed in your basement with a holding tank or are attached to the faucet in the evening, the water collected overnight being stored in a container for later use. The average amount of water produced daily ranges from $1\frac{1}{2}$ to 3 gallons a day. New units can cost from $600 to $1,800.

Solid carbon filter. These have a pre-filter to remove large particles and rust; a solid

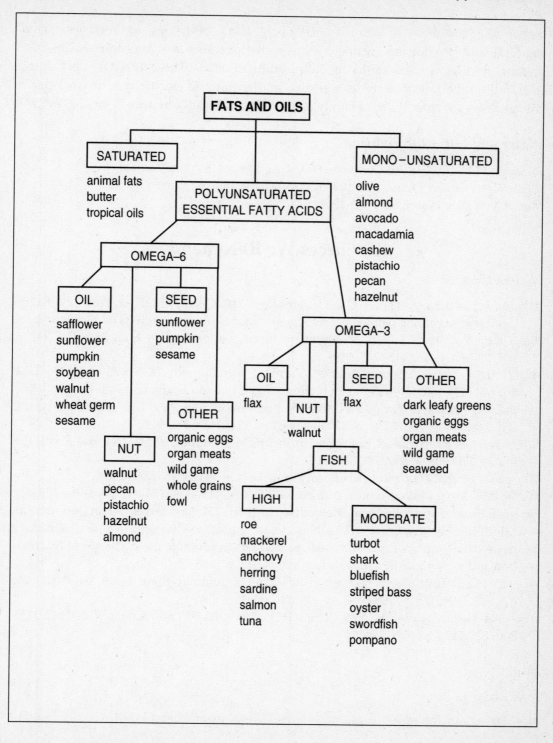

FATS AND OILS

SATURATED

animal fats
butter
tropical oils

**POLYUNSATURATED
ESSENTIAL FATTY ACIDS**

MONO–UNSATURATED

olive
almond
avocado
macadamia
cashew
pistachio
pecan
hazelnut

OMEGA–6

OIL

safflower
sunflower
pumpkin
soybean
walnut
wheat germ
sesame

SEED

sunflower
pumpkin
sesame

NUT

walnut
pecan
pistachio
hazelnut
almond

OTHER

organic eggs
organ meats
wild game
whole grains
fowl

OMEGA–3

OIL

flax

NUT

walnut

SEED

flax

OTHER

dark leafy greens
organic eggs
organ meats
wild game
seaweed

FISH

HIGH

roe
mackerel
anchovy
herring
sardine
salmon
tuna

MODERATE

turbot
shark
bluefish
striped bass
oyster
swordfish
pompano

carbon filter that removes a large variety of chemicals, pesticides, and residues, including DDT and benzine; and a micron screen that prevents lead and other toxins from passing through, while not filtering out healthful minerals. These filters are very simple to install on the faucet or under the sink, and require no electricity. The cartridge is changed every six months for a family of four. The units range in price from $200 to $500.

Water and Filter Information

Rader and Morrow Health Concepts. 800/828-9500 (ask for Jane).
Clean Water Concepts, Inc. P.O. Box 5141, North Branch, NJ 08876.
Mountain Valley Water. 800/643-1501.

Resources We Recomend

Newsletters

A Friend Indeed. Janine O'Leary Cobb, editor. Box 1710, Champlain, New York 12919-1710. Dedicated to helping women become more informed about the effects of menopause.

Breast Cancer Action. 55 New Montgomery Street, Suite 323, San Francisco, CA 94105. 415/243-9301; fax: 415/243-3996.

Health Action Network Society. 202-5262 Rumble Street, Burnaby, BC V5J2B6. 604/435-0512; fax: 604/435-1561. Newsletter and information service for health and well-being.

Health Links™. Gladys Taylor McGarey Medical Foundation. 7350 E. Stetson Drive, Suite 208, Scottsdale, AZ 85251. 602/946-4544; fax: 602/946-6902.

Health Wisdom for Women. Christiane Northrup, M.D., editor. 7811 Montrose Road, Potomac, MD 20854. 800/777-5005.

Menopause News. 2074 Union Street, San Francisco, CA 94123. 415/567-2368.

Midlife Zest. Mimi Fidlow, editor. P.O. Box 80323, Goleta, CA 93118-0323. 805-964-2252.

Women's Health Forum. Bronson Methodist Hospital, 252 East Lovell Street, Kalamazoo, MI 49007. Subscriptions: 6113 Abbey Road, Aptos, CA 95003. An interdisciplinary newsletter for physicians and medical students to promote the exchange of information and experience in women's health.

Women's Health Letter. Kerri Bodmer, editor. 2245 E. Colorado Blvd., Suite 104, Pasadena, CA 91107-3651. 818/798-0638.

Women's Health Advocate Newsletter, P.O. Box 420235, Palm Coast, FL 32142-0235. 800/829-5876.

Books

Menopause

Barbach, Lonnie, Ph.D. *The Pause.* New York: Dutton, 1993.

The Boston Women's Health Book Collective. *The New Our Bodies Ourselves.* New York: Touchstone Books, 1992.

Colbin, Annemarie. *Food and Healing.* New York: Ballantine Books, 1986.

Doress, Paula Brown, and Diana Laskin Siegal. *Ourselves Growing Older.* New York: Touchstone Books, 1987.

Fuchs, Nan Kathryn, Ph.D. *The Nutrition Detective.* Los Angeles: Jeremy P. Tarcher, 1985.

Gittleman, Ann Louise, M.S. *Super Nutrition for Menopause.* New York: Simon & Schuster, 1993.

Greenwood, Sadja, M.D. *Menopause, Naturally.* Volcano, CA: Volcano Press, 1989.

Lark, Susan M., M.D. *The Menopause Self-Help Book.* Berkeley, CA: Celestial Arts, 1992.

Love, Susan M., M.D. *Dr. Susan Love's Breast Book.* Reading, MA: Addison-Wesley, 1990.

Murray, Michael T., N.D. *Menopause.* Rocklin, CA: Prima Publishing, 1994.

Northrup, Christiane, M.D. *Women's Bodies, Women's Wisdom.* New York: Bantam Books, 1994.

Ojeda, Linda, Ph.D. *Menopause Without Medicine* Almeda, CA: Hunter House, 1992.

Parvati, Jeannine. *Hygieia A Woman's Herbal.* Berkeley, CA: Freestone Collective, 1983.

Perry, Susan, and Kathryn O'Hanlan, M.D. *Natural Menopause—Guide to a Woman's Most Misunderstood Passage.* Reading, MA: Addison-Wesley, 1992.

Reitz, Rita. *Menopause—A Positive Approach.* New York: Viking Penguin, 1977.

Weed, Susan S. *Menopausal Years.* Woodstock, NY: Ash Tree Publishing, 1992.

Wolfe, Honora. *Menopause: A Second Spring.* Boulder, CO: Blue Poppy Press, 1992.

Wolfe, Sidney M., M.D., and the Public Citizen Health Research Group with Rhoda Donkin Jones. *Women's Health Alert.* Reading, MA: Addison-Wesley, 1991.

NUTRITION REFERENCE

Appleton, Nancy, Ph.D. *Healthy Bones.* Garden City Park, NY: Avery Publishing Group, 1991.

———. *Lick the Sugar Habit.* Garden City Park, NY: Avery Publishing Group Inc, 1988.

Balch, James F., M.D., and Phyllis A. Balch, C.N.C. *Prescription for Nutritional Healing.* Garden City, NY: Avery Publishing Group, 1990.

Ballantine, Rudolph, M.D. *Diet and Nutrition.* Honesdale, PA: The Himalayan International Institute, 1978.

Dufty, William. *Sugar Blues.* New York: Warner Books, 1975.

Dunne, Lavon J. *Nutrition Almanac.* New York, NY: McGraw-Hill, 1990.

Erasmus, Udo, Ph.D. *Fats That Heal—Fats That Kill.* Burnaby, BC, Canada: Alive Books, 1993.

Gaby, Alan R., M.D. *Preventing and Reversing Osteoporosis.* Rocklin, CA: Prima Publishing, 1994.

Haas, Elson M., M.D. *Staying Healthy with Nutrition.* Berkeley, CA: Celestial Arts, 1992.

———. *Staying Healthy with the Seasons.* Berkeley, CA: Celestial Arts, 1981.

Oski, Frank A., M.D. *Don't Drink Your Milk!* Brushton, NY: TEACH Services, 1992.

COOKING

Blauer, Stephen. *The Juicing Book.* Garden City Park, NY: Avery Publishing Group, 1989.

Child, Julia. *The Way to Cook.* New York: Knopf, 1989.

Ford, Marjorie Winn, Susan Hillyard, and Mary Faulk Koock. *The Deaf Smith Country Cookbook*. New York: Collier Books, 1973.

Horsley, Janet. *Bean Cuisine*. Dorchester, England: Prism Press, 1982.

Rhoads, Sharon Ann. *Cooking with Sea Vegetables*. Brookline, MA: Autumn Press, 1978.

Stone, Sally and Martin. *The Brilliant Bean*. New York: Bantam Books, 1988.

Wittenberg, Margaret M. *Experiencing Quality*. Austin, TX: Whole Foods Market, Inc., 1987.

Organizations

Women's Health America Group: National Women's Health Hotline. 429 Gammon Place, P. O. Box 9641, Madison, WI 53715. 800/222-4767.

American Menopause Foundation, Inc. The Empire State Building, 350 Fifth Avenue, Suite 2822, New York, NY 10001. 212/475-3107.

Y-ME National Breast Cancer Organization. 800/221-2141. Hotline and referrals to local support groups.

National Women's Health Network. 514 10th St. NW, Suite 400, Wahington, DC 20004. 202/628-7814. A national public-interest membership organization and information service devoted solely to women and health.

Pesticide Hotline. U.S. Environmental Protection Agency, NPTN, Oregon State University, 333 Weniger Hall, Corvallis, Oregon 97331. Seven days a week, 6:30 a.m.–4:30 p.m. (PST).

Foods That Contain . . .

Vitamin A and Beta-Carotene

Grains: trace or none

Beans: trace or none

Vegetables:
yams
sweet potatoes
carrots
winter squash
  butternut
  acorn
  buttercup
  Hubbard
pumpkin
lamb's-quarters
shallots
spinach
dandelion greens

turnips
kale
collards
beet greens
mustard greens
chicory
red peppers
taro
bok choy
scallions
parsley
broccoli
asparagus

Fruits:
cantaloupe
mangoes
apricots

Japanese persimmon
plantains
papayas

Nuts: trace or none

Seeds: trace or none

Fish: trace or none

Poultry:
egg
liver

Meat:
liver

Oils:
fish liver

Other: butter

Thiamin (Vitamin B$_1$)

Grains:
whole rye
wild rice
whole wheat
millet
buckwheat (kasha)
bulgur
whole wheat couscous
brown rice
whole grain pasta
soba noodles
   (buckwheat)

Beans:
pinto
black
chick-peas
black-eyed peas
soybeans

Vegetables:
potatoes

green peas
Jerusalem artichokes
nori
fresh corn
okra

Fruits:
grapes
avocados
raisins
pineapple
watermelon
mangoes

Nuts:
Brazil nuts
pine nuts
pistachios
pecans
hazelnuts
cashews

Seeds:
sunflower

flax
sesame

Fish:
lobster
trout
oysters
tuna
catfish

Poultry:
duck
quail

Meat:
pork
liver
venison

Oils:
trace or none

Other:
tahini

Riboflavin (Vitamin B$_2$)

Grains:
wild rice
millet
whole wheat
bulgur
whole wheat couscous
whole grain pasta

Beans:
pinto
black

Vegetables:
yams
mushrooms
winter squash
   butternut

acorn
buttercup
Hubbard
kombu
nori

Fruits:
avocados

Nuts:
almonds
hazelnuts
chestnuts
cashews

Seeds:
pumpkin

squash
sunflower

Fish:
clams
salmon
mackerel
oysters
trout
herring

Poultry:
chicken, dark meat
liver
heart

Meat:
liver

Riboflavin (Vitamin B₂) (continued)

kidneys
caribou
antelope

goat
venison

Oils: trace or none

Other:
yogurt, plain
miso

Niacin (Vitamin B₃)

Grains:
whole wheat
brown rice
whole barley
bulgur
whole wheat
  couscous
millet
whole grain pasta

Beans:
black
pinto

Vegetables:
mushrooms
potatoes
asparagus
green peas
corn
Jerusalem
  artichokes
broccoli

summer
  squash
nori
hiziki

Fruits:
peaches
avocados

Nuts:
peanuts
almonds

Seeds:
sunflower

Fish:
tuna
swordfish
mackerel
shad
sturgeon
eel
salmon
trout

halibut
oysters
shrimp
sardines

Poultry:
chicken
turkey
pheasant
quail
liver

Meat:
liver
beef
lamb
rabbit
venison

Oils:
trace or none

Other:
miso

Pantothenic Acid (Vitamin B₅)

Grains:
all whole grains
whole grain pasta

Beans:
all legumes

Vegetables:
shiitake mushrooms
all other mushrooms

Fruits:
avocados

pomegranates

Nuts: trace or none

Seeds:
sunflower

Fish:
bluefish
abalone
trout
salmon
cod

Poultry:
liver
chicken
heart
goose

Meat:
beef liver
caribou
kidneys

Oils: trace or none

Other: trace or none

Pyridoxine (Vitamin B$_6$)

Grains:
brown rice
whole wheat
whole rye
bulgur
whole wheat
  couscous
whole grain
  pasta

Beans:
pinto
navy
lima

Vegetables:
spinach
broccoli
bok choy
potatoes

Fruits:
mangoes
watermelon
bananas
avocados
plantains
melons

Nuts:
walnuts
hazelnuts
peanuts
chestnuts

Seeds:
sunflower
flax

Fish:
tuna
trout

salmon
bluefish
octopus

Poultry:
pheasant
turkey
chicken
duck
quail

Meat:
liver
beef
pork

Oils: trace or none

Other:
blackstrap
  molasses

Vitamin B$_{12}$ (Cobalamin)

Grains: trace or none

Beans: trace or none

Vegetables: trace or
  none

Fruits: trace or none
Nuts: trace or none
Seeds: trace or none

Fish:
clams
octopus
oysters

mussels
mackerel
herring
tuna
crab
eel
snails
trout
salmon
striped bass

Poultry:
liver
heart

Meat:
liver
kidneys
beef
pork
lamb
rabbit
caribou
tongue

Oils: trace or none

Other:
yogurt, plain

Folic Acid

Grains:
whole wheat
whole barley
brown rice
bulgur
whole wheat
   couscous
whole grain
   pasta

Beans:
cranberry
lentils
mung
adzuki
chick-peas
pinto
pink
black
black-eyed peas
kidney
lupin
Great Northern
lima
navy
cannellini

Vegetables:
asparagus
beets
soybean sprouts
turnip greens
green peas
artichokes
okra
spinach
leeks
yard-long beans
mustard greens
lentil sprouts

Fruits:
avocados
boysenberries
cantaloupe
oranges
loganberries
strawberries
papayas

Nuts:
pistachios

Seeds: trace or none

Fish:
trout
oysters
tuna

Poultry:
liver
turkey
chicken
quail
eggs

Meat:
liver
beef
pork
lamb

Oils: trace or none

Other:
beer

Bioflavonoids

Grains:
buckwheat (kasha)
soba noodles
   (buckwheat)

Beans: trace or none

Vegetables:
green peppers
tomatoes
broccoli

Fruits:
oranges
lemons
limes
grapefruit
currants
grapes
plums
cherries
apricots
blackberries
papayas
cantaloupe

Nuts: trace or none

Seeds: trace or none

Fish: trace or none

Poultry: trace or none

Meat: trace or none

Oils: trace or none

Other:
rose hips

Vitamin C

Grains: trace or none

Beans: trace or none

Vegetables:
red peppers
broccoli
brussels sprouts
green peppers
kohlrabi
snow peas
mustard greens
sweet potatoes
cabbage
kale
lamb's-quarters
alfalfa sprouts
tomatoes
cassava root

potatoes
parsley

Fruits:
papayas
guavas
kiwis
lychees
oranges
lemons
limes
grapefruit
mangoes
cantaloupe
watermelon
strawberries
acerola
 cherries

black currants

Nuts: trace or none

Seeds: trace or none

Fish:
oysters

Poultry: trace or
 none

Meat:
liver

Oils: trace or none

Other:
rose hips
sauerkraut

Vitamin D

Grains: trace or none

Beans: trace or none

Vegetables:
shiitake
 mushrooms
button mushrooms

Fruits: trace or none

Nuts: trace or none

Seeds: trace or none

Fish:
kippers
mackerel
salmon
catfish
oysters
tuna
sardines
shrimp
perch
herring
cod

flounder
sole
halibut

Poultry:
egg yolks

Meat:
liver

Oils: trace or none

Other:
sunshine

Vitamin E

Grains:
millet
whole oats
whole wheat
cornmeal
bulgur
whole wheat
  couscous
whole grain
  pasta

Beans:
navy

Vegetables:
sweet potatoes
asparagus
cucumbers
kale
collards
seaweed
cabbage

Fruits:
mangoes
avocados

Nuts:
almonds
Brazil
  nuts
hazelnuts
peanuts

Seeds:
sunflower

Fish:
shrimp
haddock
mackerel
herring
salmon
oysters
perch

Poultry:
eggs

Meat:
lamb
liver
heart
kidney

Oils:
sunflower
almond
peanut
safflower
sesame
soybean
olive
flax seed
wheat germ

Other:
blackstrap
  molasses

Vitamin K

Grains: trace or none

Beans:
soybeans
lentils

Vegetables:
cauliflower
watercress
asparagus
broccoli
brussels sprouts
kale
spinach
Swiss chard
cabbage
turnip greens

endive
mustard greens
broccoli
watercress
lettuce
green peas
tomatoes
green beans
kelp
parsley
snow peas
artichokes
green peppers
cucumbers
potatoes
celery

Fruits:
chayotes
avocados
kiwis
strawberries
plums

Nuts:
pistachios

Seeds:
  trace or none

Fish:
abalone

Poultry:
egg yolks

Vitamin K (continued)

Meat:
liver
beef

Oils:
safflower
fish liver
olive

Other:
blackstrap molasses
miso
pickles

Boron

Grains:
whole rye
millet
buckwheat (kasha)
cornmeal
whole barley
whole oats
soba noodles
   (buckwheat)

Beans:
soybeans
lentils

Vegetables:
dandelion greens
spinach
potatoes
broccoli
parsley
white radishes
beets
artichokes
green peas

shallots
cabbage
carrots
onions
pumpkin
asparagus
leeks

Fruits:
apricots
figs
apples
watermelon
pears
peaches
grapes
raisins
prunes
dates
cantaloupe
nectarines
apricots
lemons
mangoes

bananas
tangerines

Nuts:
almonds
hazelnuts
peanuts
walnuts
pecans

Seeds:
flax

Fish:
shrimp

Poultry: trace or none

Meat:
kidneys

Oils: trace or none

Other:
honey
cinnamon
cider
beer

Calcium

Grains:
cornmeal
whole wheat
brown rice
bulgur
whole wheat couscous
whole grain pasta

Beans:
soybeans

kidney
pinto
chick-peas
Great Northern
navy
lima
cannellini

Vegetables:
lamb's-quarters

turnip greens
chicory
bok choy
collards
dandelion
   greens
mustard greens
kale
cabbage

Calcium (continued)

kelp
okra
acorn squash
butternut squash
rutabaga
carrots
artichokes
agar-agar

Fruits:
figs
cherimoyas
papayas
oranges
tangerines
boysenberries

Nuts:
hazelnuts
Brazil nuts
almonds

Seeds:
sesame

Fish:
sardines, with
   bones
mackerel, with
   bones
shrimp
salmon, with bones
perch

crab
soft-shell crab
clams
oysters

Poultry: trace or none

Meat: trace or none

Oils: trace or none

Other:
blackstrap molasses
yogurt, plain
goat cheese
tofu
tempeh

Chromium

Grains:
whole wheat
brown rice
whole oats
bulgur
whole wheat
   couscous
whole grain pasta

Beans: trace or none

Vegetables:
mushrooms
beets
asparagus

seaweed
potatoes
broccoli
green beans
tomatoes

Fruits:
prunes
grapes
apples
bananas

Nuts: trace or none

Seeds: trace or none

Fish:
clams
haddock

Poultry:
turkey

Meat:
liver
beef

Oils: trace or none

Other:
beer
maple syrup

Copper

Grains: trace or none

Beans:
adzuki
soybeans
chick-peas

navy
kidney
lentil
black-eyed peas
Great Northern
cranberry

Vegetables:
potatoes
shittake mushrooms

Fruits:
avocados

Copper (continued)

Nuts:
cashews
Brazil nuts
hazelnuts
pistachios
walnuts
almonds

Seeds:
sunflower
sesame

pumpkin
miso

Fish:
oysters
squid
mussels
clams
crab
octopus
crayfish

Poultry: trace or none

Meat:
liver
kidneys

Oils: trace or none

Other:
blackstrap
   molasses
chocolate, baking

Iodine

Grains:
  trace or none

Beans: trace or none

Vegetables:
kelp
spinach
potatoes
broccoli
mushrooms
asparagus

Fruits:
  trace or none

Nuts: trace or none

Seeds: trace or none

Fish:
haddock
perch
salmon
tuna
sole

oysters
shrimp

Poultry:
eggs

Meat:
liver

Oils: trace or none

Other:
yogurt, plain

Iron

Grains:
millet
brown rice
wild rice
whole rye
buckwheat (kasha)
whole wheat
bulgur
whole wheat
  couscous
whole grain pasta
soba noodles
  (buckwheat)

Beans:
black turtle
chick-peas
pinto
navy
soybeans
kidney
lentils
lima

Vegetables:
Jerusalem
  artichokes
parsley

leeks
peas
artichokes
scallions
spinach
beets
kuzu
seaweed
  agar-agar
  dulse
  wakame

Fruits:
raisins

Iron (continued)

peaches
mulberries
figs
avocados
pears
currants
boysenberries
prunes
raisins

Nuts:
pistachios
almonds
cashews
Brazil nuts
hazelnuts

Seeds:
pumpkin

sunflower
sesame

Fish:
clams
oysters
tuna
snails
abalone
shrimp
caviar
octopus
mussels

Poultry:
eggs
heart
liver
duck

Meat:
liver
venison
quail
beef
pork
lamb
heart
tongue
kidneys
caribou

Oils: trace or
    none

Other:
blackstrap
    molasses

Magnesium

Grains:
buckwheat (kasha)
whole wheat
cornmeal
bulgur
whole wheat couscous
whole rye
millet
brown rice
quinoa
bulgur
whole grain pasta
soba noodles
    (buckwheat)

Beans:
soybeans
adzuki
lima
Great Northern
cranberry
chick-peas
black

pinto
kidney
navy
cannellini

Vegetables:
spinach
beets and beet greens
broccoli
potatoes with skin
seaweed

Fruits:
figs
plantains
avocados

Nuts:
cashews
Brazil nuts
walnuts
almonds
pine nuts
hazelnuts

Seeds:
pumpkin
squash
watermelon
sesame
sunflower
flax

Fish:
shrimp
oysters
halibut
mackerel

Poultry:
egg yolks

Meat: trace or none

Oils: trace or none

Other:
blackstrap molasses
chocolate, baking
tahini
tofu

Manganese

Grains:
whole wheat
brown rice
buckwheat (kasha)
whole rye
whole oats
bulgur
whole wheat couscous
whole grain pasta
soba noodles
   (buckwheat)

Beans:
lima
chick-peas
soybeans
navy
lentils
pinto
pink
Great Northern
kidney
black-eyed peas
cannellini

Vegetables:
collards
okra
peas
seaweed

Fruits:
pineapple
bananas
loganberries
blackberries
raspberries
grapes
blueberries

Nuts:
Brazil nuts
chestnuts
hazelnuts
almonds
peanuts
walnuts
pine nuts
pecans

Seeds:
sunflower
pumpkin

Fish:
mussels
clams
bass
trout
pike
perch
smelt
oysters

Poultry: trace or none

Meat: trace or none

Oils: trace or none

Other:
chocolate, baking
carob
maple syrup
tempeh
tofu
miso

Phosphorus

Grains:
brown rice
cornmeal
whole wheat
whole oats
whole rye
quinoa
bulgur
whole wheat couscous
whole grain pasta

Beans:
chick-peas
soybeans

Vegetables: trace or
   none

Fruits:
cherimoyas
peaches
apricots
raisins
figs
prunes

Nuts:
Brazil nuts
peanuts
almonds

cashews
pistachios
walnuts

Seeds:
pumpkin
sunflower
sesame

Fish:
mackerel
lobster
bluefish
crab
carp

Phosphorus (continued)

pollock
catfish
salmon
shad
flounder

Poultry:
goose
chicken

turkey
duck
eggs
pheasant

Meat:
pork
beef
venison

liver

Oils: trace or none

Other:
butter
brewer's yeast
sheep cheese
goat cheese

Potassium

Grains:
whole rye
millet
buckwheat (kasha)
whole barley
soba noodles
   (buckwheat)

Beans:
Great Northern
lima
navy
cannellini
soybeans
pink
black
lentils
kidney
split peas
adzuki

Vegetables:
potatoes
Swiss chard
beet greens

spinach
seaweed
tomatoes
cassava root

Fruits:
raisins
papayas
plantains
figs
currants
cantaloupe
apricots
avocados
bananas

Nuts:
pistachios
almonds
peanuts
Brazil nuts
hazelnuts

Seeds:
sunflower
sesame

Fish:
dried salt cod
flounder
trout
halibut
grouper
pompano
octopus
clams
salmon

Poultry:
trace or
   none

Meat:
beef
pork
lamb

Oils: trace or
   none

Other:
sauerkraut
pickles

Selenium

Grains:
whole wheat
brown rice
bulgur
whole wheat couscous
whole grain pasta

Beans:
trace or none

Vegetables:
carrots
cabbage
mushrooms
cauliflower
fresh corn
potatoes
green beans
garlic
seaweed

Fruits: trace or none

Nuts:
Brazil nuts

Seeds:
sesame
sunflower

Fish:
shrimp
smelts
clams
lobster
crab
scallops
cod
tuna
oysters
salmon

mackerel
flounder
sole
perch
haddock

Poultry:
chicken
turkey

Meat:
liver
beef
lamb
kidneys
pork

Oils: trace or none

Other:
blackstrap molasses

Zinc

Grains:
brown rice
whole wheat
cornmeal
bulgur
whole wheat couscous
whole grain pasta

Beans:
adzuki
chick-peas
Great Northern
lima
navy
cannellini
black-eyed peas
cranberry
soybeans

Vegetables:
fresh corn

mushrooms
seaweed

Fruits: trace or none

Nuts:
Brazil nuts
cashews
pecans
peanuts

Seeds:
pumpkin
sesame
sunflower

Fish:
oysters
crab
lobster
herring

Poultry:
chicken

duck
pheasant
turkey
eggs
heart

Meat:
liver
beef
beefalo
buffalo
goat
caribou
lamb
tongue

Oils: trace or none

Other:
sauerkraut
miso

Phytohormones

Grains:
whole oats
whole barley
whole rye
brown rice
whole wheat
cornmeal

Vegetables:
potatoes
cabbage
mustard greens
sugar beets
green beans

peas
cucumbers
radishes
parsley
carrots

Beans:
soy
chick-peas
split peas
red beans

Fruit:
cherries

rhubarb
citrus

Seeds:
flax
sesame

Cooking herbs:
anise
fennel
sage

Beverages:
green tea

Nutritional Data for the vitamin and mineral charts was assembled from the following sources:

Davis, D. R., and E. H. Strickland. *NutriCircles, Version 3.0* (Computer Program). Valley Center, CA: Strickland Computer Consulting, 1993.

Dunne, Lavon J. *Nutrition Almanac,* 3rd ed. New York, NY: McGraw-Hill, 1990.

Pennington, Jean A. T. *Bowes and Church's Food Values of Portions Commonly Used.* New York, NY: Harper & Row, 1989.

INDEX

ABOUT THE AUTHORS

Lissa DeAngelis brings more than twenty years of experience as a wholefoods educator and professional wholefoods chef and baker to *Recipes for Change*. Before her ten years as associate director of the Natural Gourmet Cookery School in New York, she was the owner and operator of Good Breads, a natural-food bakery, and Conscious Catering, a home cooking service. She conducts private and corporate well-being seminars and cooking classes. She is currently completing her masters of science in nutrition, and is an active member of the International Association of Culinary Professionals. She lives in Edison, New Jersey.

Molly Siple is a registered dietitian with a masters of science in nutrition, and an experienced caterer, nutritionist, and food writer. She is the author (with Irene Sax) of *Foodstyle*, and a member of the American Dietetics Association and the American Holistic Medical Association. She travels widely, giving lectures and seminars on nutrition, and is a consultant on women's health and nutrition in both clinical and corporate settings. She lives in Los Angeles, California.